WIEDEMANN · GROSSE · DIBBERN
Characteristic Syndromes

To
David W. Smith†
Robert J. Gorlin
and
John M. Opitz,
our teachers

An Atlas of
Characteristic Syndromes
A Visual Aid to Diagnosis

for Clinicians and Practising Physicians

Professor H.-R. WIEDEMANN, Kiel
with Dr K.-R. GROSSE and
HERTA DIBBERN

Foreword by Dr H. E. BOCK
Second, fully revised and extensively enlarged edition.

English translation by Dr MARY F. PASSARGE

Wolfe Medical Publications Ltd

General Editor, Wolfe Medical Atlases:
G. Barry Carruthers, MD(London)

This book is one of the titles in the series of
Wolfe Medical Atlases, a series which brings
together probably the world's largest systematic
published collection of diagnostic photographs.

For a full list of Atlases in the series, plus
forthcoming titles and details of our surgical,
dental and veterinary Atlases, please write to
Wolfe Medical Publications Ltd, Wolfe House,
3 Conway Street, London W1P 6HE

Printed by Hazell Watson and Viney Limited, Aylesbury, England

FOREWORD

Most physicians rely heavily on visual cues. The impressive pictures of the important malformation syndromes presented here will engage their attention – as will the concise text. And rightly so, because the aberrations which in the past were found in curio cabinets or in pathologists' collections are now appearing in practices and clinics as part of the daily routine. Bernfried Leiber calculated that, at a rate of 3 to 5 per cent, at least 35 000 are born* with malformations every year, with at least 4000 showing severe or complex syndromes; to these must be added the numerous inborn errors of metabolism. Thus the physician is obliged to concern himself with the myriad aberrations, whether obvious or hidden, which may manifest themselves congenitally or later in life.

Magic spells, the evil eye, and a 'shock' during pregnancy have become obsolete as precipitating factors (they always were to embryologists on temporal grounds), rubella embryopathy and the thalidomide catastrophe having taught us the 'calendar and clock' characteristics of the pathogenesis of exogenous malformation syndromes. The systematic study of malformations was begun by Ernst Schwalbe and later extended by Georg Gruber (*Allgemeine Mißbildungslehre*). Thus the knowledge of teratogenetic termination phases is 75 years old. Forty-five years ago, Hans Spemann opened new conceptional realms for teratogenesis by presenting evidence of an organiser effect. The rubella embryopathies and the thalidomide syndrome revealed the significance of the placenta for the entrance of infectious and chemical noxae. The Büchner school demonstrated that anoxaemia is an important disruptive factor in embryogenesis. Scientific as well as accidental 'experiments' have disclosed the correct course of the genetic clock in teratogenesis.

The old maxim that one should avoid all possible harm during pregnancy and thus shun unhealthy habits and refrain from ingesting toxicants has been borne out in the malformation syndrome caused by nicotine, and more recently in those caused by alcohol and phenylhydantoin. This should serve as a warning – hopefully, finally, an effective one. 'Nest warmth', the significance of which we recognise in the bosom of the family and in the social womb of society, should begin before implantation of the egg in the uterus.

The apparently increasing number of malformations should alarm all those responsible for the toxicity of the environment, and should provoke the earliest possible defensive efforts. Physicians are obliged to learn even more about malformations, since medicine long ago progressed from the descriptive to the pathophysiological phase, with aetiological knowledge now making medical treatment possible.

The suffering laid on a family and on society by a malformed child is great, and the ability of the affected to cope within their limited surroundings is generally admirable. But has society provided adequate preventive measures and offered the handicapped sufficient support and opportunities for assimilation?

A book that presents the most important syndromes resulting from past events belongs not only in the hands of paediatricians and obstetricians, but in the library of every physician. In addition, geneticists, embryologists, and endocrinologists, and especially toxicologists and pharmacologists, should be moved and stimulated, since they have at their disposal the knowledge and the means to trace aetiologies and devise help.

Hans Erhard Bock
Prof. Dr med., Dr med. h. c.
Tübingen

---

* In West Germany

PREFACE TO THE SECOND EDITION

'Characteristic Syndromes' aroused great interest and approval; the first reprinting was required in only two years, and foreign-language editions have appeared. The reviewers have all commended the atlas, not only for its basic format and the 'information density' of its texts, but also for the quality of the illustrations. Having been thus encouraged and stimulated by frequently expressed wishes to include other syndromes, we present a new edition. The purpose and task of this book and its organisation have remained unchanged: It is intended to be *practical*. (Please refer to the Preface to the first edition!)

At the time of the first edition the photographic material almost without exception came from the archives of the Paediatrics Department of the University of Kiel or from the private files of the first author. In this edition we illustrate 204, instead of 97, syndromes – thus more than doubling the contents of the book. This has required 'material help' on the part of kind colleagues. We wish to thank the contributors listed below for the photographs and clinical data of more than 50 of the newly included malformation complexes and hereditary syndromes.

Along with the now more than 170 recognised and more or less familiar syndromes which have been presented in this volume with the aim of 'visual recognition of syndromes' (*Blickdiagnose von Syndromen*), or at least of suggesting diagnoses from appearance, about 30 further distinctive, apparently unknown clinical pictures have been included. They have come almost exclusively from the collected observations of the first author and for the time being represent single cases or 'personal syndromes'. In our experience, the study of this kind of presentation by colleagues frequently leads to 'recognition' of earlier analogous observations they themselves have made or to helpful associations from other fields – and thus to closer definition and classification. The inclusion of these cases is thus 'for the good of the cause'.

The text of the first edition has also been revised; some of the original photographs have been rearranged. In addition to a table of contents, the present edition offers a diagnostic survey (which has been expanded to include new groups), an alphabetical index of the syndromes (including important synonyms), and a table of particularly·unusual signs.

In conclusion, clinical genetics has become greatly differentiated, and continues to become more so at an accelerated rate. As a result, a book such as this one contains many, naturally well-deliberated, simplifications. This was unavoidable in staying within the prescribed framework.

We are grateful for the help and support especially of the following colleagues:

I. Anton Lamprecht, Heidelberg
H. Bartels, Bremen-Würzburg
M. Bauer, Gießen
F. A. Beemer, Utrecht
G. Beluffi, Pavia
G. Bennholdt-Thomsen †, Cologne
A. Blankenagel, Heidelberg
G. R. Burgio, Pavia
O. Butenandt, Munich
Cl. Fauré, Paris
J. P. Fryns, Leuven
A. Fuhrmann-Rieger, Gießen
W. Fuhrmann, Gießen
J. Gehler, Mainz
E. Gladtke, Cologne
R. J. Gorlin, Minneapolis
H.-G. Hansen, Lübeck
R. Happle, Münster i. W.
H. Helge, Berlin
U. Hillig, Marburg a. d. L
H. Kemperdick, Düsseldorf
D. Knorr, Munich
J. Kunze, Berlin
B. Leiber, Frankfurt a. M.
W. Lenz, Münster i. W.
F. Majewski, Düsseldorf
P. Maroteaux, Paris
P. Meinecke, Hamburg
C. Mietens, Bochum
H. Moll, Papenburg
J.-D. Murken, Munich
G. Neuhäuser, Gießen
J. W. Oorthuys, Amsterdam
J. M. Opitz, Helena
E. Passarge, Essen
A. K. Poznanski, Chicago
H. Reich, Münster i. W.
A. Rett, Vienna
A. Rütt, Cologne
H. Schönenberg, Aachen
M. Seip, Oslo
J. Spranger, Mainz
G. B. Stickler, Rochester
U. Wendel, Düsseldorf
G. Wendt, Marburg a. d. L.

We are no less grateful to our colleagues K. Aeissen, E. Christophers, E. Dieterich, H. Doose, H. Hauss, P. Heintzen, Kl. Heyne, Ch. v. Klinggräff, A. Proppe, J. Schaub, E. Stephan, M.-E. Tolksdorf, and W. Blauth in Kiel, and not the least to my secretary

Mrs Maria Fliedner for her constant lively interest and dedicated, untiring assistance. We appreciate the care taken by the publisher and printer in producing the book. It was a pleasure to work with them. We offer special thanks to Prof. Dr Dr h. c. P. Matis and Mr H. Schwer of Schattauer Verlag and their co-workers for being considerate of our wishes and for their personal interest. In conclusion we acknowledge the slide collection 'Syndromes' ROCOM/ Roche 1982, which supplemented the present atlas edition.

Kiel, summer 1982   in the name of all the authors,
Hans-Rudolf Wiedemann

From the PREFACE to the First Edition 1976

Was ist das Schwerste von allem? Was dir das
    Leichteste dünket,
Mit den Augen zu sehn, was vor den Augen dir
    liegt.*
(J. W. v. Goethe, Xenie** from the literary remains)

'Syndromes' abound in modern medicine. According to G. Fanconi, more than six times as many syndromes can be tabulated now than could be at the beginning of the century. This is mainly an effect of advances in research and, therefore, may be viewed positively.

The early diagnosis of syndromes is important, as it is to draw the necessary conclusions from the diagnosis. Many syndromes are easy to recognise if the physician has a trained eye. To aid in this training is the intention of this book. Almost one hundred such syndromes, which can be partially or totally visually comprehended, have been presented here, each in an illustrated plate. Most of them represent so-called dysmorphosis syndromes, whereby the manifestations may be present at birth, but also may not appear until later. Since this book was meant to be of practical use, the authors have neither followed the strict definition of a syndrome nor limited themselves to a sharply delineated category of syndromes.

Blickdiagnosen (diagnoses from appearances) are not to be understood here generally as 'prima vista' or 'at-a-glance' diagnoses. To be sure, most of the syndromes presented can be identified by an experienced observer with a physician's eye alone, and do not require more or less extensive laboratory tests, which unfortunately and unjustifiably are often put first by the young physician. But, of course, in many cases a careful history will supplement the impression, with a thorough clinical examination being necessary to underpin the tentative diagnosis. The text accompanying each of the photographic plates gives the essence and additional information, both concisely formulated.

The frequencies of the syndromes are to be understood within the framework of the frequency of dysmorphosis syndromes in general. Several stand out, especially the Down's syndrome (1: approx. 650 births), but also neurofibromatosis, Noonan syndrome, Prader–Willi syndrome, Turner syndrome, and several others, perhaps including the newly recognised 'fetal alcohol syndrome'. For the given patient and his family it is of no particular consolation that his condition is rare. For he himself, the frequency of his disorder is always '100%'; accordingly, he expects his physician to be well informed about it. In addition, we might observe: 'The rare things in medicine are *not rare*; only observers are rare' (H. R. Clouston, 1939).

Patients with the syndromes presented here will be taken to general practitioners and to colleagues of the most diverse specialties – ophthalmologists and radiologists, dermatologists and psychiatrists, human geneticists and otologists, internists and orthopaedic surgeons, paediatricians and neurologists. This atlas would like to serve all of them. The Diagnostic Survey following the Table of Contents should facilitate locating syndromes which come into question.

Kiel, October 1976   in the name of all the authors,
                                Hans-Rudolf Wiedemann

---

* Roughly:
  What is the hardest of all? What you as easiest would deem,
  To see with your eyes, what lies before your eyes.

** Satirical epigrams

Contents

Diagnostic Survey

but see also:

II. Syndromes in Which Tall Stature is a (Possibly Transient) Prominent Feature

but see also:

III. Syndromes with Prominent Growth Retardation (Primordial and/or Postnatal Proportionate or Disproportionate)

IV. Syndromes With Prominent Aged Appearance

V. Syndromes with Prominent Thinness or Emaciation

VI. Syndromes with Prominent Obesity

XI. Syndromes with Prominent Haemangiomatous and/or Vascular Anomalies of the Skin or Soft Tissues

XII. Syndromes with Prominent 'Connective Tissue Weakness'

XIII. Syndromes with Prominent 'Spontaneous' Fractures

XIV. Syndromes with Prominent Anomalies of the Extremities

But see also:

XV. Syndromes with Prominent Cartilaginous or Bony Excrescences or Protrusions of the Skeleton or Soft Tissues

XVII. Syndromes with Triphalangeal Thumbs (Fingerlike Thumbs)

XVIII. Syndromes with Hypo- or Aplasia of the Thumbs

XIX. Syndromes with Shortening of the Big Toes

XX. Syndromes with Marked Dental and/or Jaw Anomalies

XXI. Syndromes with Dysplastic or Dystrophic Nails

But see also:

XXII. Syndromes with Abnormalities of the Hair or Its Amount, with Ichthyosis or Epidermolysis

XXIV. Syndromes with Haematological Signs and Symptoms

See under:

XXV. Syndromes with Marked Muscular Hypotonia and/or Neurological Signs
(apart from seizures or seizure disorder and from isolated mental retardation)

But see also:

XXVI. Syndromes with Obligatory or Possible Impaired Vision

But see also:

XXVII. Syndromes with Possible Hearing Impairment or Deafness

See under:

XXVIII. Syndromes with Regular or Possible Mental Retardation and/or Behavioural Disorders

See under:

Table of Unusual Signs

(Syndromes referred to by their title number in the text)

Acanthosis nigricans: 101, 119

Adipose tissue hernias of the skin: 125

Buccal cleft, transverse: 20

Coloboma of the eyelids: 18, 19, 20, (21), 158

Ear: Indentations on the lobe and/or on the helix: 41
Swelling of the pinnae in early infancy due to cystic masses: 83

Ectopia lentis: 44, 46, 136

Eye: Accessory lacrimal points: 144
Blepharophimosis: 17, 50, 51, (67), 81, 145, 190, 191
Coloboma of the eyelid: 18, 19, 20, (21), 158
Dermoids; lipodermoids, epibulbar: 20, (21), 108, 115, 117
Iridodonesis, luxation of the lens: 44, 46, 136

Hemihypoplasia, total: 49, (125), 126

Iridodonesis: 44, 46, 136

Luxation of the lens: 44, 46, 136

Macroglossia: 30, 37, (38), 39, 41

Mouth: Cleft mouth (cleft cheek), transverse: 20
Difficulties in opening: 17, 50, 190
Frenula, hyperplastic intraoral: (5), 23, (24), 86, 143, 157
Gingival fibromatosis: 113
Hamartoma of the tongue: 23, (24), (115)
Lobulation of the tongue: 23, 157
Macroglossia: 30, 37, (38), 39, 41
Teeth, congenital: 86, 98, 201

Nose: Bony tori, paranasal: 33
Indentation, bilateral, of the tip: 78
Indentation or cleft, median: 14, (63), 157

Oedema in childhood, of the distal lower extremities: (47), 64, 66, (134), 176

Pterygium colli: 64, 66, (72), (161), 176, (191)

'Scored' ears: 41

Scrotal folds, shawl-like, enclosing penis: 65

Skin: Acanthosis nigricans: 101, 119
Hernias of fatty tissue: 125
Oedema of the legs in childhood: (47), 64, 66, (134), 176
Pterygium colli: 64, 66, (72), (161), 176, (191)

'Tail' (median sacral rudimentary tail): 85

Thumbs: Abduction (at the proximal phalanx): 83
Deviation (at the interphalangeal joint): 52

Tongue: Enlargement: 30, 37, (38), 39, 41
Hamartoma: 23, (24), (115)
Lobulation: 23, 157

Syndromes

1. Crouzon Syndrome

(Craniofacial Dysostosis)

A characteristic hereditary syndrome with acrocephaly
(tower head).

Main Signs:
1. Acrocephaly with a high wide forehead, sometimes with a decided bulge at the anterior fontanelle region; flat occiput (**1–3, 5** and **6**).
2. Exophthalmos of the widely spaced eyes (with flat orbits). Slight antimongoloid slant of the palpebral fissures. Convergence of the globes difficult or impossible; divergent strabismus. Ptosis in some cases (**1–6**).
3. Maxillary hypoplasia with 'parrot-beak' nose, short upper lip, high narrow palate, narrowly spaced teeth; prognathism (**2, 3c, 6a, c** and **7b**).

Supplementary Findings: Frequently slight to moderate mental retardation. In some cases, signs of craniostenosis and also of optic atrophy with decreased visual acuity. Exceptionally, defective hearing.

Radiologically, craniosynostosis, especially of the coronary and lambdoid sutures; short anterior, deep middle and posterior cranial fossae; often very pronounced digital markings of the skull (**7a** and **c**).

Manifestation: At birth.

Aetiology: An autosomal dominant hereditary condition with high penetrance, but various degrees of expressivity.

Frequency: Low (in 1966 somewhat more than 100 published cases were counted).

Course, Prognosis: Essentially dependent on the presence and degree of mental impairment and/or optic nerve damage.

Differential Diagnosis: Chotzen syndrome (p.4).

Treatment: Symptomatic. Early craniotomy, performed in the first months of life, even in the absence of signs of craniostenosis, suited to the individual's problem and revised at regular intervals. Cosmetic surgery may be indicated eventually to mitigate facial deformity.

Illustrations:
1 A newborn;
2 An infant;
3 and 5 Young pre-school children;
4 and 7b A 6-year-old and
6 A 10-year-old girl.
7a and c Digital markings on the skull X-rays of the child in **4** and **7b** at age 10 years.

Some of these children represent definite hereditary cases; the others, sporadic cases (interpreted as new mutations).

References:
Vulliamy D. G., Normandale P. A.: Craniofacial dysostosis in a Dorset family. Arch. Dis. Childh. *41*: 375 (1966)
Kushner J., Alexander E., Davis jr C. H., et al Crouzon's disease (craniofacial dysostosis). Modern diagnosis and treatment J. Neurosurg. *37*: 434 (1972)

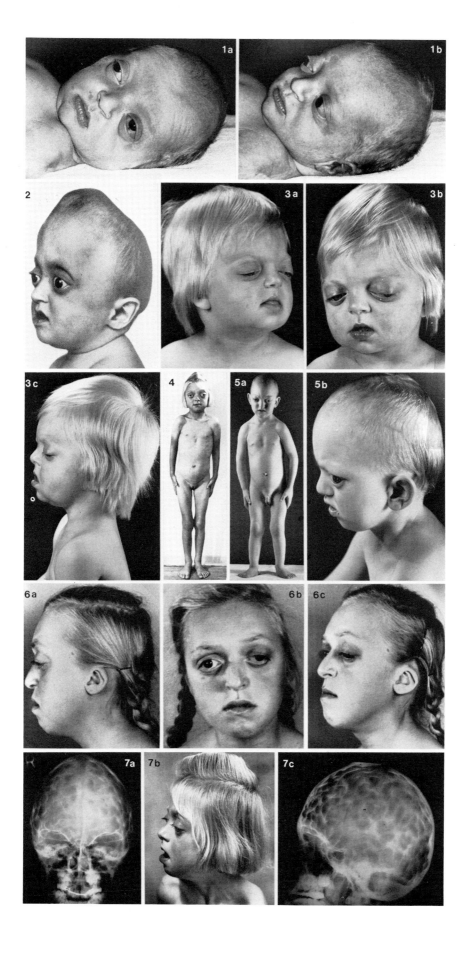

2. Chotzen Syndrome

(Acrocephalosyndactyly Type Chotzen, Saethre–Chotzen Syndrome)

A hereditary syndrome comprising acrocephaly, quite characteristic facies, mild to moderate syndactyly of the hands and feet, and possible mental retardation.

Main Signs:
1. Relatively mild acrocephaly and a broad forehead (**1-3**).
2. Face: Often markedly asymmetric. Frequently low anterior hairline. Hypertelorism, wide flat root of the nose, antimongoloid slant of the palpebral fissures, eyebrows often raised, possible slight exophthalmos. Ptosis, strabismus. Narrowing of the tear ducts possible, dystopia canthorum. Beak-like curve of the nose with deviated septum. In some cases low-set ears. Hypoplasia of the upper jaw, narrow palate; prognathism (**1-3, 4,** and **6**).
3. Relatively short and stubby fingers (often with inturned little fingers); exclusively soft-tissue syndactyly between the proximal segments principally of digits II and III of the hands (**5**), but also of other digits. Normal number of fingers and toes; normal thumbs and big toes. Cutaneous syndactyly of the toes.

Supplementary Findings: Occasional mental retardation. Frequent mild hearing impairment.
    Small stature.
    Possible cryptorchidism.
    Radiologically, premature synostosis of the coronal sutures.

Manifestation: At birth.

Aetiology: An autosomal dominant hereditary disorder.

Frequency: Low, but substantially higher than that of the Apert syndrome (p.8).

Course, Prognosis: Principally dependent on whether there is mental retardation.

Differential Diagnosis: Crouzon syndrome (p.2).

Treatment: Early neurosurgical intervention may considerably improve the patient's eventual appearance.

Illustrations:
1–6 An affected boy at ages 4 months (above) and 2 years (below). Acrocephaly with premature synostosis of the coronal sutures. Characteristic facies (including slight ptosis, right convex scoliosis of the face, deviated septum, and low-set ears). Short, stubby fingers with bridges of soft tissue between digits II and III (**5**), radial deviation of the little fingers; soft tissue syndactyly between toes III and IV bilaterally. Slight shortness of stature. Psychomotor retardation.

References:
Kreiborg S., Pruzansky S., Pashayan H.: The Saethre–Chotzen syndrome. Teratology 6: 287 (1972)
Pantke O. A., Cohen jr M. M., Witkop jr C. R.: The Saethre–Chotzen syndrome. Birth Defects *11*: 190 (1975)

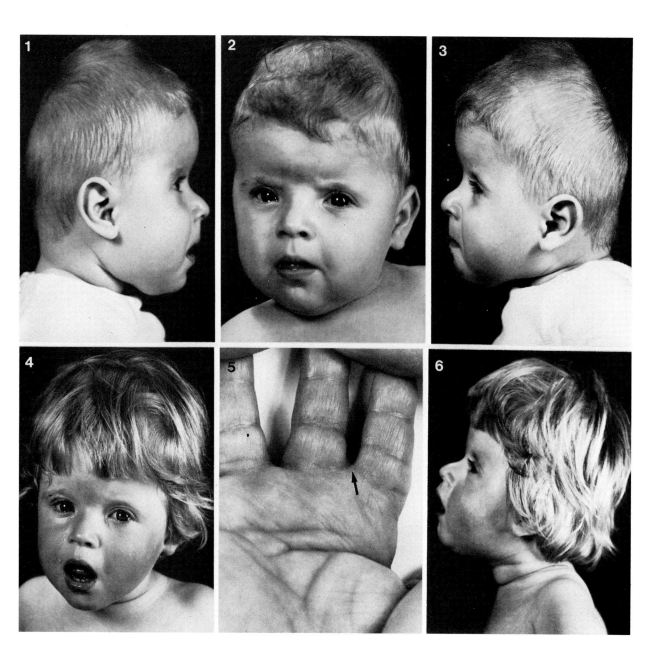

3. Pfeiffer Syndrome

(Acrocephalosyndactyly Type Pfeiffer)

A hereditary syndrome of acrocephaly; facial dysmorphism; broad, stocky thumbs and halluces; and syndactyly of mild to moderate severity.

Main Signs:
1. Acrobrachycephaly (**1-3**).
2. Face: Broad with a flat profile; hypertelorism; broad, low-set nasal root; antimongoloid slant of the palpebral fissures; high arched palate, and small upper and, in some cases, lower jaw. (**1** and **2**).
3. Big toes (**4**) and thumbs coarse, broad, short, and usually deviated. Various degrees of soft tissue syndactyly.

Supplementary Findings: Possible small stature.
   On X-ray, the anterior fontanelle may be enlarged (**3**), with premature synostosis especially of the coronal suture.
   Various malformations, particularly of the bones of the first rays of the hands and feet.

Manifestation: At birth.

Aetiology: Autosomal dominant hereditary disease.

Frequency: Low.

Course, Prognosis: On the whole, favourable.

Differential Diagnosis: Other acrocephalosyndactyly syndromes. Whether the Pfeiffer syndrome and Apert syndrome (p.8) represent different grades of severity of the same hereditary defect is still an open question.

Treatment: Corrective surgical measures for the cranium and/or hands in some patients.

Illustrations:
1–5 A 2-month-old girl. Acrobrachycephaly with steep cranial base; distinct interparietal bone; wide open anterior fontanelle with premature ossification of the coronal suture and part of the sagittal suture (**3**). Hypertelorism, antimongoloid slant of the palpebral fissures, strabismus. Broad, stubby thumbs and halluces with mild cutaneous syndactyly.
   Unremarkable female chromosome complement. The mental development of this girl, who underwent early cranial surgery and has been followed up for years, is within normal limits.

References:
Naveh S., Friedman A.: Pfeiffer syndrome: report of a family and review of the literature. J. Med. Genet. *13*: 277 (1976)
Bull M. J., Escobar V., Bixler D., et al: Phenotype definition and occurrence risk in the acrocephalosyndactyly syndromes. Birth Defects *15*:65 (1979)
Sanchez J. M., de Negrotti T. C.: Variable expression in Pfeiffer syndrome. J. Med. Genet. *18*:73 (1981)

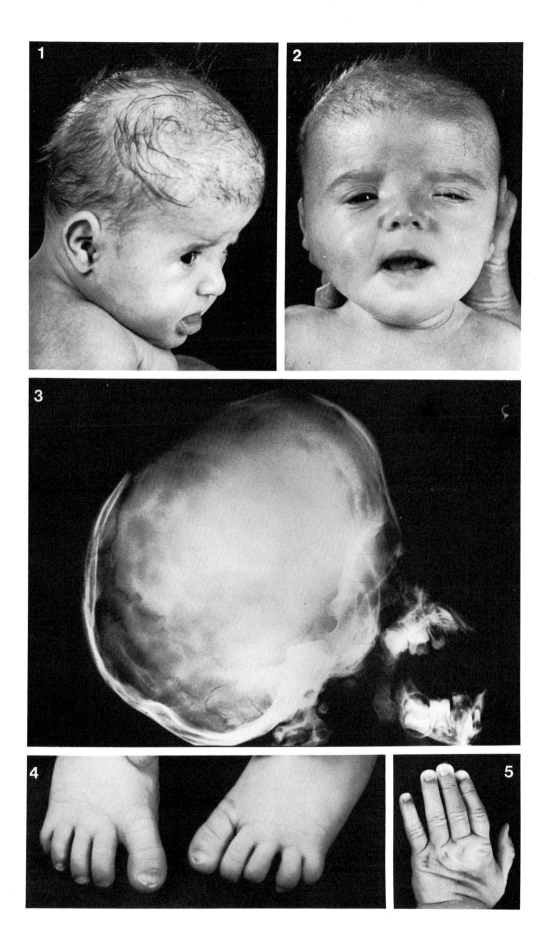

7

4. Apert Syndrome

(Acrocephalosyndactyly Type I)

A characteristic hereditary syndrome comprising acrocephaly, facial dysmorphism, and extensive symmetrical syndactyly of the fingers (including osseous) and toes.

Main Signs:

1. Acrocephaly with high 'full' forehead, flat occiput (**1, 2, 4,** and **6**).
2. More or less flat face with a supraorbital horizontal groove, widely spaced eyes, flat orbits with exophthalmos, strabismus, slight antimongoloid slant of the palpebral fissures, and often small turned-up (sometimes beaklike) nose and low-set ears. Hypoplasia of the upper jaw. Narrow palate (sometimes cleft); narrowly spaced teeth (**1, 2, 4,** and **6**).
3. Extensive syndactyly to more or less complete spoon-like deformity of the hands (**4-7**), generally with bony fusion of the 2nd to 4th fingers (**10**), which often share a common nail (**5**). Fingers often short (**4**). Ends of the thumbs frequently broad and misshapen (**7**). Soft tissue syndactyly of many or all toes. Big toes stubby and deformed (**8, 9, 11,** and **12**).

Supplementary Findings: Abnormally short upper extremities (**4**), impaired mobility of the elbow and shoulder joints, anomalies of the shoulder girdle.

Not infrequently mental retardation, which may be severe.

Radiologically, irregular craniosynostosis, especially of the coronal sutures and often of the lambdoid suture; short anterior and deepened middle and posterior cranial fossae; hypoplasia of the upper jaw, possible digital markings of the skull on X-ray (**3**).

Numerous other possible associated malformations (gastrointestinal or urinary tract, heart, etc.).

Manifestation: At birth.

Aetiology: Autosomal dominant hereditary disease. However, the vast majority of cases are sporadic and represent new mutations (such as occur more frequently with increased paternal age).

Frequency: Low (150 published cases were counted in 1960).

Course, Prognosis: Essentially dependent on the severity of the typical malformations, the presence or development of mental impairment, and the possible manifestation and consequences of additional defects in other organ systems. Relatively high mortality in the first years of life.

Treatment: Symptomatic. Early neurosurgical intervention for acrocephaly (first months of life), even in the absence of signs of craniostenosis. Corrective surgery of the extremities should be undertaken sufficiently early, at a time determined in consultation with the hand surgeon. Psychological guidance and all necessary aids for the handicapped.

Illustrations:

1–8 A 5-month-old boy. Microdolichotrigonocephaly (**1–4**). Bilateral buphthalmos. Anteverted nostrils. Long philtrum. Macrostomia (**1** and **2**); high narrow palate; preauricular dimples (**5**). Short neck, malformed thorax, ventricular septal defect; cryptorchidism. Laxity of skin and musculature. Short hands, with bilateral clinodactyly V and simian crease (**6** and **7**); club feet with hypoplasia of rays III to V. Unremarkable male chromosome complement.

References:

Spranger J. W., Langer jr L. O., Wiedemann H.-R.: Bone Dysplasias. An Atlas of Constitutional Disorders of Skeletal Development, Stuttgart and Philadelphia, G. Fischer and W. B. Saunders, 1974

Stewart R. E., Bixon G., Cohen A.: The pathogenesis of premature craniosynostosis in acrocephalosyndactyly (Apert's syndrome). Plast. Reconstr. Surg. *59*:699 (1977)

Beligere N., Harris V., Pruzansky S.: Progressive bone dysplasia in Apert syndrome. Radiology *139*:593 (1981)

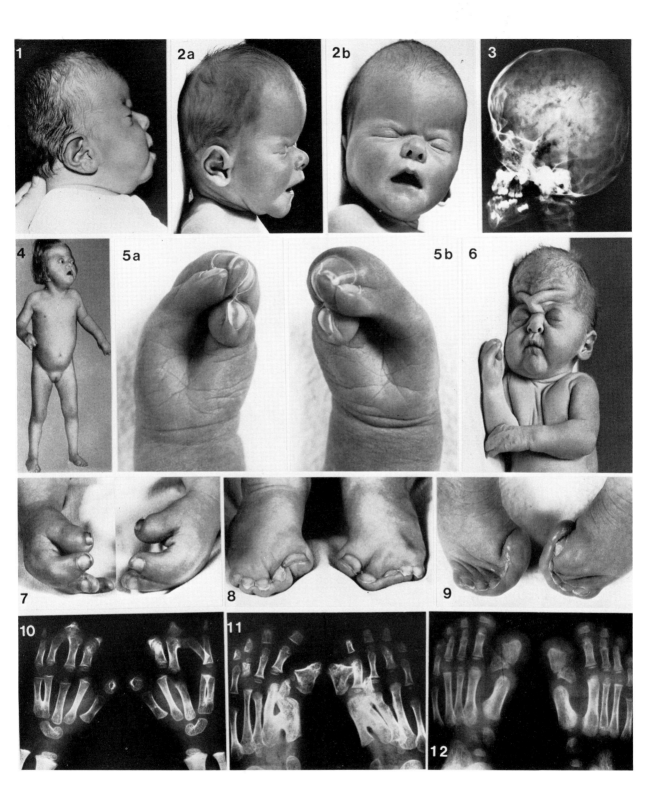

5. Opitz Trigonocephaly Syndrome

(C Syndrome – after the initial of the family name of the first cases described)

A hereditary syndrome with characteristic facies, unusual formation of the palate, loose skin, joint disorders, microcephalic mental retardation, and possible polysyndactyly.

Main Signs:
1. A somewhat triangular-shaped cranium, narrowing toward the top (trigonocephaly), with the forehead showing a prominent medial ridge and, in some cases, bitemporal depressions (**1** and **4**). Low nasal root, mongoloid slant of the palpebral fissures, strabismus, epicanthal folds (**1** and **2**), and various anomalies of the external ears. Very narrow palate, especially anteriorly, between abnormally wide-appearing alveolar ridges (sometimes with mucous membrane bridges between the latter and the buccal mucous membrane).
2. Loose skin, sometimes quite marked at the neck. Hyperextensibility, dislocation, or contractures of the large joints.
3. Failure to thrive. Muscular hypotonia. Increasing tendency to microcephaly with corresponding impairment of mental development.
4. In some cases short hands and/or fingers, club feet, postaxial hexadactyly and cutaneous syndactyly.

Supplementary Findings: Possible cardiac defect. Deformities of the thorax, genital anomalies, short extremities, small size.
Normal findings on chromosome analysis.

Manifestation: At birth.

Aetiology: Autosomal recessive hereditary defect.

Frequency. To date scarcely a dozen cases have been described. However, the syndrome is probably not extremely rare.

Course, Prognosis: Initially failure to thrive, with death frequently occurring in early infancy. Surviving children are usually severely retarded.

Treatment: Conservative, symptomatic.

Illustrations:
1–8 A 5-month-old boy. Microdolichotrigonocephaly (**1–4**). Bilateral buphthalmos. Anteverted nostrils. Long philtrum. Macrostomia (**1** and **2**); high narrow palate; preauricular dimples (**5**). Short neck, malformed thorax, ventricular septal defect; cryptorchidism. Laxity of skin and musculature. Short hands, with bilateral clinodactyly V and simian crease (**6** and **7**); club feet with hypoplasia of rays III to V. Unremarkable male chromosome complement.

References:
Oberklaid F., Danks M.: The Opitz trigonocephaly syndrome. Am. J. Dis. Child. *129*:1348 (1975)
Antley R. M., Sung Hwang D., Theopold W., Gorlin R. J., Steeper T., Pitt D., Danks M., McPherson E., Bartels H., Wiedemann H.-R., Opitz J. M.: Further delineation of the C (trigonocephaly) syndrome. Am. J. Med. Genet. *9*:147 (1981)

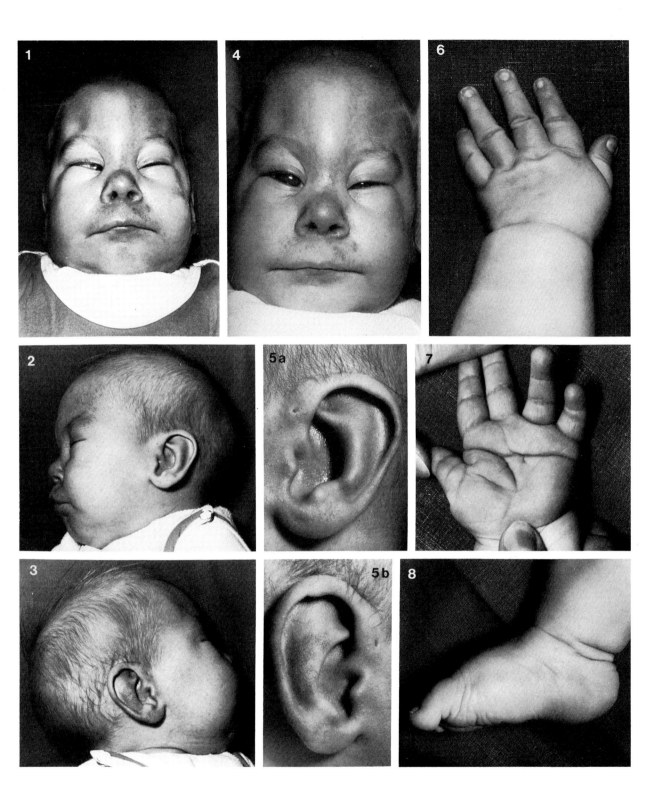

6. Carpenter Syndrome

(Acrocephalopolysyndactyly Type Carpenter)

A hereditary syndrome comprising acrocephaly, facial dysmorphism, brachyclinosyndactyly of the hands, and polysyndactyly of the feet.

Main Signs:
1. Oxy- or acrobrachycephaly with a bulging fontanelle (1). In some cases marked protrusion of the temporal areas, symmetrically or asymmetrically (1 and 3), somewhat resembling the changes of a cloverleaf skull (p.14).
2. Broad, flat face with exophthalmos, hypertelorism, possible mongoloid or antimongoloid slant of the palpebral fissures and epicanthus, low-set and posteriorly rotated auricles, high arched palate, and microgenia (1 and 2). Short neck.
3. Short hands; brachydactyly; broad thumbs; cutaneous syndactyly between the middle and ring fingers, in some cases more extensive (1 and 2). Short and very wide big toes, more or less obviously doubled, with various degrees of syndactyly of the toes.

Supplementary Findings: Frequent cardiac defects, mental retardation. Obesity of the trunk; also small size, hypogenitalism.

Radiologically, characteristic configuration, malpositioning, and duplication in the thumb and big toe regions (4 and 5).

Manifestation: At birth.

Aetiology: Autosomal recessive hereditary disorder.

Frequency: Low (by 1980, somewhat over 30 cases had been reported).

Course, Prognosis: Essentially dependent on the presence and severity of primary mental retardation and on early surgical treatment of the cranium and, in some cases, the heart.

Diagnosis, Differential Diagnosis: Greig's polysyndactyly craniofacial dysmorphism syndrome (p.312) can be easily ruled out by the mild cranial dysmorphism; in addition, it is transmitted by autosomal dominant inheritance.

A Laurence–Moon syndrome (p.210), suggested by the obesity, hypogenitalism, mental retardation, and polydactyly, can be excluded by the shape of the skull, the facies, the doubling of the halluces and syndactylies of the Carpenter syndrome, and by the absence of tapetoretinal degeneration.

Treatment: Surgical treatment of the cranium, the extremities, and in some cases, the heart.

Illustrations:
1–5 A female infant with the Carpenter syndrome. Cutaneous syndactyly of the 3rd and 4th fingers and of the 1st-3rd toes bilaterally; broad, stubby thumbs and halluces. Radiologically, deviation of the hypoplastic proximal phalynx of the thumb and hypo- and aplasia of various middle phalanges. Coarse broadening of the 1st ray in both feet, with duplication of the proximal and distal phalanges of the big toes. (By kind permission of Prof. H. Schönenberg, Aachen, FRG.)

Reference:
Pfeiffer R. A., Seeman K. B., Tünte W., et al: Akrozephalo-polysyndaktylie. Klin. Pädiatr. *189*:120 (1977)

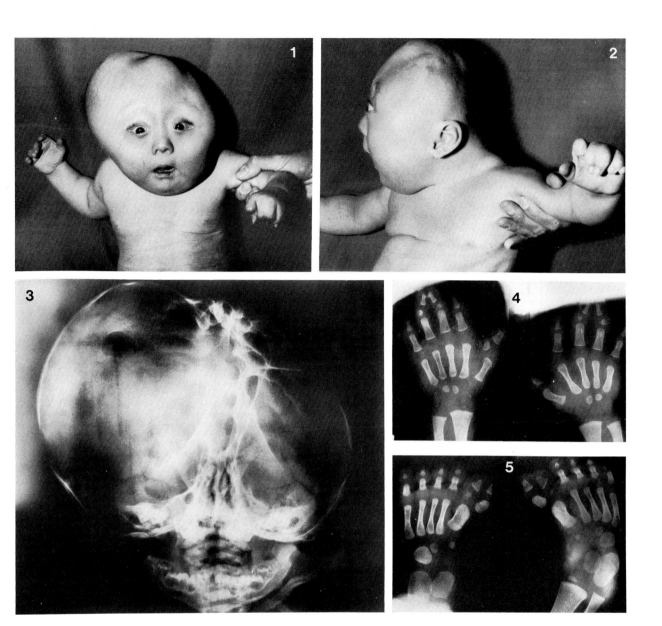

7. Cloverleaf Skull Syndrome Kleeblattschädel Syndrome

According to a new provisional definition a syndrome of cloverleaf-like deformity of the skull with normally proportioned trunk and extremities and the absence of other apparent malformations.

Main Signs: Marked bubble-like outpouching of the cranium upwards and bilaterally outwards at the temporal areas, with downwards displacement of the ears to an almost horizontal position, depressed nasal root, and protrusio bulborum (1 and 2). Hydrocephalus (3).

Supplementary Findings: Increased cranial pressure, dystrophy, impaired psychomotor development.

Manifestation: At birth.

Aetiology: Uncertain; probable genetic basis.

Frequency: Very low.

Coarse, Prognosis: Unfavourable; early death.

Differential Diagnosis: Cloverleaf skull associated with systemic skeletal dysplasia of the thanatophoric dwarfism type (p.150). Cloverleaf skull as may occur in other syndromes with craniosynostosis (Apert, Carpenter, Crouzon and Pfeiffer syndromes).

Treatment: Symptomatic neurosurgical measures may be indicated.

Illustrations:
1 and 2 A 2-month-old infant with cloverleaf skull syndrome. Normally proportioned trunk and extremities. At examination, no anomalies apart from the cranial. No joint deformities.
3 Pneumoencephalogram showing markedly dilated lateral ventricles in the temporal areas. (Death of the child at age 5 months.)

References:
Holtermüller K., Wiedemann H.-R.: Kleeblattschädel-Syndrom. Med. Monatschr. *14*:439 (1960)
Wiedemann H.-R., Ostertag B.: Kleeblattschädel und allgemeine Mikromelie. Klin. Pädiatr. *186*:261 (1974)
Aksu F., Mietens C.: Kleeblattschädel-Syndrom. Klin. Pädiatr. *191*:418 (1979)

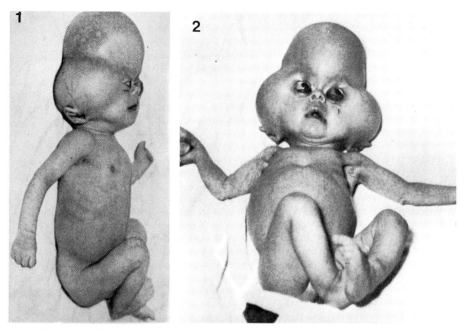

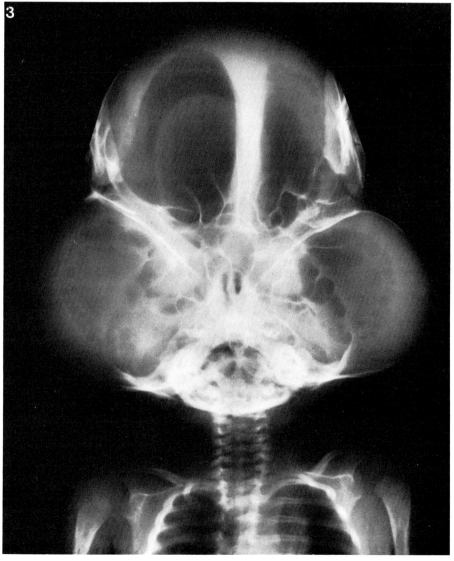

15

8. Oto-palato-digital Syndrome

A malformation syndrome with typical facial dysmorphism; signs of bone dysplasia, particularly in the form of 'frog hands and frog feet'; cleft palate; and impaired hearing.

Main signs:
1. Characteristic facies with broad prominent forehead, hypertelorism, antimongoloid slant of the palpebral fissures, marked supraorbital bulges, broad root of the nose, flat midface, and microstomia with down-turned corners of the mouth (3, 4, 11, and 12). Median cleft palate.
2. Broadening and shortening of the distal phalanges of the hands and feet with accentuation of the 1st ray, the shortness of which is due mainly to hypoplasia of the metacarpal or the metatarsal I and the proximal phalanx. Shortening and radial deviation of the little finger also frequent. Partial syndactylies. All in all, reminiscent of a 'frog hand' or 'frog foot' (5–8). Deformity and limited motion of the large joints.
3. Frequently moderate conductive hearing impairment. Tendency to otitis, sinusitis, and mastoiditis. Frequent mild mental retardation.

Supplementary Findings: Slight shortness of stature.
Anomalies of the teeth.
Fusions and deformities at the metacarpal and metatarsal levels with additional ossification centres and ossicles. Incomplete fusion of the neural arches generally involving several vertebral bodies. Vertically positioned clivus.

Manifestation: At birth.

Aetiology: Hereditary disorder, with the mode of inheritance not yet definitely established. X-chromosomal recessive as well as X-chromosomal dominant has been considered; more recently, autosomal dominant with incomplete penetrance and various degrees of expressivity has been suggested. Females tend to be less severely affected.

Frequency: Including the children shown here, 69 cases in males and 34 in females were known up to 1981.

Course, Prognosis: Normal life expectancy.

Diagnosis, Differential Diagnosis: Other syndromes featuring broad, short halluces and thumbs, such as the Münchmeyer (p.340) or the Rubinstein–Taybi syndrome (p.104), etc., can easily be excluded by the total picture. The same should be true for the Larsen syndrome (p.304), which also includes flat facies and joint deformities.

An X-ray of the feet is especially valuable in establishing the diagnosis of oto-palato-digital syndrome.

Treatment: Symptomatic.

Illustrations:
1–6 The index case at age 7 years. Birth measurements and present size within normal limits. After total correction of tetralogy of Fallot. Bipartite uvula, slightly impaired hearing, frequent otitis. Intellect in the low normal range. Limited motion at the large joints; thenar hypoplasia. Anomalies in the carpal and tarsal regions, with synostoses in the latter. Wide defect in the neural arches from the lower thoracic to the sacral vertebrae.
7–12 The brother of the index patient at age 12 years. Birth measurements and present size within normal limits. Essentially the same somatic findings, however: complete median cleft of the soft palate (post-operative), no cardiac defect; no X-rays of the vertebral column.
13 and 14 The sister of the two brothers at age 13 years. On the basis of the similarity of her facial features, she may be regarded as a gene carrier. Except for slightly limited motion at the wrists, no further anomalies.

References:
Spranger J. W., Langer jr L. O., Wiedemann H.-R.: Bone Dysplasias. An Atlas of Constitutional Disorders of Skeletal Development, Stuttgart and Philadelphia, G. Fisher and W. B. Saunders, 1974.
Salinas C. F., Jorgenson R. J., Lorenzo R. L.: Variable expression in otopalatodigital syndrome; cleft palate in female. Birth Defects 15:329 (1979)

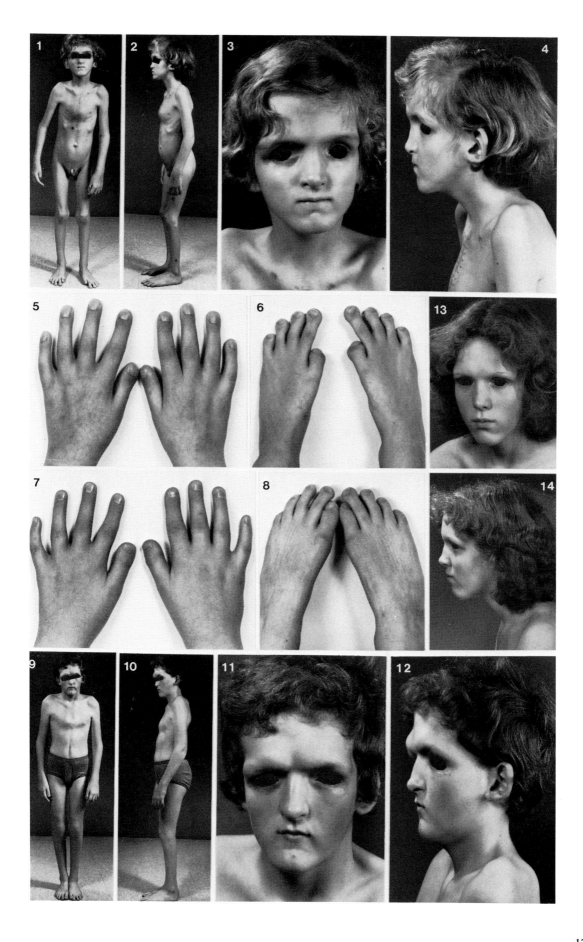

17

9. Coffin–Lowry Syndrome

A hereditary syndrome comprising unusual coarse facies, mental retardation, small stature, generalised hypotonia, and characteristic hands – with males more severely affected than females.

Main Signs:
1. Facies: Coarse supraorbital arches; hypertelorism; antimongoloid slant of the palpebral fissures; thick upper eyelids or ptosis; broad nasal root; coarse, broad nose with thick septum and alae nasi and anteverted nostrils; mouth often held open; pouting lower lip; unusual ears. (2 and 4–7).
2. Considerable mental retardation in males (IQ usually under 50), (milder in females).
3. Small stature, height possibly less than the 3rd percentile.
4. Clumsy, soft hands with tapering, hyperextensible fingers (8). Short halluces.

Supplementary Findings: Laxity of the joints and ligaments. Loose skin and muscular weakness (1). Frequent kyphoscoliosis (3), pectus carinatum or excavatum and pes valgus. Clumsy wide-based gait. (These findings especially pronounced in males.)

Radiologically, ungual phalanges of the fingers, short and distally tufted, coarse middle phalanges, short rays of the big toes in the feet, coxae valgae, and other deformities. Possible cerebral seizures.

Manifestation: At birth or later.

Aetiology: Hereditary disorder with mode of inheritance not yet definitely established (primary sex-linked recessive, but sex-limited autosomal dominant inheritance has been considered as has autosomal dominant with various grades of expressivity).

Frequency: Rare; 17 observations had been reported up to 1977.

Course, Prognosis: The signs and symptoms increase with age.

Differential Diagnosis: Further forms of mental retardation and growth deficiency with coarse facies.

Treatment: Symptomatic. Handicap aids. Genetic counselling for the parents.

Illustrations:
1–8 A proband with typical signs of the syndrome. (By kind permission of Prof. W. Lenz, Münster i. W., FRG.)

References:
Tentamy S. A., Miller D., Hussels-Maumenee I.: The Coffin–Lowry syndrome: An inherited faciodigital mental retardation syndrome. J. Pediatr. *86*:724 (1975)
Fryns J. P., Vinken L., van den Berghe H.: The Coffin syndrome. Hum. Genet. *36*:271 (1977)

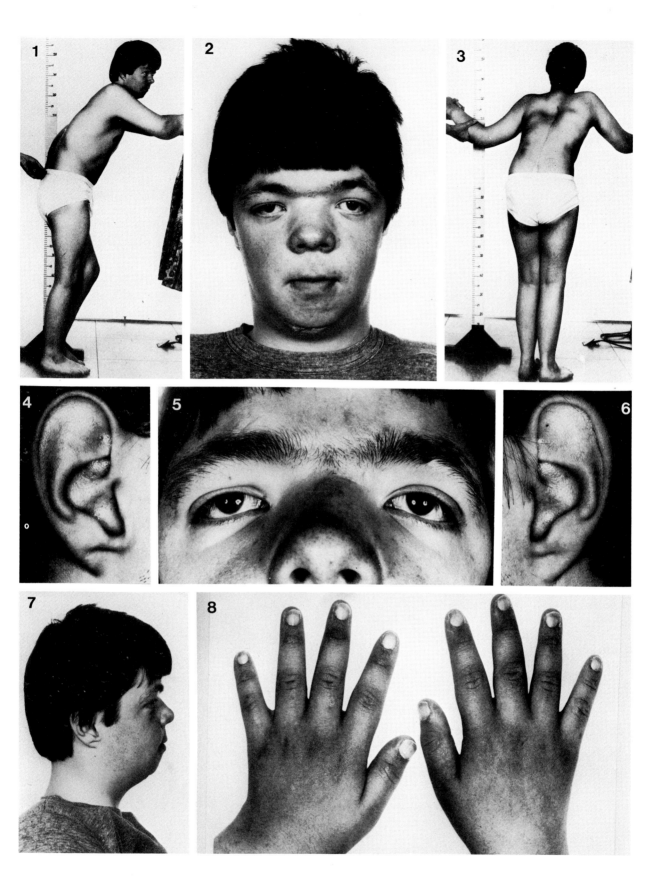

10. Melnick–Needles Syndrome

(Osteodysplasty)

A highly characteristic hereditary syndrome of the osseous system, with typical facial appearance.

Main Signs:
1. Relatively large cranium with high prominent forehead and more or less marked delay in closure of the anterior fontanelle. Facial part of the skull small, with exophthalmos, hypertelorism, fleshy nose and full cheeks, relatively large ears, malalignment of the teeth, malocclusion (1).
2. More or less distinct bowing of the arms and legs with cubitus valgus and genu valgum positions. Slight shortening of the distal phalanges of the hands and feet, especially of the thumbs.
3. Bizarre, characteristic changes on X-rays (especially: constrictions of the diaphyses and cortical irregularities) of the long bones (2), the ribs (4), clavicles, shoulder blades and the pelvis (5): severe coxa valga; other areas affected as in a generalised skeletal dysplasia.

Supplementary Findings: Hip dysplasia not infrequent; club feet. Mental development not affected.

A possible hearing defect or anomalies of the urinary tract must be ruled out.

Manifestation: Pre- and postnatal. Apart from the abnormal facies and delayed closure of the anterior fontanelle, the patients usually come to attention because of their abnormal gait and 'bowed limbs'.

Aetiology: Monogenic hereditary disorder, autosomal dominant. Considerable variability of penetrance and expressivity. Majority of the described cases female. The question of heterogeneity is still open. Basic defect unknown.

Frequency: Very low (scarcely 50 cases have been described in the literature).

Course, Prognosis: Not infrequently initial failure to thrive as well as increased susceptibility to infections of the upper respiratory tract and the middle ear in the first years of life. As a rule, normal adult height. Normal life expectancy. Possible difficulties with child bearing due to pelvic deformity. Premature arthroses.

Diagnosis, Differential Diagnosis: Prenatal recognition of skeletal changes on X-ray possible. Some superficial resemblance to, e.g., pyknodysostosis (p.136), craniometaphyseal dysplasia (p.66), or the Engelmann–Camurati syndrome (p.390), which can be immediately ruled out radiologically. Weakly expressed forms of the syndrome may be recognised only by chance.

Treatment: Symptomatic. Orthopaedic treatment, as required, for the spinal column, the hips, or the feet. Dental and orthodontic care.

Illustrations:
1–5 An 8-year-old patient with the fully expressed syndrome. Note in addition the related sclerosis of the base of the skull (3). (Kindly provided by Dr J. P. Fryns, Löwen.)

References
Spranger J. W., Langer jr L. O., Wiedemann H.-R.: Bone Dysplasias. An Atlas of Constitutional Disorders of Skeletal Development, Stuttgart and Philadelphia, G. Fischer and W. B. Saunders, 1974.
Leiber B., Olbrich G., Moelter N., et al: Melnick–Needles-Syndrom. Monatschr. Kinderheilkd. *123*:178 (1975)
Fryns J. P., Maertens R., van den Berghe H.: Osteodysplastia – a rare skeletal dysplasia. Acta Paediatr. Belg. *32*:65 (1979)

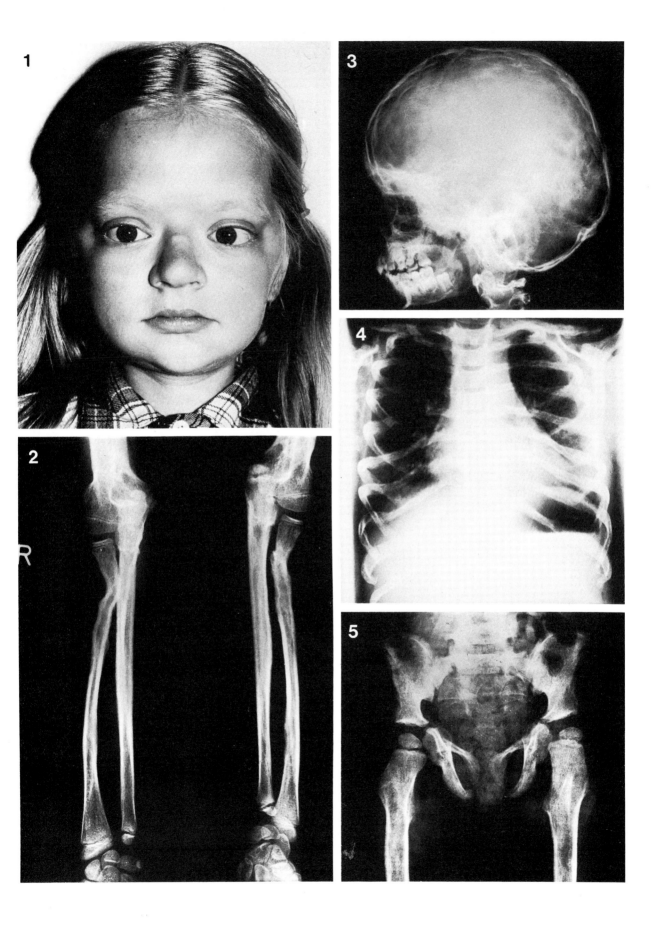

21

11. Syndrome of Cleidocranial Dysplasia

(Scheuthauer–Marie Syndrome)

A characteristic hereditary syndrome especially of the skeleton (cranium, clavicle, pelvis) with typical physical appearance.

Main Signs:
1. Large, broad and short cranium with frontal and parietal bossing and a supraglabellar depression (**1** and **3**), persistence of the fontanelles and sutures for years (**7**); facial part of the cranium relatively small with increased interocular distance; broad, depressed nasal root; in some cases anteverted nares (**2**) and mild exophthalmos.
2. Upper thorax narrow with absent or poorly defined superior and inferior clavicular depressions and drooping, angular shoulders (**2**, **4**, and **5**) with a-, hypo-, or dysplasia of the clavicles (**8**). Hypermobility of the shoulders (**3** and **6**)!

Supplementary Findings: Narrow pelvis, slender extremities, slight shortness of stature possible after infancy. Dysodontiasis (delay of both dentitions, supernumerary teeth) (**9**). Sometimes hypoplastic-brittle nails (**10**). Radiologically, numerous wormian bones (**7**), markedly delayed ossification of the bony pelvis, especially the pubic bones.

Manifestation: At birth.

Aetiology: Monogenic hereditary disorder, autosomal dominant, with quite variable expressivity. Isolated occurrence of a case in a kindred with no signs of the condition suggests a new mutation. However, the occurrence of an autosomal recessive hereditary form has recently been under discussion.

Frequency: Not so rare. By 1962, about 700 cases in the literature.

Course, Prognosis: Life expectancy not at all or scarcely affected. In many cases there are defects of the teeth and jaws. Disposition to luxation. Narrowness of the pelvis may necessitate caesarean deliveries.

Differential Diagnosis: In newborn and young infants, possible erroneous initial diagnosis of hydrocephalus or osteogenesis imperfecta. Later, possible confusion with the much less frequently occurring pyknodysostosis (p.136; having distinct growth deficiency, absence of the supraglabellar depression, clavicular ridges usually normal, no comparable defect of ossification of the pelvic bones; but, above all, osteosclerosis, tendency to fractures, poorly defined submaxillary angle. Autosomal recessive transmission).

Treatment: Early, qualified dental and orthodontic care. Orthopaedic treatment in some cases.

Illustrations:
1 A 2½-year-old.
2 and 3 A 5-year-old.
4–6 A 1½-year-old child.
7 Skull X-ray of a 4-year-old child: Open fontanelles and sutures, markedly widened frontal suture, numerous wormian bones.
8 Chest X-ray of an 8-year-old child: Aplasia of the clavicles and abnormally positioned scapulae.
9 Supernumerary incisors in both the upper and lower jaws between persisting deciduous teeth in a 9-year-old child.
10 Hypoplastic and brittle nails in a 5-year-old child.

References:
Wiedemann H.-R.: Gestörte Ossifikation besonders der bindegewebig präformierten Belegknochen: Die Dyostosis cleidocranialis. Handbuch der Kinderheilkunde, Bd. 6, p.128ff., Heidelberg, Springer 1967
Spranger J. W., Langer jr L. O., Wiedemann H.-R.: Bone Dysplasias. An Atlas of Constitutional Disorders of Skeletal Development, Stuttgart and Philadelphia, G. Fischer and W. B. Saunders, 1974
Goodman R. M., Tadmor R., Zaritsky A., et al: Evidence for an autosomal recessive form of cleidocranial dysostosis. Clin. Genet. 8:20 (1975)

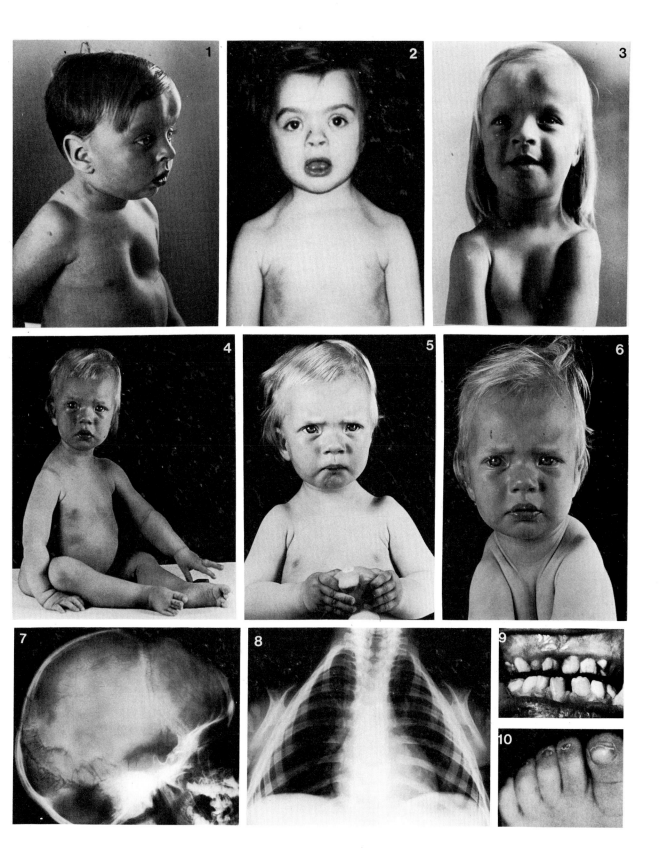

23

12. Syndrome of Increasing Macrocephaly with Signs of Cardiac Overload from Intracranial A-V Shunt

A clinical picture of progressive macrocephaly (with or without definite hydrocephalus) and signs of cardiac overload (in the absence of congenital heart defect) with intracranial A-V fistula (usually an aneurysm of the vein of Galen).

Main Signs:
1. An abnormally expanding cranium (**1** and **2**) with development of more or less distinct dilatation of the ventricular system and with minimal to definite signs of increased intracranial pressure.
2. Signs of cardiac strain without demonstrable congenital heart disease.
3. In most (but not all) cases a continuous or systolic vascular murmur is present over all or part of the cranium; in some cases increased vascular patterns, pulsations, etc. Usually conspicuously strong pulses of the cervical vessels, with thrills and murmurs.

Supplementary Findings: Demonstration of an intracranial A-V fistula (A-V aneurysm, generally involving the great vein of Galen) (**3** and **4**).

Manifestation: Macrocephaly apparent congenitally or postnatally. Signs of cardiac overload manifest sooner or later depending on the size of the shunt.

Aetiology: Uncertain.

Frequency: Not so rare; probably not a few go unrecognised.

Course, Prognosis: In view of the precarious cerebral and cardiac problems, always dubious.

Diagnosis: Initially, computer tomography; subsequently bilateral carotid and vertebral artery angiograms indicated.

Treatment: The myocardial insufficiency may not respond to medical therapy. In given cases, ultimate surgical correction at a time carefully chosen by the neurosurgeon and cardiologist.

Comment: 1. When of a corresponding size, an extra-cardiac A-V shunt in any location of the body can lead to signs of cardiac overload and possibly to life-threatening decompensation.
2. Intracranial shunts of a given size are frequently manifest immediately post partum with severe cyanotic cardiac insufficiency. When not manifest until later in infancy or thereafter, developing hydrocephalus and convulsions or subarachnoid haemorrhages and neurological defects may dominate the picture. The 'craniomegaly' form presented here is one particular, unusual clinical form.

Illustrations:
1 and 3 A 5-year-old boy with congenital, progressive macrocephaly (at birth, 39 cm; 11 months, 52.8 cm; 13 months, 54 cm; 4 years, 58 cm). Signs of cardiac overload, without evidence of congenital heart defect, due to an extracardial left-to-right shunt. Continuous vascular murmur along with increased venous markings on the cranium; low voltage EEG, dilated ventricles, and papilloedema. Otherwise normal development for age, with no neurological deficits. On angiogram, a large aneurysm of the great vein of Galen; aneurysmic enlargement of the confluence of the sinuses and adjacent vessels due to A-V shunts to both posterior cerebral arteries; numerous angiomas.
2a, b, c Another patient at ages 5, 7, and 8 years. Congenital, progressive macrocephaly (at birth 38 cm, at 5 years 60 cm). Signs of cardiac overload, without evidence of congenital heart defect, due to an extracardial left-to-right shunt. Continuous vascular murmur and increased vascular markings and pulsations on the cranium; low voltage EEG, secondary internal hydrocephalus (Pudenz–Heyer catheter). Otherwise normal development for age, with no neurological deficits. On angiogram, large aneurysm of the great vein of Galen with some angioma-like enlargement of adjacent vessels due to A-V shunts with both posterior cerebral arteries.
4. Successful operative closure of most of the pathological anastomoses without neurological sequelae at age 7 years (Prof. Yasargil, Zürich).
(By kind permission of Prof. P. Heintzen and Dr E. Stephan, Kiel.)

References:
Gold A. P., Ransohoff J., Carter S.: Vein of Galen malformation. Acta Neurol. Scand. *40*: (Suppl 11):1 (1964)
Amacher A. L., Shillito jr J.: The syndromes and surgical treatment of aneurysms of the great vein of Galen. J. Neurosurg. *39*: 89 (1973)
Cuncliffe P. N.: Cerebral arteriovenous aneurysm presenting with heart failure. Br. Heart J. *36*:919 (1974)
Kelly jr J. J., Mellinger J. F., Sundt jr T. M.: Intracranial arteriovenous malformations in childhood. Ann. Neurol. *338*:314 (1978)

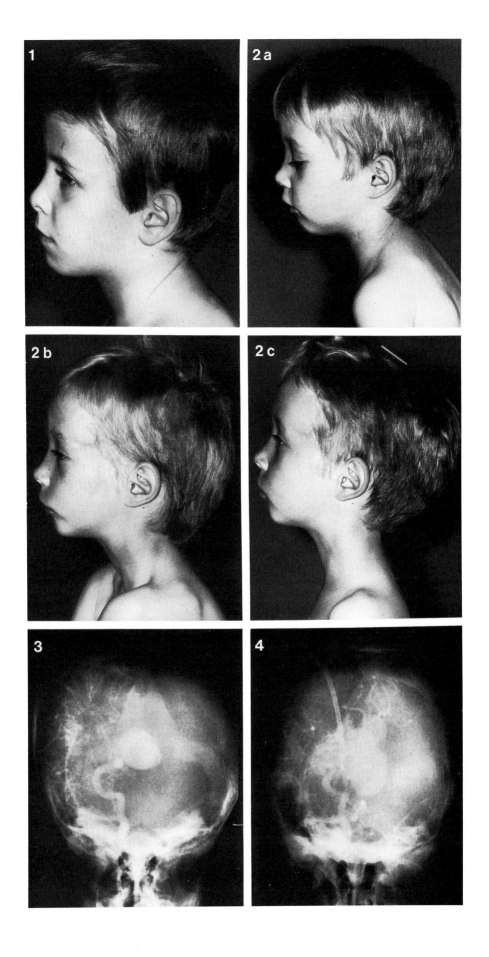

25

13. Syndrome of Megalencephaly, Distinctive Facies, and Developmental Retardation

A syndrome of primary megalencephaly, unusual facies, primary developmental retardation, and cardiac anomaly.

Main Signs:
1. Macrodolichocephaly (head circumference increasingly greater than the 98th percentile starting at a young age). Protrusion of the back part of the head, markedly prolonged closure of the anterior fontanelle, which is neither tense nor bulging, protruding forehead. Strikingly deep-set eyes, broad nose, and pointed chin (**1** and **2**).
2. Primary, obvious psychomotor retardation.

Supplementary Findings: Normal height. Short neck; thickset, bulky trunk and limbs (**1** and **2**). Heart murmur. Large genitalia (**1a**); testicular volume of the older boy at 20 months 3–4 ml, at 4 years and 5 months 5–6 ml.

No evidence of intracranial vascular malformation nor of hydrocephalus (normal cerebral ventricles on repeated echo-encephalograms; diaphanoscopy negative; cerebral angiography negative bilaterally). Ophthalmological examination negative. Exhaustive neurological examinations negative. Endocrinological investigations negative. Specific tests for storage diseases and other hereditary degenerative diseases negative. Chromosome analysis negative.

Skull X-rays: Elongated cranium, marked delay in closure of the fontanelles, somewhat poorly defined and deeply serrated sutures, elongated flat sella turcica, numerous bony islands in the lambdoid suture (**3** and **4**). Further X-rays of the skeleton: Dissociated bone maturation (definitely delayed ossification in addition to partially accelerated ossification). Normal size heart with left-sided prominence in both brothers; suspected atrial septal defect and idiopathic dilatation of the pulmonary artery in the older boy.

Manifestation: Birth or shortly thereafter.

Aetiology: Genetic factors very likely; possibly autosomal dominant transmission with development of signs much more likely in males.

Course, Prognosis: Principally determined by the primary mental impairment in these children. No evidence of mental deterioration.

Diagnosis, Differential Diagnosis: The known conditions accompanied by increased intracranial pressure and the syndrome described on p.24 must be ruled out. Macrocranium without signs of cerebral compression and with normal neurological and sometimes developmental behaviour of the child should, especially in familial cases, suggest megalencephaly and can obviate the use of invasive methods of examination.

Treatment: Symptomatic.

Illustrations:
1–4 The 2nd and 3rd children of young, healthy, nonconsanguineous parents after a girl and 2 abortions. Others with large heads in the family! The first born is – to a lesser degree – likewise macrodolichocephalic (at 5½ months, 44 cm; at 4 years 5 months 55 cm) and has congenital heart disease (persistent ductus arteriosis, repaired; ventricular septal defect; anomalies of the pulmonary artery); completely normal psychomotor development, slight adiposity. Normal pregnancy and delivery with both brothers. Birth measurements of the older: 4.3 kg, 59 cm, 38.5 cm. Head circumference of the younger (**2**) at 13 months, 53 cm (**3**); the older at 10 months, 52 cm; 20 months, 57 cm; 2½ years, 59 cm; and 3 years 2 months (**4**), 61.5 cm. Obesity in the older brother. Resemblance of the brothers increasing. (In part, by kind permission of Prof. P. Heintzen and Prof. H. Doose, Kiel.)

References:
DeMyer W.: Megalencephaly in children. Neurology 22:634 (1972)
Jennings M.T., Hall J.G., Kukolich M.: Endocardial fibroelastosis, neurologic dysfunction and unusual facial appearance in two brothers, coincidentally associated with dominantly inherited macrocephaly. Am. J. Med. Genet. 5:271 (1980)
Petit R. E., Kilroy A. W., Allen J. H.: Macrocephaly with head growth parallel to normal growth pattern. Arch. Neurol 37:518 (1980)
Priestly B. L., Lorber J.: Primary megalencephaly. Z. Kinderchirur. 31:335 (1980)

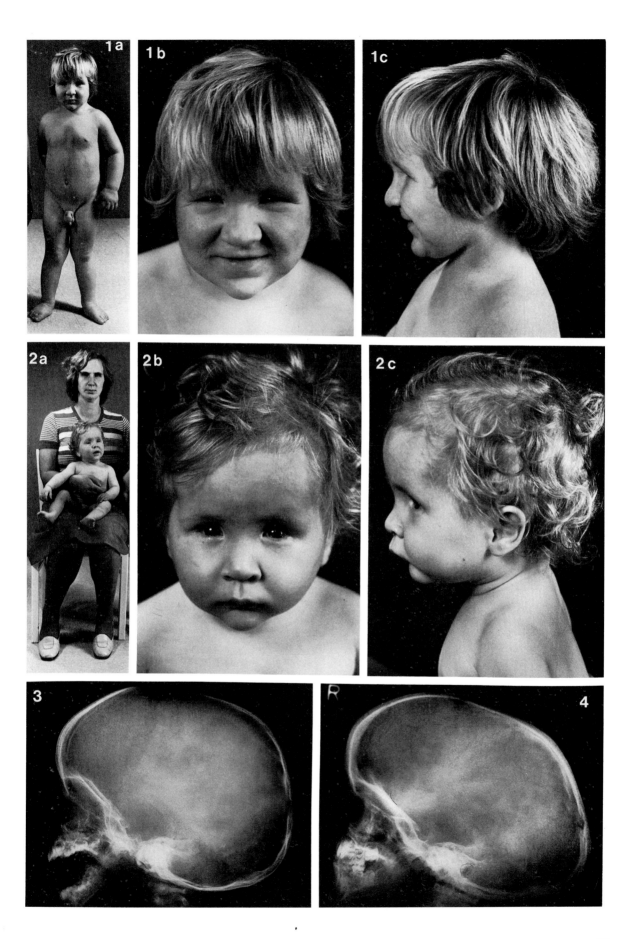

14. Hypertelorism Syndrome

(Greig's Hypertelorism Syndrome, Median Cleft Face Syndrome, Syndrome of Frontonasal Dysplasia)

A syndrome of ocular hypertelorism (abnormally increased interorbital distance), its concomitant signs and sequelae in the head region, and various other associated anomalies.

Main Signs:
1. Hypertelorism up to lateralisation of the eyes in extreme cases. Divergent strabismus. Low, wide bridge of the nose (**1** and **2**), sometimes indented sagittally (**3**) or even cleft (in such cases frequent cranium bifidum occultum and/or schistoprosopia). Broad cranium with wide open anterior fontanelle and open frontal suture, even in milder cases.
2. Cleft lip and palate, high wide palate, diastematic dentition.
3. Relatively infrequent mental retardation.

Supplementary Findings: Frequent association of various extracranial malformations such as heart defects, kidney malformations, anomalies of the extremities such as brachydactyly, clinodactyly, and others.

Manifestation: At birth.

Aetiology: Predominantly sporadic occurrence. As an exception, autosomal dominant transmission has been observed.

Frequency: Low (somewhat more than 70 cases described in the literature up to 1970).

Course, Prognosis: Life expectancy normal except in very severe cases.

Differential Diagnosis: Hypertelorism occurs as a mere con-comitant sign in numerous other malformation syndromes.

Treatment: In some cases operative measures for strabismus or, possibly, plastic surgery.

Illustrations:
1–3 Cases of different grades of severity in infants. Patient 1 had a heart defect as associated anomaly.

References:
Sedano H. O., Cohen M. M., Jirasek J., Gorlin R. J.: Frontonasal dysplasia. J. Pediatr. 76:906 (1970)
DeMyer W.: Median facial malformations and their implications for brain malformations. Birth Defects *11* (no 7):155 (1975)

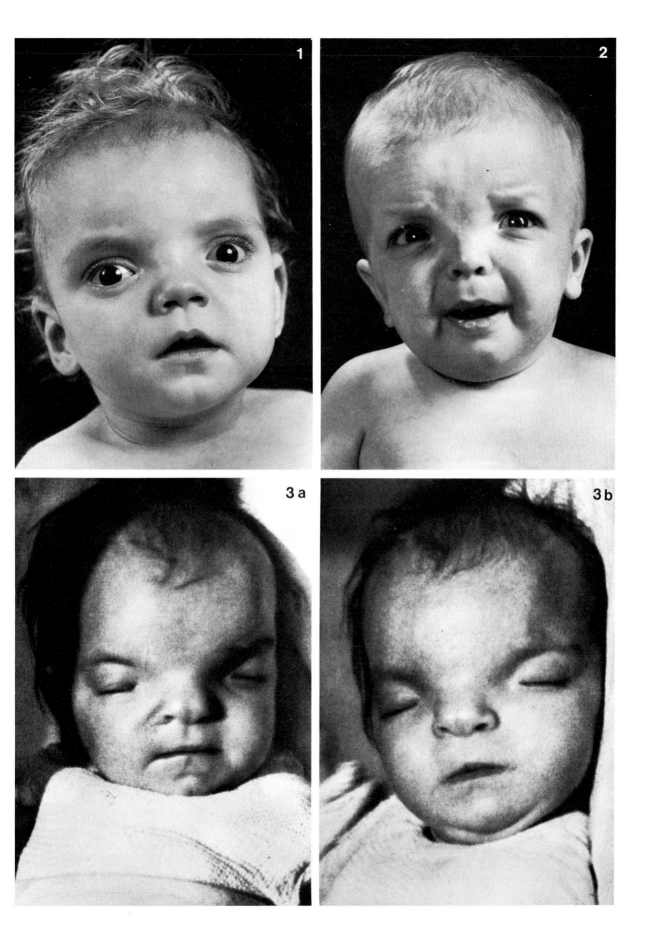

15. Holoprosencephaly Syndrome

(Arhinencephaly Syndrome)

A syndrome of markedly decreased interocular distance, hypoplasia of the nose, and maldevelopment of the prosencephalon.

Main Signs:

1. Abnormally decreased interorbital distance with cyclopia in extreme cases and corresponding narrowing and flattening of the nose, frequently with choanal atresia and absence of the septum (1–3). In the extreme case of cyclopia, the orbits and eyes fuse to produce monophthalmia, with the nose as a rudimentary 'sausage-like' organ located above the eye.

2. Bilateral cleft lip and palate, seldom in cases of cyclopia, occurring frequently in the less severe cases (1–3).

3. Primordial growth deficiency.

4. Microcephaly, sloping forehead, exophthalmos (2 and 3); trigonocephaly, occasionally hydrocephalus.

Supplementary Findings: Incomplete or lack of differentiation of the prosencephalon into hemispheres and a corresponding ventricular system, so that in the extreme case a single large ventricle is enclosed by pallium without a sagittal division. Generaly absence of the corpus callosum, septum pellucidum, and hypophysis; arhinencephalia in the narrower sense. Severity of the brain deformity corresponds essentially to that of the facial.

Poikilothermia, spasticity, seizures, respiratory disorders.

No psychomotor development.

Manifestation: At birth.

Aetiology: Heterogeneous; there is evidence for autosomal dominant (mostly new mutations) and recessive inheritance. Teratogenic influences are also likely. The general risk of recurrence is about 6%.

Frequency: Ca. 1:16000 live births.

Prognosis: Practically all children die before 1 year of age.

Differential Diagnosis: The holoprosencephaly syndrome may be part of the trisomy 13 syndrome (p.56), of the syndrome of deletion of the short arm of chromosome 18, or of other chromosomal syndromes. In these cases multiple extra-cranial anomalies are usually present.

Treatment: Conservative, symptomatic.

Illustrations:

1–3 A 7-day-old child. Birth measurements 46 cm, 2800 g, 28 cm (head circumference). Seizures, fluctuating temperature, tachypnoea, dysphagia. Death at age 5½ months (weight 5500 g) from bronchopneumonia. Monoventricular prosencephalon, synostoses of the cranial sutures.

References:

DeMyer W., Zeman W., Palmer C.: The face predicts the brain: diagnostic significance of median facial anomalies in holoprosencephaly (arhinencephaly). Pediatrics 34:256 (1964)

Roach E., DeMyer W., Conneally P.M., et al: Holoprosencephaly: birth data, genetic and demographic analyses of 30 families. Birth Defects XI/2:294 (1975)

Burck U.: Genetic counselling in holoprosencephaly. Helv. Pediatr. Acta 37:231 (1982)

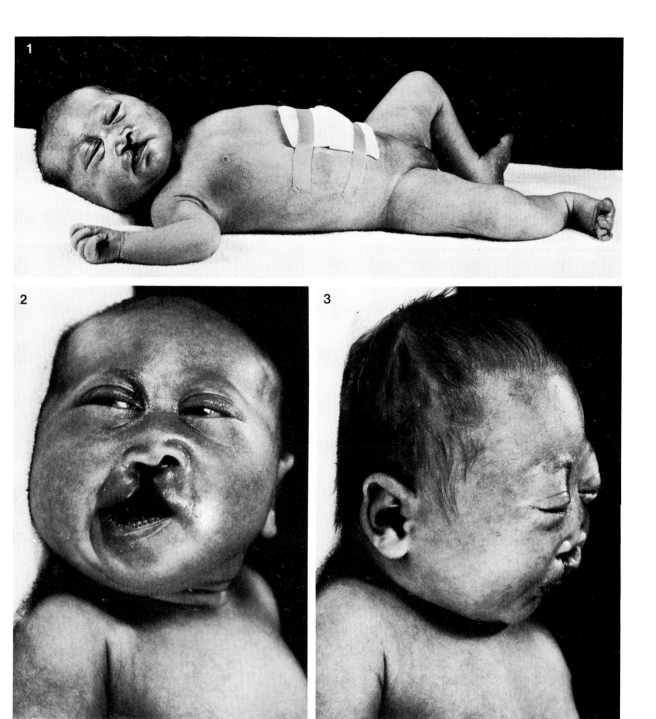

31

16. An Unfamiliar Syndrome with Cleft Lip and Palate

A syndrome of cheilognathopalatoschisis, severe psychomotor retardation, and internal malformations.

Main Signs:
1. Bilateral cleft lip; complete cleft of the upper jaw and palate on the left, incomplete cleft of the jaw on the right (1–5). Cranial deformities: head somewhat oxycephalic with marked bulging of the forehead on the right (1–5); delayed closure of the sutures and fontanelles. Low-set, dysplastic auricles (5–8). Complete paralysis of the right facial nerve (2, 3, and 5). Abnormal hairline.
2. Severe psychomotor retardation.
3. Congenital heart defect.

Supplementary Findings: Short neck with loose skin at the back of the neck. Barrel-shaped chest. Limited mobility of the shoulder joints. Retarded bone age.

Left-sided inguinal hernia; bilateral undescended testicles.

Manifestation: At birth.

Aetiology: Undetermined.

Course: Early death of the child due to renal insufficiency (see below).

Illustrations:
1–8 The child described above at ages 7 and 8½ months. The boy was the 2nd child of healthy young parents (1st child healthy); no evidence of parental consanguinity. Child born 6 weeks prematurely (2130 g, 43 cm). Early manifestation of renal insufficiency; persistent anaemia; no evidence of tubulopathy. Normal, unremarkable male karyotype on chromosome analysis (banding technique). Death at age 1½ years. At autopsy, *diffuse angiomatosis of the leptomeninges over the frontal lobes* of both cerebral hemispheres. No hydrocephalus. Ectasia of the pulmonary artery. Right-sided *renal aplasia*.

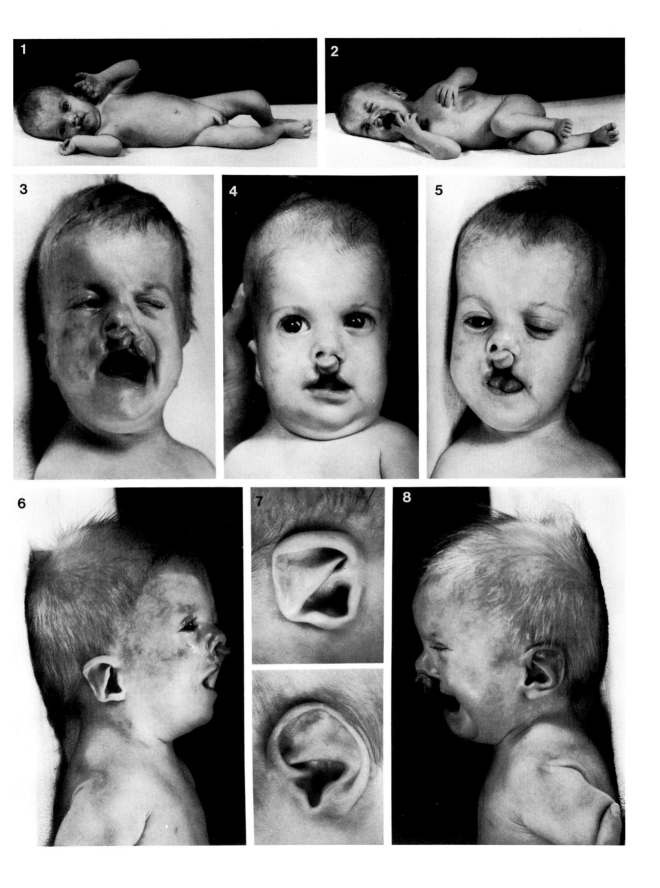

17. Freeman–Sheldon Syndrome

(Craniocarpotarsal Dysplasia; Whistling Face Syndrome)

A highly characteristic hereditary syndrome with mask-like 'whistling' face, hypoplastic alae nasi, ulnar deviation of the hands, flexion contractures of the fingers, and club feet.

Main Signs:
1. Face: Round, full-cheeked; mask-liked immobility with deep-set, relatively widely spaced eyes, narrow palpebral fissures with slight antimongoloid slant, convergent strabismus; wide, low-set root of the nose; epicanthus; small nose with hypoplastic alae; long philtrum and small mouth, which is difficult to open, with – more or less distinctly – lips pursed as though for whistling. Paramedian creases or dimples between the lower lip and the tip of the chin (1–3).
2. Ulnar deviation of the hands and flexion contractures of the fingers, especially the thumbs (4). Club feet resistant to therapy, contractures of the toes.

Supplementary Findings: Transverse ridge below the forehead or furrow in the supraorbital soft tissue (3). In some cases ptosis; high palate, usually not cleft; occasionally defective hearing.

Short neck (sometimes slight pterygium). Usually considerable growth deficiency. Frequently development of marked scoliosis.

Manifestation: At birth.

Aetiology: Hereditary defect with autosomal dominant transmission. Apparent occurrence of an autosomal recessive type also, i.e., heterogeneity.

Frequency: Low; approximately 65 cases have been described.

Course, Prognosis: Life expectancy not affected.

Diagnosis, Differential Diagnosis: Exclusion of arthrogryposis (p.302) should not cause problems. In children beyond infancy, Catel–Schwartz–Jampel syndrome (p.380) may be difficult to rule out. There is considerable symptomatologic overlap – thus, in 'true' cases of Freeman–Sheldon syndrome, extra-facial disturbance in muscle tone may be seen at an early age; later on, frequent contractures of the large joints observed, and also less severe skeletal dysplasias determined. However, as a rule, congenital manifestations absent, demonstrable myotonia (EMG), and recessive inheritance in the Catel–Schwartz–Jampel syndrome.

Treatment: Adequate corrective treatment of club feet, of the fingers, of strabismus, of the mouth, etc. Psychological guidance. Genetic counselling of the family.

Illustrations:
1–4 A 1-year-old boy from a healthy family (new mutation) with the full clinical picture at birth. Unremarkable psychomotor development. Extreme malpositioning of all fingers (4). The left 2nd and right 4th toes are displaced proximally (shortened metatarsals). (By kind permission of Prof. A. Rett, Vienna.)

References:
Antley R. M., Uga N., Burzynski N. J., et al: Diagnostic criteria for the whistling face syndrome. Birth Defects *11* (5):161 (1975)
Vaitiekaitis A. S., Hornstein L. Neale H. W.: A new surgical procedure for correction of lip deformity in cranio-carpotarsal dysplasia (whistling face syndrome). J. Oral Surg. *37*:669 (1979)
Kousseff B. G., McConnachie P., Hadro T. A.: Autosomal recessive type of whistling face syndrome. Pediatrics 69:328 (1982)

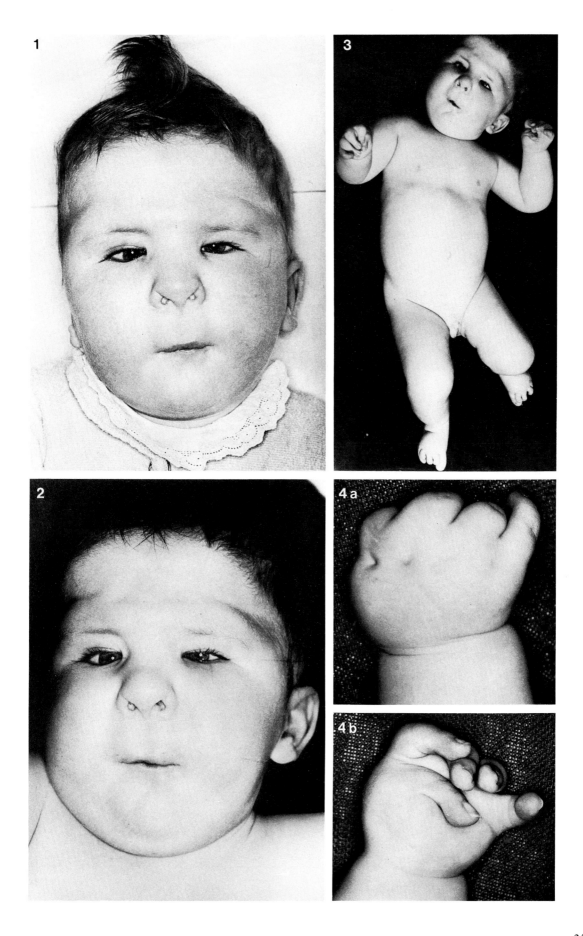

18. Syndrome of Mandibulofacial Dysostosis

(Franceschetti–Zwahlen Syndrome; Treacher Collins Syndrome)

A hereditary syndrome with very characteristic facial dysmorphism.

Main Signs:
1. Antimongoloid slant of the (possibly abnormally short) palpebral fissures with more or less distinct coloboma (possibly only indentation) in the lateral half of the lower eyelids (from which the eyelashes may be more or less absent) – rarely also of the upper lids (**1–4**).
2. Frontonasal angle often flat (**1–3**). Possibly beak-like and/or large-appearing nose, sometimes with narrow nares (**1–4**).

Hypoplasia of the zygomata and of the upper and lower jaws with the cheeks appearing sunken in (see especially **3a**); narrow, receding chin.

In many cases macrostomia (**1b**) with high narrow or cleft palate and malocclusion.
3. More or less marked malformation of the external ear (microtia, stenosis or atresia of the auditory canal) (**1–4**). Not infrequently defects of the middle and/or inner ear; these are more likely, the more severe the external ear deformity. Possibly atrophic areas of skin, blind fistulas, or skin tags between the corner of the mouth and the ear (**1c**). (The appearance has been described as fish- or bird-like facies) (**1** and **2**).
4. Frequent conductive hearing impairment or deafness.

Supplementary Findings: Abnormal growth of the hair from the temples on to the cheeks, toward the corners of the mouth (**1a, 3b** and **4a**). Occasionally, the facial anomalies can be asymmetric or even unilateral.

Malformations of the eyes such as microphthalmos or coloboma of the iris are unusual. Choanal atresia in isolated cases.

Diverse extracranial malformations, e.g., congenital heart defect, may occur. Intelligence normal as a rule (in cases of doubt, allowance should be made for the patient's psychological handicap and the possibility of hearing impairment).

Manifestation: Birth; hearing impairment later, if present.

Aetiology: Autosomal dominant hereditary disorder with high penetrance, but variable expressivity. Large proportion of new mutations.

Frequency: Not so rare (in 1964 it was possible to compare 200 cases from the literature).

Course, Prognosis: With growth of the facial skeleton during childhood, some improvement in appearance is possible.

Differential Diagnosis: Exclusion of the Goldenhar syndrome (p.40), the Hallermann–Streiff–François syndrome (p.402), hemifacial microsomia (p.42), Nager's dysostosis acrofacialis (p.38), postaxial acrofacial dysostosis syndrome (p.316), and the Wildervanck syndrome (p.216) should not be particularly difficult.

Treatment: Symptomatic. Early evaluation of hearing and prompt use of appropriate aids as required. Possibly plastic surgery as well as orthodontic and dental treatment.

Illustrations:
1 and 3 Two different newborn infants.
2 and 4 Two 3-month-old infants.

The child in **3** represents a hereditary case (father: full clinical picture of the syndrome); the other three children apparently represent new mutations. The infants in **1**, **2**, and **4** show bilateral atresia of the auditory canal; the latter child does not react at all to noises. Child in **1**: cleft palate. Child in **2**: bifid uvula, heart defect.

References:
Rogers B. O.: Berry–Treacher Collins syndrome: a review of 200 cases. Br. J. Plast. Surg. *17*:109 (1964)

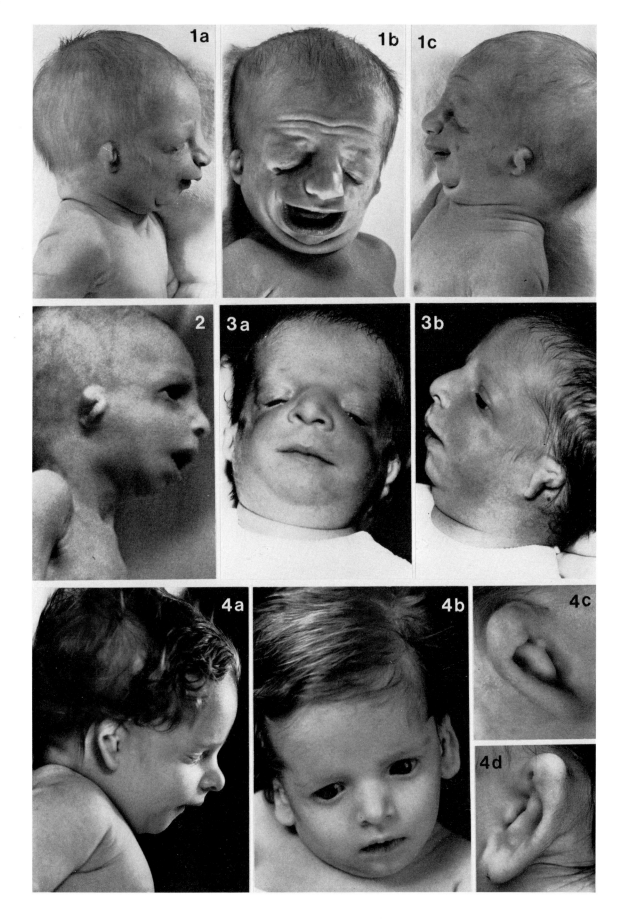

37

19. Nager Dysostosis Acrofacialis

(Nager–de Reynier Syndrome of Acrofacial Dysostosis)

A mandibulofacial hereditary dysostosis with hypoplasias of the extremities, especially of the 1st rays of the upper limbs.

Main Signs:
1. Facial dysmorphism in the pattern of dysostosis mandibulofacialis (p.36) (**1** and **2**). Frequently conductive hearing impairment.
Additionally:
2. Anomalies of the thumbs (triphalangism, hypoplasia, aplasia), in some cases of the neighbouring rays also, and possibly of the bones of the forearms (radial hypoplasia, radioulnar synostosis, etc.) (**3** and **4**). Occurrence of hypoplasias of the lower limbs also.

Supplementary Findings: Initial sucking and swallowing difficulties (as with the Robin anomaly, p.52) not unusual.

Growth deficiency apparently frequent. Occurrence of cryptorchidism and dysplastic mamillae.

Possible mild to moderate mental retardation.

Manifestation: Birth; hearing defect later, if present.

Aetiology: A genetic basis certain, but the precise situation not completely clear. Predominantly autosomal recessive inheritance with autosomal dominant transmission apparently also possible. Thus, heterogeneity likely. Basic defect unknown.

Frequency: Low (about 30 cases described).

Course, Prognosis: Growth processes in the facial skeleton during childhood may bring about some improvement in appearance.

Differential Diagnosis: The syndrome of the absent 5th ray (p.316) should not be difficult to rule out on the basis of the other localisation of the defects.

Treatment: Symptomatic. Early evaluation of hearing, thereafter prompt use of special hearing and speech aids as required.

Hand, orthopaedic, and/or cosmetic surgery and orthodontic therapy as indicated.

Illustrations:
1–4 A child of healthy nonconsanguineous parents. Bilateral triphalangism of the thumbs, no radial dysplasia. High palate without cleft, considerable mandibular hypoplasia on X-ray too; hearing apparently not affected. Heart and lower extremities negative.

References:
Burton B.K., Nadler H.L.: Nager acrofacial dysostosis. J. Pediatr. *91*:84 (1977)
Meyerson M.D., Jensen K.M., Meyers J.M. et al: Nager acrofacial dysostosis: Early intervention and long term planning. Cleft Palate J. *14*/1:35 (1977)

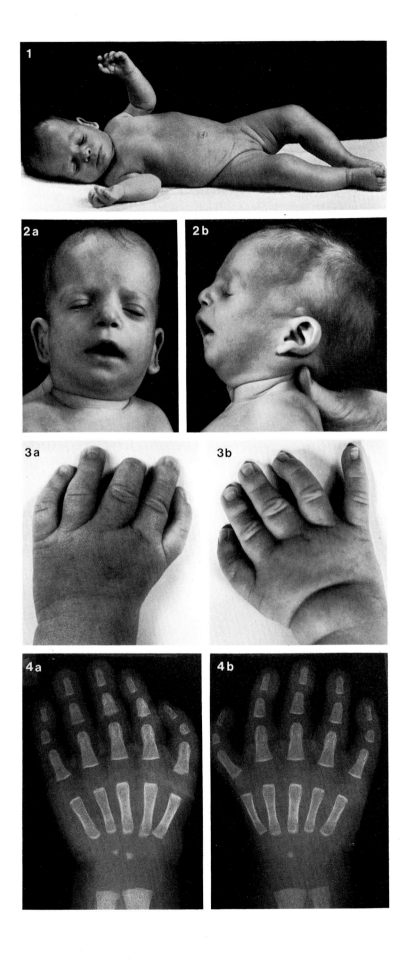

39

20. Goldenhar Syndrome

(Syndrome of Oculoauricular Dysplasia or Oculoauriculovertebral Dysplasia; Goldenhar–Gorlin syndrome)

A relatively characteristic complex of malformations including anomalies of the eye, ear, buccal, and possibly the vertebral regions.

Main Signs:
1. More or less pronounced facial asymmetry due to unilateral hypoplasia (**2** and **4**); usually prominence of the forehead (**1** and **4**), hypoplasia of the zygomatic region, sloping chin.
2. Epibulbar dermoid or lipodermoid (mostly bilaterally, at the lateral corneoscleral junction); coloboma of the upper lid (generally unilateral). Occurrence of other ocular anomalies also.
3. Preauricular tags, single or multiple, uni- or bilaterally on a line between the tragus and the corner of the mouth (**1**, **3**, **4**, and **7**). Similarly located blind fistulas also possible. Occasionally dysplasia of the external ear (**7a**).
4. In many cases unilateral macrostomia as a result of transverse fissure of a cheek (**2** and **4**).
5. More or less marked dysplasia in the (especially upper) vertebral column, often demonstrable by X-ray only (**5**); occasionally scoliosis.

Supplementary Findings: Frequent anomalies of the teeth.

Possible conduction deafness.

Occasional mental retardation.

Cardiac, pulmonary, and other deformities may occur.

Manifestation: At birth; possible hearing defect, later.

Aetiology: Probably heterogeneous. Mostly sporadic occurrence. Isolated cases indicate possible autosomal dominant, and some, autosomal recessive transmission.

Frequency: Not so rare.

Course, Prognosis: Favourable.

Diagnosis, Differential Diagnosis: No single sign is obligatory. Differentiation from mandibulofacial dysostosis (p.36) should not pose any particular problems, but differentiation from hemifacial microsomia (p.42) and from Wildervanck syndrome (p.216) may be practically impossible.

Treatment: Removal of preauricular tags and larger dermoids. Closure of a buccal fissure if present (**6**). Plastic–cosmetic surgery in some cases. Dental care.

Early evaluation of hearing in all cases. If needed, hearing aids from early childhood on.

Illustrations:
1–3 and 6 Male infant at ages 8 and 9 months. Macrocephaly, slight facial asymmetry favouring the left side with evident hypoplasia of the right mandible. Lipodermoid on the right bulb laterally, right palpebral fissure narrower than the left. On the right, preauricular tag; on the left, three small tags, one of which is located between the ear and the corner of the mouth. Transverse buccal fissure on the right. Capillary angiomas of the midface and occiput. Scoliosis; 13 pairs of ribs. Mental development and hearing apparently unaffected.
4 and 5 Newborn girl. Facial asymmetry; three right-sided preauricular appendages; hypoplasia of the zygoma; macrostomia as a result of a small right-sided transverse buccal fissure, receding chin; vertebral body anomalies.
7a and b Newborn girl with epibulbar dermoid on the left, low-set auricles, microtia on the right with atresia of the auditory canal (left auditory canal narrowed), bilateral preauricular tags, macrostomia (without a buccal fissure), and vertebral body anomalies (hemi- and block vertebrae) as well as 10 ribs on the right, 11 on the left.

References:
Shokeir M.H.K.: The Goldenhar syndrome: A natural history. Birth Defects *13*/3C: 67 (1977)
Feingold M., Baum J.: Goldenhar's syndrome. Am.J.Dis.Child. *132*:136 (1978)
Setzer E.S., Ruiz-Castenada N., et al: Etiologic heterogeneity in the oculoauriculovertebral syndrome. J.Pediatr. *98*:88 (1981)
Regenbogen L., Godel V., Goya V. et al: Further evidence for an autosomal dominant form of oculoauriculovertebral dysplasia. Clin.Genet. *21*:161 (1982)

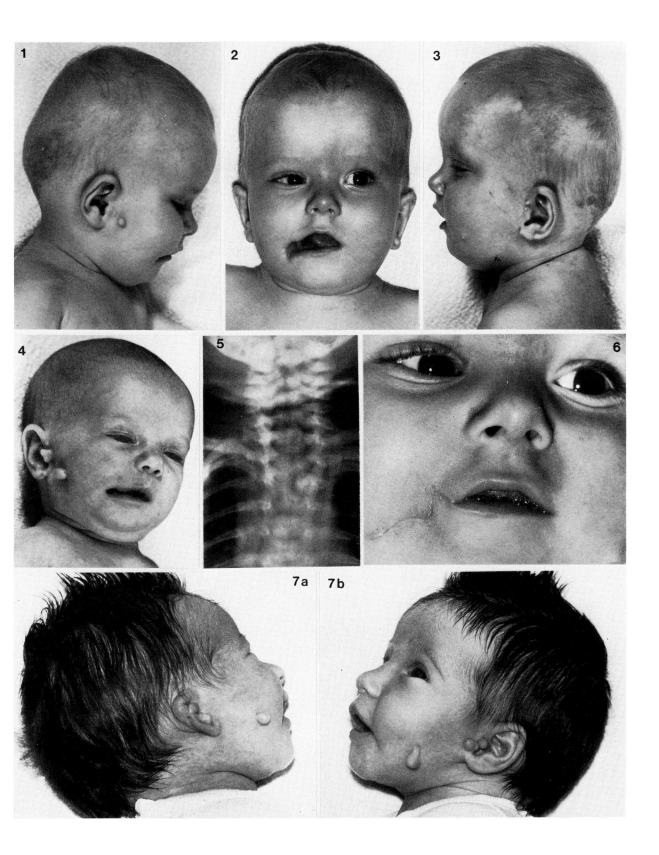

21. Hemifacial Microsomia

A clinical picture consisting of unusual facial asymmetry with unilateral ear deformity and ipsilateral hypoplasia especially of the ramus and condyle of the mandible.

Main Signs:
1. More or less marked facial asymmetry due to unilateral hypoplasia of the jaw; receding chin (1–3).
2. Preauricular appendages or dysplasia of the outer ear (2). In some cases aplasia.
3. Malocclusion on the affected side.

Supplementary Findings: Rather as an exception, anomalies of the eyes on the affected side (and generally *no* dermoids, lipodermoids, or colobomas of the upper lid).
   Possibly defective hearing.

Manifestation: At birth; hearing impairment later, if present.

Aetiology: Probably not uniform. Sporadic occurrence as a rule.

Frequency: Not so rare.

Course, Prognosis: Favourable.

Diagnosis, Differential Diagnosis: Differentiation from mandibulofacial dysostosis (p.36) easy; differentiation from Goldenhar syndrome (p.40) may be difficult or impossible.

Treatment: Plastic–cosmetic surgery in some cases. Dental care. Early evaluation of hearing. Hearing aids from early childhood in some cases.

Illustrations:
1–3   A 5-year-old boy from a healthy family. Malformation of the right ear (2: appearance after two operations to reconstruct a less conspicuous right ear) and hypoplasia of the right mandible.
   Marked, probably combined hearing defect on the right. Normal psychomotor development. Additional abnormalities: Limited ability to turn the head to the extreme right, low posterior hairline, hypoplastic accessory mamilla on the right.

References:
Pashayan H., Pinsky L., Fraser F.C.: Hemifacial microsomia: Oculo-auriculo-vertebral dysplasia: A patient with overlapping features. J. Med. Genet. 7:185 (1970)
Stewart R.E.: Craniofacial malformations. Pediatr. Clin. North America 25:500 (1978)
Feingold M.: Hemifacial microsomia. In: Birth Defects Compendium, 2nd Edn., p.511 (1979)

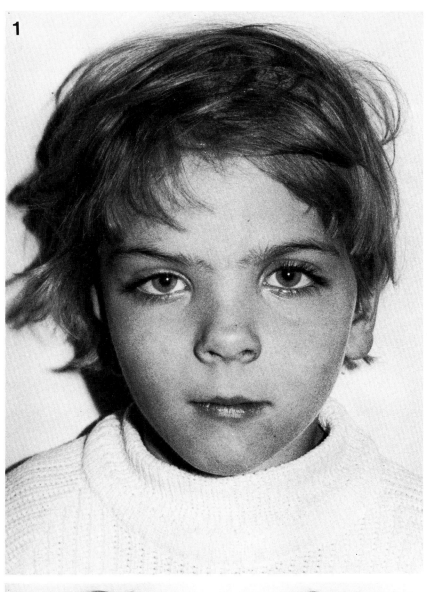

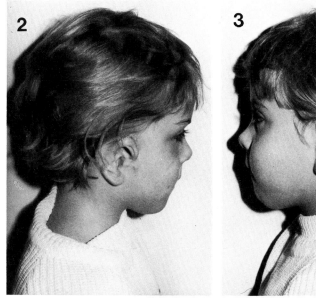

22. Syndrome of Progressive Hemifacial Atrophy

(Romberg Syndrome)

Localised facial atrophy, possibly associated with heterochromia iridis complicata.

Main Signs:
Progressive atrophy of some or all of the tissues on one side of the face. The whole side of the face may be involved (early stage shown in **1**; meanwhile further progression). Or patchy or stripe-like areas are affected, such that the changes – 'en coup de sabre' – resemble a sword-cut wound (**2**).

Supplementary Findings: Frequent pigmentation changes in the affected skin areas; similarly, discoloration and eventually loss of hair (eyebrows, eyelashes, etc.). Sensation remains intact on the affected side of the face; motor function barely affected despite involvement of the musculature.

In some cases involvement of the eye: sinking in of the eyeball; heterochromia iridis with cyclitis; strabismus.

Possible headache or facial neuralgia. In some cases contralateral disturbance of neurological function (e.g., focal epilepsy with contralateral expression).

Manifestation: Mainly in the first two decades of life.

Aetiology: Uncertain. Uniformity of the syndrome questionable. Occasional familial occurrence suggests genetic factors in these cases.

Frequency: Low.

Course, Prognosis: The atrophic process frequently subsides after a few years.

Differential Diagnosis: Hemifacial microsomia (p.42) and possibly Goldenhar syndrome (p.40).

Treatment: Symptomatic. Eventual cosmetic–plastic surgery in some cases.

Illustrations:
1 A 2½-year-old girl, normally developed for her age and from a healthy family. Since the end of her first year of life, increasing 'sinking in' of the whole right side of her face, including soft tissue, bony parts, and the eye, with unaltered toddler-like fullness of the left side of the face.

Occasional strabismus on the right. Tongue negative; no depigmentation of the integument; no heterochromia; no neurological findings. Symmetrical development of the remainder of the body as judged by appearance and measurements.

2 A 7¼-year-old boy, tall and slightly obese, from a healthy family: underdevelopment of the left side of the face noted since infancy; distinct underdevelopment of the maxillary sinuses and teeth on the left as compared with the right. On the forehead, two parallel, longitudinal pigmented atrophic areas of skin, ca. 4 cm long and barely a fingerbreadth wide, with bony involvement as in localised scleroderma of the 'en coup de sabre' type, the one median, the other 2 cm to the left. Development of these areas in the last few years. Occasional left-sided headache. Signs of a mild right-sided spastic hemiparesis with left-sided focal findings on EEG; no seizure disorder. Mild retardation. Ophthalmological investigations negative to date.

References:
Franceschetti A., Koenig H.: L'importance du facteur hérédo-dégénératif dans l'hémiatrophie faciale progressive (Romberg). Étude des complications oculaires dans ce syndrome. J. Génét. Hum. *1*:27 (1952)
Fulmek R.: Hemiatrophia progressiva faciei (Romberg-Syndrom) mit gleichseitiger Heterochromia complicata (Fuchs-Syndrom). Klin. Mbl. Augenheilkd *164*:615 (1974)
Muchnick R. S., Sherrel J. A., Rees Th. D.: Ocular manifestations and treatment of hemifacial atrophy. Am. J. Ophthalmol. *88*:889 (1979)
Asher St. W., Berg B. O.: Progressive hemifacial atrophy. Arch. Neurol. *39*:44 (1982)

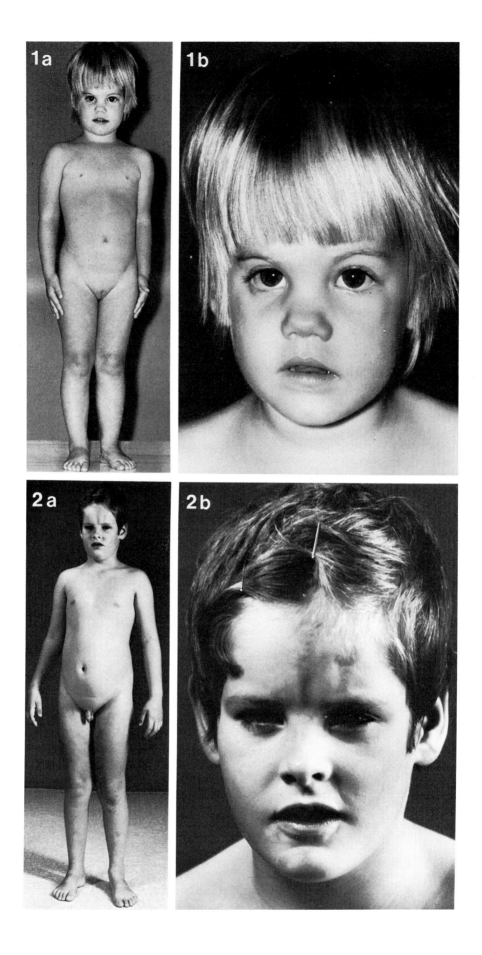

23. Oro-facio-digital Syndrome I

(OFD Syndrome I, Papillon = Léage-Psaume Syndrome)

A hereditary syndrome in females with lobulation of the tongue, hyperplastic frenula, notched alveolar processes, unusual facies, and anomalies of the hands and feet.

Main Signs:

1. Lobulation of the tongue into two or more lobes (**5**). Multiple hyperplastic intraoral frenula often with extensive fixation of the tongue and/or upper lip. Lateral notching of the alveolar process of the upper jaw (**8**), possible notches anteriorly in the alveolar process of the lower jaw. Cleft palate.

2. Unusual facies (**1–3**): broad root of the nose, asymmetry of the alae nasi, hypoplasia in the jaw area with dysodontiasis (lower lateral incisors frequently absent), possible median cleft lip. Milia on the face and around the ears during early infancy, later receding. Dry skin and alopecia of the scalp possible.

3. Clino-, brachy-, and syndactyly of the hands and feet (**7** and **9**, **10–12**).

Supplementary Findings: About half of the cases mentally retarded (then, average IQ of 70); dysraphism not uncommon. Hamartoma of the tongue in about 50% of the cases.

Manifestation: At birth.

Aetiology: An X-chromosomal dominant hereditary disorder. Since the gene is completely lethal in males, only females are affected clinically (exception: Klinefelter syndrome).

Frequency: Low; estimated frequency 1:50000.

Course, Prognosis: Practically normal life expectancy. Dependent on the mental development of the patient.

Differential Diagnosis: The oro-facio-digital syndrome II (p.314) occurs in both sexes (autosomal recessive inheritance); the main differentiating characteristics are bilateral polydactyly of the feet medially, broad notched tip of the nose, and absence more frequently of the middle than of the lateral incisors.

Treatment: Closure of clefts, removal of hypertrophic frenula, orthodontic and dental care, possibly corrective surgery of the hands, special schooling if required, etc. Genetic counselling.

Illustrations:

1–12 A 10-year-old girl with the fully expressed syndrome (appearance after operative correction of the inner canthi, upper lip, tongue, palate, and hands). Mild mental retardation. Small stature, below the 10th percentile. Flat midface. Thin hair. (By kind permission of Prof. B. Leiber, Frankfurt a. M.)

Reference:
Melnick M., Shields E. D.: Orofaciodigital syndrome, type I: A phenotypic and genetic analysis. Oral. Surg. *40*:599 (1975)

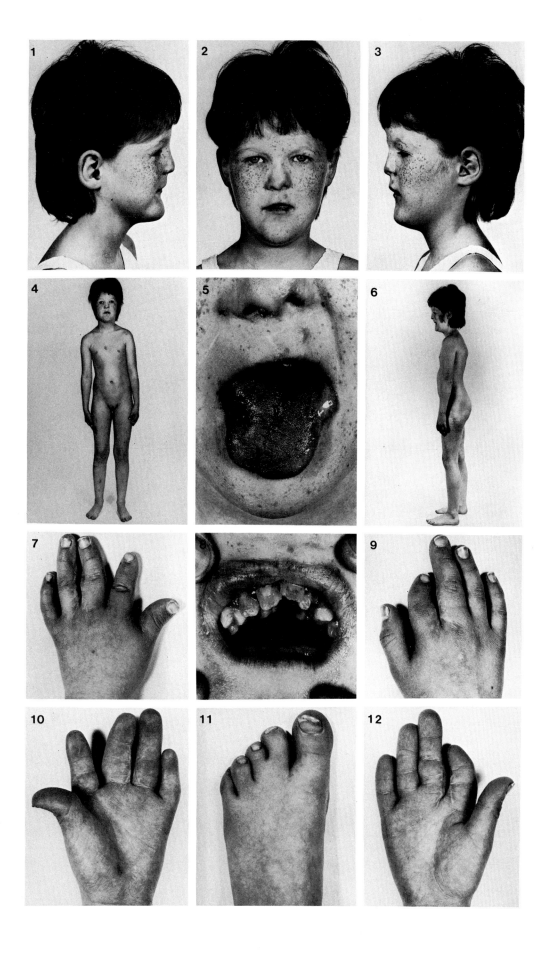

24. Syndrome of Microcephaly and Intraoral (Fibro-)Lipomatoid Hamartomatosis

A syndrome of congenital microcephaly, polypoid (fibro-)lipomatous hamartomas of the oral mucous membranes, and mild mental retardation.

Main Signs:

1. Congenital microcephaly (head circumference of the younger child at birth 33 cm, with birth length of 51 cm; head circumference thereafter always below the third percentile; at 3½ years, 45 cm; in the older sibling, 48 cm at 5 years) (1–5). Closure of fontanelles normal for age.

2. Congenital polypoid (fibro-)lipomatous hamartomas of the oral mucosa (multiple tumourlike, whitish to yellow-brown growths, rounded to lobular, on the tip, back, and edges of the tongue as well as on the alveolar processes, some removed surgically shortly after birth and some later in infancy; no recurrence). In addition, long tongue, which is furrowed, especially in the younger child (1, 2, 4, and 5); in 6, residua on the tongue of the older girl.

3. Slight delay of statomotor development of the older (walking unsupported at 18 months), considerable delay in the younger child (walking without support, still somewhat unstable, at 3 years); relatively good mental development of the younger sister and practically normal mental development of the older.

Supplementary Findings: Small stature (older sister below the 10th percentile, younger below the 3rd).

In both girls a fossette cutanée above the knee joint bilaterally (1). Bluish sclera and hyperextensible joints; hypotonia. External integument, ocular fundi, neurological examination (in the younger child including CCT, echo-EG, EEG), dental processes, dentition, as well as hands and feet unremarkable. Blood chemistries, endocrinological examinations (and chromosome analysis in the younger child) normal.

Manifestation: At birth.

Aetiology: Unknown; genetic basis probable.

Frequency: Unknown.

Course, Prognosis: Apparently relatively favourable.

Comment: In the differential diagnosis, an atypical oro-facio-digital syndrome type I (p.46) especially had to be considered, which however does not fit in this case. It appears to be a 'new syndrome'.

Illustrations:

1–6 The only children to date of young, healthy, nonconsanguineous parents.

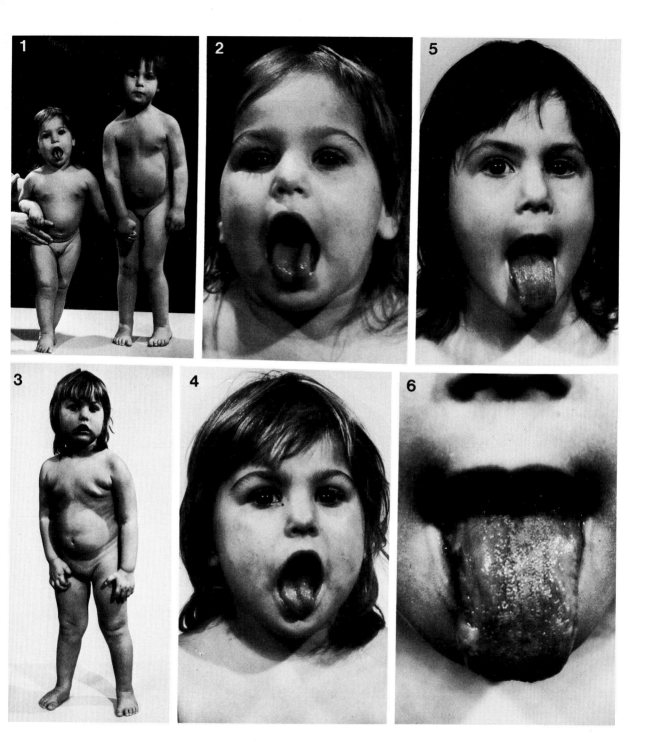

25. Cat-Eye Syndrome

(Coloboma–Anal Atresia Syndrome)

A syndrome of unusual facies, preauricular appendages and/or fistulas, coloboma of the iris, anal atresia, as well as other malformations and mental retardation.

Main Signs:
1. Facies characterised by hypertelorism, antimongoloid slant of the palpebral fissures, low root of the nose (**1** and **2**). Preauricular tags and/or fistulas (**3** and **4**). Generally bilateral coloboma of the iris (retina, choroid) (**2**). Possible microphthalmos.
2. Anal atresia with or without recto-vaginal or recto-perineal fistula.
3. Mental retardation not unusual, but generally mild.

Supplementary Findings: Various malformations of the kidneys and the urinary tract.
Cardiac defects.
Chromosome complement shows an extra small chromosome that has not yet been identified with absolute certainty.

Manifestation: At birth.

Aetiology: The above-mentioned extra chromosome can probably be regarded as the cause. Increased risk of occurrence for the affected family.

Frequency: Rare. To date, about 40 cases have been described.

Prognosis: Dependent on the presence and degree of mental retardation and on the severity of heart and kidney malformations and whether they are correctable.

Differential Diagnosis: There is a further 'cat-eye syndrome' with normal chromosomes, position anomalies of the hands and feet, and strikingly large thumbs.

Treatment: Operative correction of the anomalies amenable to surgical treatment and all appropriate handicap aids. Genetic counselling for the parents.

Illustrations:
1–4 A 5½-year-old girl who has had surgery for anal atresia as well as partial removal of preauricular appendages. Doubling of the renal pelves and ureters on pyelography. Development delayed only initially. IQ at 3½ years, 118.

Reference:
Schinzel A., Schmid W., Fraccaro M., et al: The 'Cat Eye-Syndrome':.... Hum.Genet. 57:148 (1981)

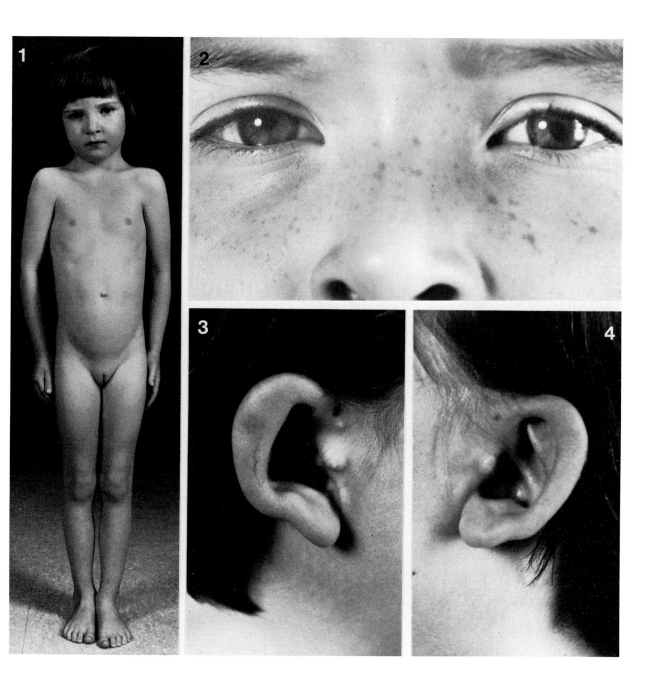

26. Robin Anomaly

(Pierre Robin Syndrome, Robin Syndrome)

A characteristic combination of hypoplasia of the lower jaw, glossoptosis, and cleft palate.

Main Signs:
1. Usually marked, sometimes extreme, micrognathia (**1, 2,** and **4**). In addition, retroglossia with narrowing of the airway, corresponding stridor, and in some cases signs of hypoxia.
2. Median cleft palate (**3**), possibly only a very high palate or bipartite uvula.

Supplementary Findings: Bulging of the upper rib cage (**5**) as a result of impeded respiration. Mental retardation not infrequent in patients with a history of hypoxic episodes.

Reports in the literature describe the Robin triad associated with anomalies of various other organs. Some of these cases can be further classified, e.g., as trisomy-18 syndrome (p.58), oro-acral syndrome (p.286), Möbius syndrome (p.372), and others; some cases will not fit into other groups. Because of this and of the various aetiologies, the Robin triad is viewed as an anomaly, which can occur alone or as part of a syndrome. In every newborn with the Robin anomaly, arthro-ophthalmopathy (Stickler syndrome p.404) must be ruled out, especially when there is a positive family history of hereditary myopia with or without retinal detachment, cleft palate, and spondylo-epiphyseal dysplasia. Examination by an ophthalmologist.

Manifestation: At birth.

Aetiology: Genetically nonuniform, with the majority of cases occurring sporadically. The primary defect is probably failure of the mandible to attain the proper size during the second fetal month, so that the tongue is not brought down and forward and closure of the palate is impeded.

Frequency: Not rare.

Prognosis: Dependent on the severity of the malformation. Danger of asphyxiation and of hypoxaemic brain damage. After survival of the first two months of life, prognosis good as a result of development of the mandible (**4** and **5**, a child at age 6 weeks and later, at age 1½ years).

Treatment: Abdominal position, glossopexy, extension of the lower jaw; tracheostomy should be reserved for desperate cases. Tube feeding, possibly gastrostomy. Surgery for cleft palate.

Illustrations:
1–3 A 4-week-old infant. Frequent asphyxial episodes. Aspiration pneumonias. Treated by abdominal position and tube feedings.
4–5 A patient at ages 6 weeks and 1½ years. Dyspnoea, stridor, frequent episodes of asphyxia in the first three weeks of life. Treatment by abdominal position and tube feedings. Note development of the mandible!

References:
Grimm G., Pfefferkorn A., Taatz H.: Die klinische Bedeutung des Pierre Robin-Syndroms und seine Behandlung. Dtsch Zahn-, Mund-, Kieferheilkd 43:169 (1964)
Opitz J.M.: Familial anomalies in the Pierre Robin syndrome. Birth Defects 5: 119 (1969)
Cohen jr M.M.: The Robin anomaly – its nonspecificity and associated syndromes. J.Oral Surg. 34:587 (1976)
Williams A.J. Williams M.A., Walker C.A., et al: The Robin anomalad (Pierre Robin syndrome) – a follow-up study. Arch.Dis.Child. 56:663 (1981)
Heaf D.R., Helms P.J., Dinwiddie R., et al: Nasopharyngeal airways in Pierre Robin syndrome. J. Pediatr. 100:698 (1982)

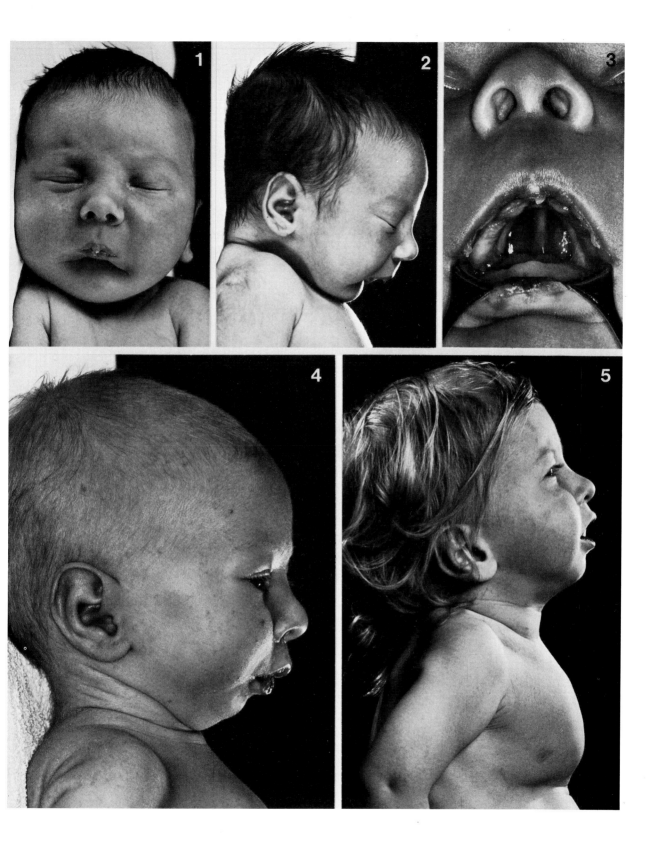

27. Cryptophthalmos Syndrome

Syndrome comprising absence of the palpebral fissure(s) – in most cases with eyelids and eyebrows missing to various degrees and with defects of the eyes, especially of the anterior portions – combined with anomalies of the external ear, the extremities, the genitalia, or of other areas.

Main Signs:
1. Uni- or bilateral absence of the palpebral fissure, usually with defects of the eyelids and eyebrows and anomalies of the eyes (defects of the anterior segment, microphthalmos, anophthalmos). Clumps of hair growing from the low temporal regions to the lateral parts of the eyebrows. Broad root of the nose, hypoplasia and notching of the alae nasi. Various degrees of dysplasia of the external (possibly also middle and inner) ears (1–3, 4, and 6).
2. Partial cutaneous syndactyly and more extensive anomalies of the extremities (7–9).
3. Malformation of the genitalia (hypospadias, vaginal atresia, pseudohermaphroditism) (5).

Supplementary Findings: Possible anomalies of the dome of the cranium, encephalocele, facial clefts, stenosis or atresia of the larynx, anal atresia, heart and/or kidney malformations.

Manifestation: At birth.

Aetiology: Presumably a nonuniform syndrome. Frequent sporadic occurrence. A type transmitted by autosomal recessive inheritance may be considered certain.

Frequency: Rare (about 50 cases described up to 1969).

Course, Prognosis: Dubious to poor with regard to visual acuity. Otherwise dependent on the type and severity of accompanying defects.

Treatment: 'Rehabilitating' measures, also of a cosmetic nature, where possible. Genetic counselling.

Illustrations:
1 and 2, 4–9 A newborn, the third child of healthy parents after two healthy children. Palpable bulbus oculi bilaterally; median notch of the nose; syndactyly of the hands and feet with hypoplasia of the distal phalanges; ambiguous external genitalia (normal female karyotype); malformations of internal organs. (By kind permission of Dr A. Fuhrmann-Rieger, Prof. W. Fuhrmann, and Dr M. Bauer, all of Giessen a. d. Lahn.)

3 A 10-year-old girl, the second child of consanguineous parents (two healthy siblings). Small bulbus oculi palpable on the left; combined hearing impairment and stenosis of the auditory canal bilaterally; partial cutaneous syndactyly of the hands and feet; vaginal atresia. (By kind permission of Prof. H. Schönenberg, Aachen.)

Reference:
Schönenberg H: Kryptophthalmus-Syndrom. Klin. Pediatr. *185*:165 (1973)

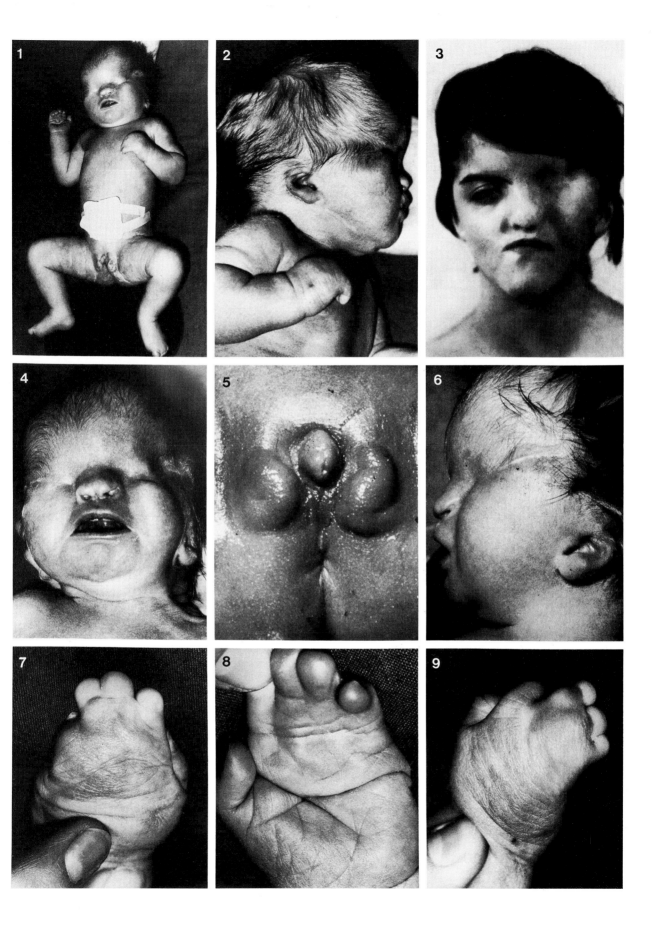

28. Trisomy 13 Syndrome

(D₁ Trisomy Syndrome, Pätau Syndrome)

A malformation syndrome with characteristic facies, hexadactyly, primordial growth deficiency, profound psychomotor retardation, and multiple other anomalies.

Main Signs:
1. Typical facies with sloping forehead, hypo- or hypertelorism, mongoloid slant of the palpebral fissures, microphthalmos to anophthalmos, cleft lip and palate, and micrognathia (**1, 2, 5,** and **6**).
2. Microcephaly, profound psychomotor impairment, seizures; muscular hypotonia, rarely hypertonia.
3. Postaxial hexadactyly, mainly of the upper extremities, hyperextensible thumbs; narrow, hyperconvex fingernails (**3**). Simian crease. Protruding calcaneus.
4. Localised skin defects in the occipital area (**7**). Capillary haemangiomas.
5. Cryptorchidism, partial fusion of the penis and scrotum, hypospadias.

Supplementary Findings: Omphalocele.

Heart defects of various types, especially ventricular septal defect and persistent ductus arteriosis.

Polycystic kidneys and anomalies of the urinary tract.

Holoprosencephaly-type malformation of the brain (p.30), anomalies of the cerebellum.

Manifestation: At birth.

Aetiology: Disturbance of genetic balance due to trisomy of chromosome no. 13 or to a three-fold dose of the genetic material located on this chromosome. The extra chromosomal material almost always exists independently; very rarely it is attached to another chromosome.

Frequency: Approximately 1:5000 live births.

Course, Prognosis: Practically no psychomotor development. About 85% die before reaching 1 year of age.

Treatment: Symptomatic. Prenatal diagnosis after birth of the index case, especially in older mothers or in the case of a balanced translocation in one of the parents.

Differential Diagnosis: Meckel syndrome, which usually shows occipital encephalocele and cystic kidneys in addition to the otherwise similar signs. Chromosomes normal.

Illustrations:
1 Patient 1 on the first day of life. Birth measurements: 2230 g, length 48 cm, head circumference 26 cm. Death on the first day of life. Holoprosencephaly, microphthalmos, ventricular septal defect, renal cortical cysts, duplication of the renal pelvis and ureter bilaterally.
2–4 Patient 2 on the first day of life: ninth child of a 40-year-old woman. Birth measurements within normal limits. Death at age 9 days. Omphalocele, coloboma of the iris, renal cortical cysts, duplication of the renal pelvis and ureter bilaterally, undescended testicles, hypospadias, hypoplasia of the mitral and aortic valves.
5 and 6 Patient 3 at age 7 days. Death on the 19th day of life. Hexadactyly of the hands, microphthalmos, high-arched palate, bifid uvula, persistence of the left superior vena cava, ventricular septal defect, persistent ductus arteriosis, horse-shoe kidneys, bicornate uterus.
7 and 8 Patient 4 at age 3 days. Birth measurements: 2000 g, length 44 cm, head circumference 31 cm. Death at age 2 days. Holoprosencephaly, hexadactyly of both hands, club feet, bilateral cleft lip and palate. Atresia of the pulmonary valve, ventricular septal defect, overriding aorta, patent ductus arteriosis, bicornate uterus.

Reference:
Hamerton J. L.: Human Cytogenetics, vol II. Academic Press, New York and London 1971

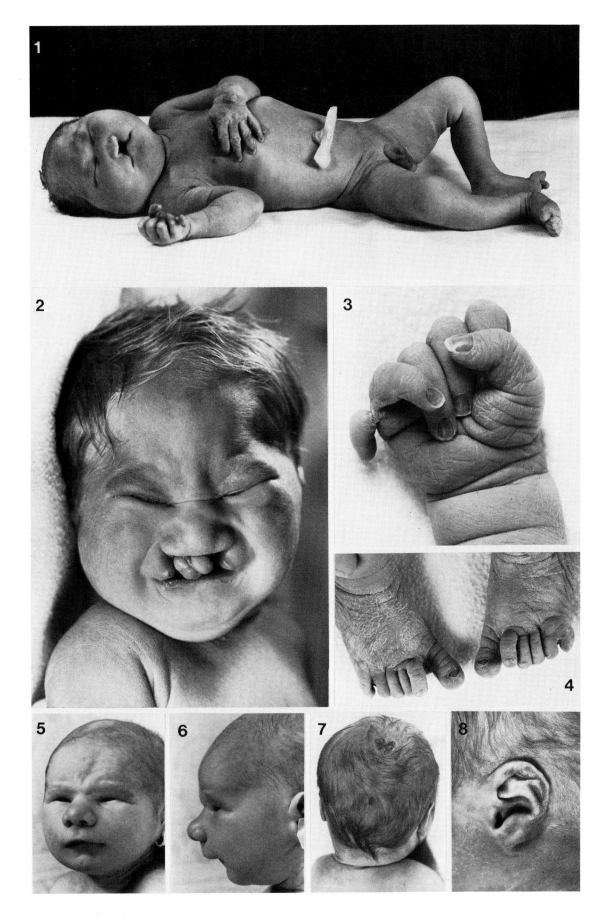

29. Trisomy 18 Syndrome

(Edwards' Syndrome)

A syndrome of primordial growth deficiency, typical facial dysmorphism, profound psychomotor retardation, and multiple other anomalies.

Main Signs:
1. Characteristic facies, distinguished especially by protruding forehead, short – sometimes upward-slanting – palpebral fissures, micrognathia, microstomia, short philtrum, not infrequently cheilognathopalatoschisis or components thereof,. Narrow microcephalic skull with prominent occiput, dysplasia of the auricles of the ears (**4–8**).
2. Pronounced pre- and postnatal growth deficiency.
3. Profound psychomotor retardation, seizures; muscular hypertonia after initial hypotonia (**1**).
4. Flexion contractures of the finger joints with overlapping of the 2nd and 5th over the 3rd or 4th finger (**2**); hypoplastic nails, especially of the feet; generally partial syndactyly, short dorsiflexed big toes; protruding calcanei, rockerbottom feet (**3**).
5. Short sternum; small, relatively widely spaced nipples; umbilical and inguinal hernias, cutis laxa.

Supplementary Findings: Aplasia of the radius, polydactyly.

Anomalies of the central nervous system such as hydrocephalus and myelomeningocele.

Cardiac defects, especially ventricular septal defect and persistent ductus arteriosis.

Diaphragmatic hernia.

Hypospadias, cryptorchidism, bifid uterus, ovarian hypoplasia, renal anomalies (hydronephrosis, renal cysts, etc.).

Manifestation: At birth.

Aetiology: Genetic imbalance due to trisomy of chromosome no. 18 or to a three-fold dose of the genetic material located on this chromosome. Almost without exception, the extra chromosomal material exists as an independent entity (and not translocated to another chromosome).

Frequency: Ca. 1:5000 live births. Predominance of females over males.

Course, Prognosis: Practically no psychomotor development. 90% of the cases die before 1 year of age.

Treatment: Symptomatic. Prenatal diagnosis in mothers who have previously borne such a child, especially older mothers, or in the case of a balanced translocation in one of the parents.

Illustrations:
1–3 Patient 1: birth measurements 2220 g, length 45 cm, head circumference 31 cm. Death at age 4 weeks. Hypertrophy of the clitoris, stenosis of the aortic isthmus, patent ductus arteriosis, bicuspid pulmonary and aortic valves, ventricular septal defect with overriding aorta, elongated kidneys with doubling of the renal pelvis on the left.
4–5 Patient 2: birth measurements 2260 g, length 45 cm, head circumference 32 cm. Death at age 3 days. Partial syndactyly between all fingers and toes, ventricular septal defect with overriding aorta, diaphragmatic hernia.
6–8 Patient 3: birth measurements 1690 g, length 40 cm, head circumference 31.5 cm. Death at age 8 weeks. Syndactyly, camptodactyly, hypoplastic labia majora, horse-shoe kidneys, Meckel's diverticulum, diaphragmatic hernia, atrial and ventricular septal defects, bicuspid aortic valve, hypoplasia of the left pulmonary vein.

References:
Hamerton J.L.: Human Cytogenetics, vol II. Academic Press, New York and London 1971
Schinzel A., Schmid W.: Trisomie 18… Helv. Pediatr. Acta 26:673 (1971)

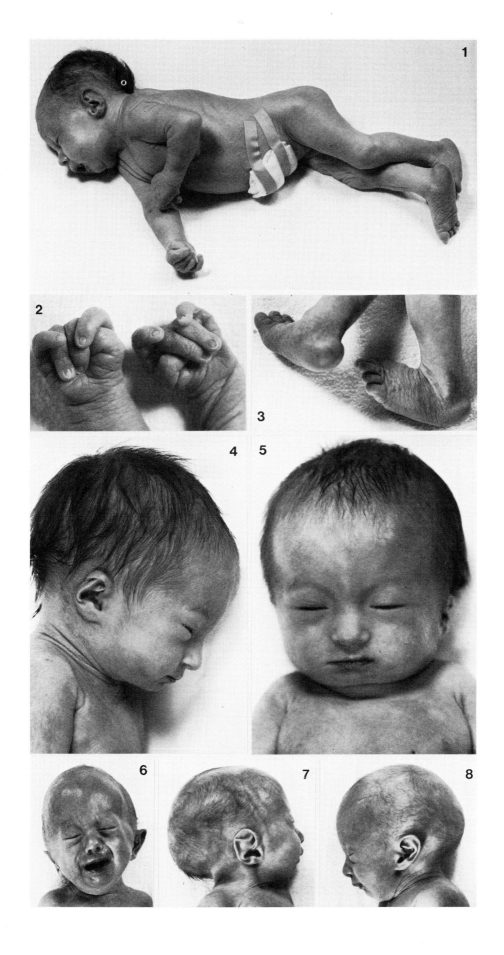

30. Down's Syndrome

(Trisomy 21 Syndrome, Mongolism, Mongoloidism)

A malformation syndrome with mental retardation and very characteristic physical appearance.

Main Signs:
1. 'Flat face' with mongoloid slant of the palpebral fissures, epicanthal folds, low nasal root, small nose, and dysplastic external ears (**1–8 and 12–14**). Short cranium with steeply sloping occiput (**14**). Macroglossia (often with fissured tongue); dysodontiasis.
2. Short-appearing neck with loose skin (more apparent in younger children). Relatively short stature, short stubby hands and fingers, frequently with radial deviation of the little fingers and simian crease of the palms (**15**); widely spaced big and second toes (**13 and 16**).
3. Hypotonia and generalised hypermobility of the joints with laxity of the ligaments (**9–11**).
4. Mental retardation in the severe to moderate range.

Supplementary Findings: Cardiac defect in almost half of the cases (mostly septal defects).

Slight exophthalmos; strabismus, nystagmus; small white 'porcelain' (Brushfield) spots in the light iris of the young infant; occasionally cataracts.

Hypoplasia of the pelvis with flaring of the ilia and abnormally small angle between the ilium and the roof of the acetabulum on X-ray. Relatively short penis and frequently undescended testicles (**10**).

Tendency to localised redness of the cheeks and nose (**6**), to dryness of the skin, and to cutis marmorata. Obstipation.

Manifestation: At birth.

Aetiology: This syndrome is the expression of a chromosomal aberration, namely, trisomy of chromosome 21 or the disturbance of genetic equilibrium caused by a three-fold dose of the genetic material located on this chromosome. In over 95% of cases the extra chromosomal material exists independently; infrequently (about 3% of cases), it is attached to another chromosome (translocation).

Frequency: One case in about 650 births. More than 5% of all mentally retarded children have Down's syndrome.

Course, Prognosis: Very dependent on the presence and severity of a heart defect. Distinctly increased susceptibility to respiratory tract ailments. Increased disposition to acute leukaemia.

Psychomotor performance in infancy rather apathetic and sluggish; later, hyperagile conduct. Infertility of affected males.

Treatment: Cardiac surgery in some cases. Paediatric physiotherapy. Educational guidance. Genetic counselling of the parents and preventive measures in case of increased risk of occurrence.

Illustrations:
1–8 Facial appearance of, respectively, a 4-week-old, 7-month-old, 10-month-old, 1¼-year-old, 1¾-year-old, 2¾-year-old, 6½-year-old, and 15-year-old child.
9–11 Hypotonia and hyperextensibility of a 10-month-old and of a 1½-year-old child.
12–14 Typical flaccid and doltish posture of a 6½-year-old and a 9½-year-old child.
15 and 16 Simian crease and 'prehensile' foot in, respectively, a 6-month-old and a 1-month-old child.

References:
Wiedemann H-R.: Pathologie der Vererbung und Konstitutionspathologie. In:Lehrbuch der Kinderheilkunde, 24th edn. G. Joppich and F. Schulte (eds.). G. Fischer, Stuttgart 1980
Burgio G.R., Fraccaro M., Tiepolo L. (eds.): Trisomy 21. Springer, Heidelberg 1981

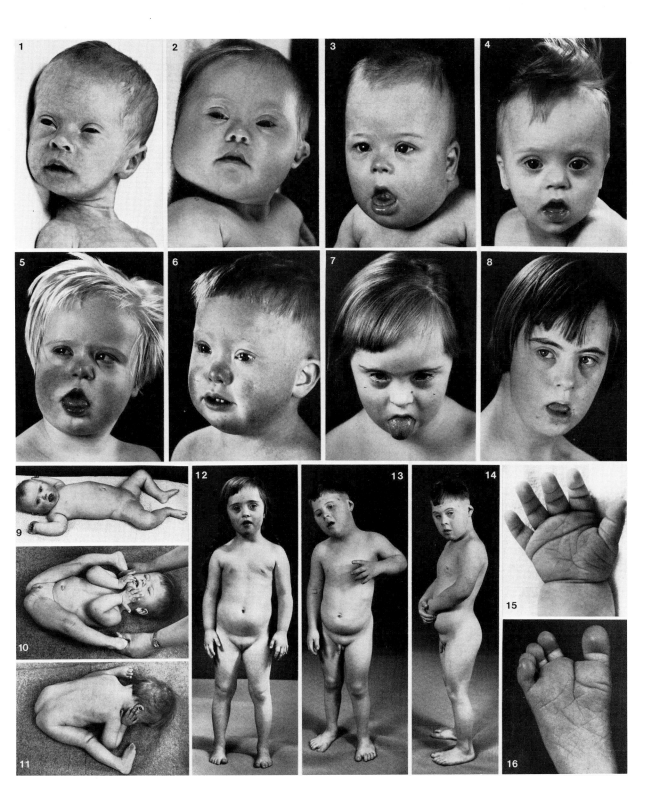

31. Cri Du Chat Syndrome

(Chromosome 5p− Syndrome, Cat Cry Syndrome)

A syndrome of typical facial dysmorphism, primordial growth deficiency, psychomotor retardation, and cat-like crying in early infancy.

Main Signs:

1. Face in infancy round and usually flat. Hypertelorism, epicanthal folds, usually antimongoloid slant of the palpebral fissures, strabismus, low wide root of the nose, and micrognathia (**1–3**).

2. Primordial growth deficiency.

3. Microbrachycephaly and severe psychomotor retardation.

4. Cat-like cry (strikingly plaintive, high-toned, weak) as characteristic anomaly in early infancy.

5. Connate stridor.

Supplementary Findings: Frequently dysplasia or at least remarkable configuration (**3**) of the external ears. Short neck; scoliosis at a later age.

Malocclusion, high palate, bipartite uvula.

Partial syndactyly, short metacarpal and metatarsal bones, simian crease.

Hypotonia, inguinal hernia, diastasis recti abdominis.

Manifestation: At birth.

Aetiology: Loss of a piece of the short arm of chromosome 5. As long as neither of the parents has a corresponding translocation, no increased risk of recurrence.

Frequency: Low, about 1:50000 newborns; up to 1980, about 400 observations had been reported.

Course, Prognosis: Decreased life expectancy. The characteristic cry is lost during the first months of life.

Differential Diagnosis: Wolf syndrome (deletion of the short arm of chromosome 4); here, 'fish mouth', cleft lip and palate, coloboma, heart defect, hypospadias.

Treatment: Symptomatic. Prenatal diagnosis in cases of increased risk of recurrence.

Illustrations:

1–3 Two affected girls, aged 2 months and 6 months.

References:

Niebuhr E.: The cri du chat syndrome... Hum. Genet. *44*:227 (1978)

Wilkens L.E., Brown J.A., Wolf B.: Psychomotor development in 65 home-reared children with cri-du-chat syndrome. J. Pediatr. 97:401 (1980)

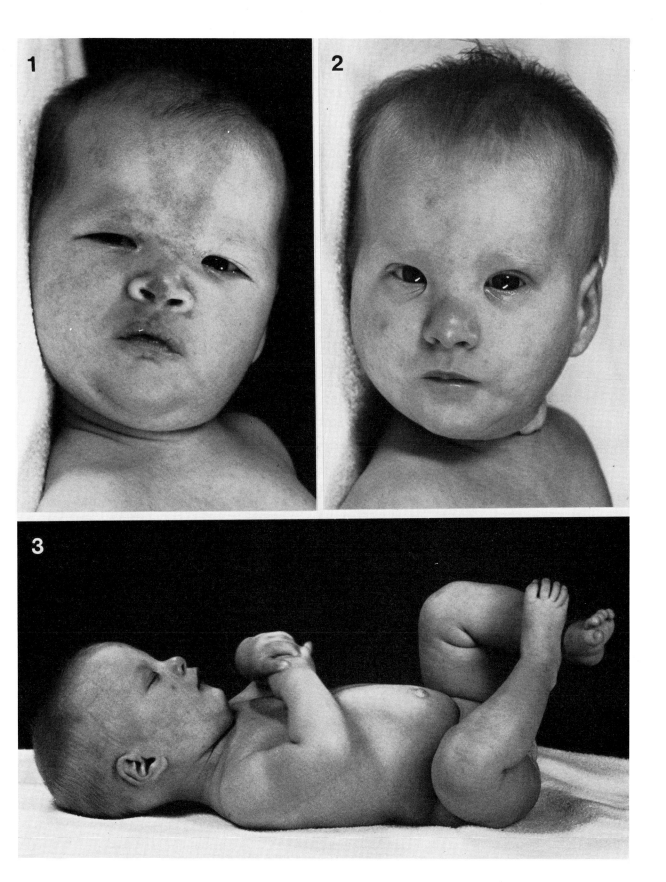

63

32. Syndrome of Infantile Cortical Hyperostosis

(Caffey Syndrome; Caffey–Silverman Syndrome)

A clinical picture occurring chiefly in young infants as firm, frequently asymmetric soft-tissue swellings generally of the face or jaw and parts of the extremities, with marked osseous swelling on X-ray and usually eventual complete recovery.

Main Signs:

1. Painful, firm, often asymmetric soft-tissue swellings located on the face and/or regions of the extremities and accompanied or heralded by fever and general irritability (**1 and 3**).
2. X-rays show periosteal hyperostosis, often severe, usually affecting several areas of the skeleton; preferentially the mandible, clavicle, scapula, ribs, and long bones (**2, 4,** and **5**).

Supplementary Findings: Occasionally pseudoparesis of part of an extremity during the acute swelling phase. Leucocytosis, elevated ESR, and possible thrombocytosis during the acute phase. Frequently moderately elevated serum alkaline phosphatase.

Manifestation: Early infancy. (Prenatal onset has also been demonstrated repeatedly on X-ray.) The hyperostosis is usually detectable within weeks of the onset of the external swelling.

Aetiology: Unknown. Familial occurrence is not unusual especially in siblings, but also in successive generations. Genetic factors probable.

Frequency: Low (about 150 observations reported in the literature in 1967).

Course, Prognosis: Occasionally intermittent course, i.e., with several phases or exacerbations. In isolated cases a more chronic course may lead to distinct bowing or to overgrowth of the long bones and to marked delay of the statomotor development. Prognosis as a rule quite favourable. Usually complete clinical, followed after several months by radiological, recovery.

Differential Diagnosis: Traumatic, inflammatory, and toxic conditions and (C-, D-)avitaminosis must be ruled out.

Treatment: Symptomatic. Administration of corticosteroids during the acute stage.

Illustrations:

1 A 9-week-old infant with asymmetric, firm soft-tissue swellings of both lower legs and of the upper extremities.
2 Hyperostosis of the lower edge of the body of the mandible in an infant of 10 months.
3 Soft-tissue swelling and convex forward bowing of the tibiae in a 1-month-old boy.
4–5 Marked cortical hyperostosis of the tibia and bones of the arm of the infant in **1**.

References:
Spranger J. W., Lange jr L. O., Wiedemann H.-R.: Bone dysplasias. An Atlas of Constitutional Disorders of Skeletal Development. Stuttgart and Philadelphia, G. Fischer and W. B. Saunders, 1974
Finsterbusch A., Rang M.: Infantile cortical hyperostosis. Follow-up of 29 cases. Acta Orthop. Scand. 46:727 (1975)
Fried K., Manor A., Pajewski M., et al: Autosomal dominant inheritance with incomplete penetrance of Caffey disease (infantile cortical hyperostosis). Clin. Genet. 19:271 (1981)

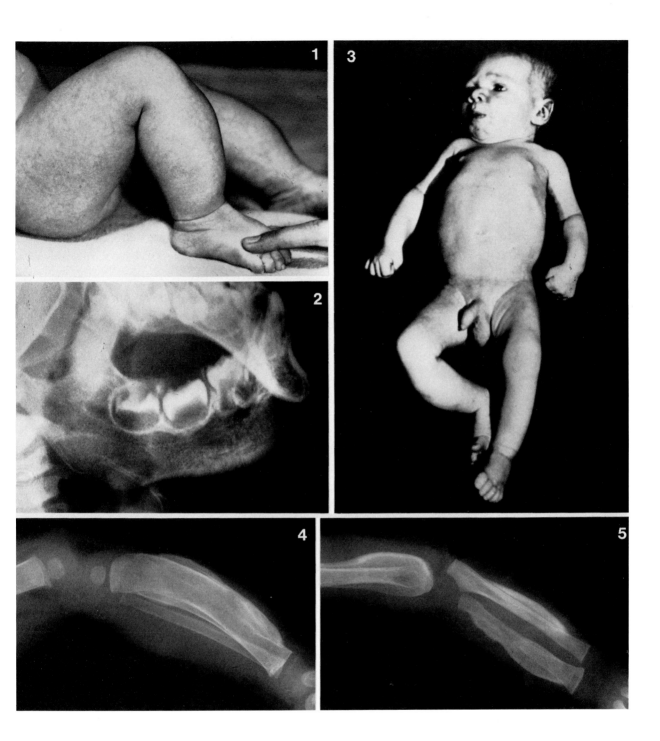

33. Syndrome of Craniometaphyseal Dysplasia

A hereditary systemic defect of ossification with widening of the metaphyses, thickening of the skull bones, and frequent impaired hearing.

Main Signs:
Hypertelorism (2) with paranasal bony ridges (1 and 2) and bulging of the broad nasal root and the glabella (3), which together with a large, occipito-frontally protruding cranium produces a characteristic appearance. Narrowing of the nasal meatuses with mouth breathing.

Supplementary Findings: Compression of the auditory, optic, and facial nerves not unusual. Involvement of dentition possible. On X-ray, hyperostosis of the cranial bones (4); abnormally shaped long bones with flask-shaped flaring of the metaphyses (5).

Manifestation: Possibly as early as the first year of life, more frequently later in childhood.

Aetiology: Monogenic hereditary disease with variable expressivity. Heterogeneous. Autosomal dominant form more frequent than a – perhaps more severely progressive – recessive type.

Frequency: Low.

Course, Prognosis, Treatment: Life expectancy normal as a rule. Good development of height. Symptomatic treatment of neural, dental, and other complications.

Illustrations:
1–6 A 6-year-old boy, normally developed for his age but with defective hearing, and his X-rays (4–6). 6 shows typical mild changes.

References:
Spranger J. W., Langer L. O., jr, Wiedemann H.-R.: Bone Dysplasias. An Atlas of Constitutional Disorders of Skeletal Development. Stuttgart and Philadelphia, G. Fischer and W. B. Saunders 1974
Beighton P., Hamersma H., Horan F.: Craniometaphyseal dysplasia – variability of expression within a large family. Clin. Genet. *15*:252 (1979)
Penchaszadeh V. B., Gutierrez E. R., Figueroa P.: Autosomal recessive craniometaphyseal dysplasia Am. J. Med. Genet. *5*:43 (1980)

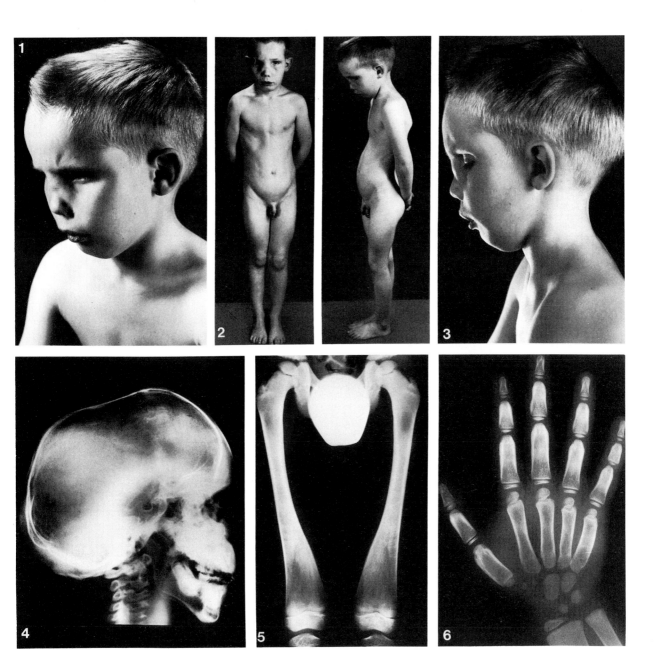

34. Cherubism Syndrome

A hereditary syndrome involving almost exclusively the bones of the jaw, with typical facial dysmorphism.

Main Signs:
1. Generally bilateral, symmetrical, indolent distension of the submandibular or malar regions (1–4) due to more or less extensive replacement of the jaw bones (mandible and/or maxilla; maxilla especially) by fibrous tissue. When the floor of the orbit is involved, displacement of the bulbi cranially, with the sclera being visible below the rim of the iris (1–3), the 'heavenward' glance and the 'cherubic' cheeks giving the syndrome its name.
2. Hypertelorism as a rule.
3. Severely affected primary dentition with many malpositioned or exfoliated teeth (2 and 5); hypodontia of the secondary dentition.

Supplementary Findings: During the stage of markedly increasing swelling, possible enlargement of the regional lymph nodes and elevation of the serum alkaline phosphatase.

X-ray examination of the skeleton may demonstrate slight cystic translucence of other areas also (e.g., bones of the hands).

Manifestation: First years of life.

Aetiology: Hereditary condition with autosomal dominant transmission, variable expressivity, and incomplete penetrance in females.

Frequency: Low; up to 1980 apparently only somewhat more than 100 cases were reported.

Course, Prognosis: The tumourlike dysplasia affects dental germs and odontogeny, and their natural consequences; it may impair nasal breathing and function of the tongue. After years of progression, cessation of the swelling before, during, or soon after puberty, then gradual retrogression. Thus, self-limiting and benign. Complete healing, but with atrophy of the alveolar processes after reossification of the basal areas of the jaw.

Diagnosis: From appearance, X-rays (5), and in some cases, histological findings on biopsy (proliferative loose fibrous tissue with spindle cells and multinucleated giant cells; sparse membranous bone formation).

Treatment: In some cases curettage of tissue hindering nasal breathing or function of the tongue. X-ray therapy contraindicated. Timely prosthetic measures. Possibly a modelling osteotomy after adolescence.

Illustrations:
1–4 Physically and mentally normally developed 4-year-old boy with cherubism (mother and sister of the boy similarly affected – the former now in the healing stage). Broad, low midface with a very wide nasal root, slight hypertelorism, prominent zygomatic arches, small and flat nose with anteverted nostrils; bulbi rotated slightly 'heavenwards'. Distension of the lower half of the face. Palate strongly arched forward; child unable to close his mouth because of distension of the alveolar processes; severe anodontia.
5 Vast multicystic distension of the upper and lower jaws with marked thinning of the cortex. Maxillary sinuses cannot be delineated with certainty; zygomatic arches displaced cranially; orbits narrowed; nasal bone almost horizontal; position anomalies of the tooth buds.

References:
Hoppe W., Spranger J., Hansen H. G.: Cherubismus. Arch. Kinderheilkd. *174*:310 (1966)
Khosla V. M., Korobkin M.: Cherubism. Am. J. Dis. Child. *120*:458 (1970)
Peters W. J. N.: Cherubism: A study of 20 cases from one family. Oral Surg. Oral Med. Oral Pathol. *47*:307 (1979)
Hoyer P. F., Neukam F.-W.: Cherubismus…Klin. Pädiatr. *194*:128 (1982)

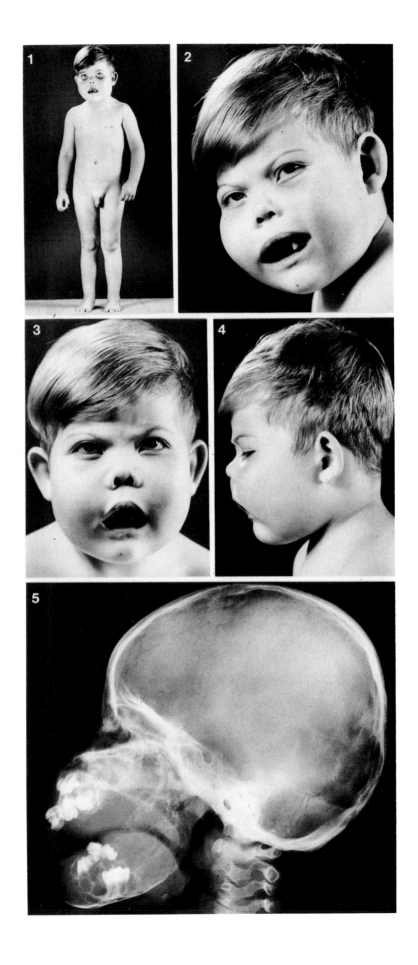

35. Menkes Syndrome

(Kinky Hair Syndrome, Steely Hair Syndrome, Syndrome of Trichopoliodystrophy)

A disease of copper metabolism in boys with depigmented monilethrix hair, relatively typical facies, growth retardation, psychomotor retardation, seizures, and a poor prognosis.

Main Signs:
1. Sparse, kinky, short, brittle hair, still pigmented during the first weeks of life, thereafter depigmented. Microscopically, twisting in the long axis, varying thickness of the shaft. Sparse eyebrows (**2** and **3**).
2. Face puffy due to full cheeks, 'carp-like mouth', micrognathia, low root of the nose, and short philtrum (**1** and **2**). High palate, broad dental lamina. Posteriorly rotated, poorly modelled ears.
3. Skin pale, doughy, with seborrhoeic changes (**3**).
4. Psychomotor retardation; microcephaly. Seizures. Spasticity alternating with hypotonia.
5. Growth deficiency. Flaring, increased density, and spur-like extensions of the metaphyses of the long bones, rachitic rosary, pectus excavatum (**1**), possible club feet.

Supplementary Findings: Not infrequently small size at birth; early failure to thrive, dystrophy.

Tendency to hypo-, less frequently hyperthermia. Frequent infections.

Skeleton: Wormian bones along the sagittal suture. After the 2nd month of life, goblet-shaped widening of the metaphyses, which gradually regresses during the latter part of infancy (**4** and **5**). Osteoporosis, periosteal bone formation. Vacuolated promyelocytes in the bone marrow. On angiography, characteristic corkscrew twisting, elongation, and varying calibre of the cerebral, visceral, and soft tissue vessels. Subdural haemorrhages. Low levels of copper in serum and tissues, but elevated levels in the mucosa of the small intestine ('defect of copper distribution').

Manifestation: In the first months of life.

Aetiology: X-linked recessive hereditary disorder; thus, males affected.

Frequency: From the first report in 1962 until 1980, about 75 cases were recognised.

Course, Prognosis: With the onset of cerebral seizures in the 2nd to 3rd months of life, cessation of psychomotor development and soon thereafter loss of attained milestones, on to decerebration. Death usually in the second year of life.

Treatment: Symptomatic. Neither oral nor parenteral copper administration has proved effective in modifying the clinical picture to date. Genetic counselling. Prenatal diagnosis.

Illustrations:
1–5 Photographs and X-rays of an 8-month-old patient. Normal development up to the first seizure at age 2½ months, then standstill of development and shortly thereafter regression. Frequent infections, frequent hypothermia. Death at 12 months from meningitis.

References:
Heyne Kl., Dörner K., Graucob E., Wiedemann H.-R.: Monophyle Vakuolisierung von Promyelozyten bei
Menkes-Syndrom... Klin. Pädiatr. *190*:576 (1978)
Grover W. D., Johnson W. C., Henkin R. I.: Clinical and biochemical aspects of trichopoliodystrophy. Ann. Neurol. *5*:65 (1979)
Dobrescu O., Larbrisseau A., Dubé L.-J., et al: Trichopoliodystrophie... CMA Journal *123*:490 (1980)
Taylor C. J., Green S. H.: Menkes' syndrome (trichopoliodystrophy): Use of scanning electron-microscope in diagnosis and carrier identification. Develop. Med. Child Neurol. *23*:361 (1981)

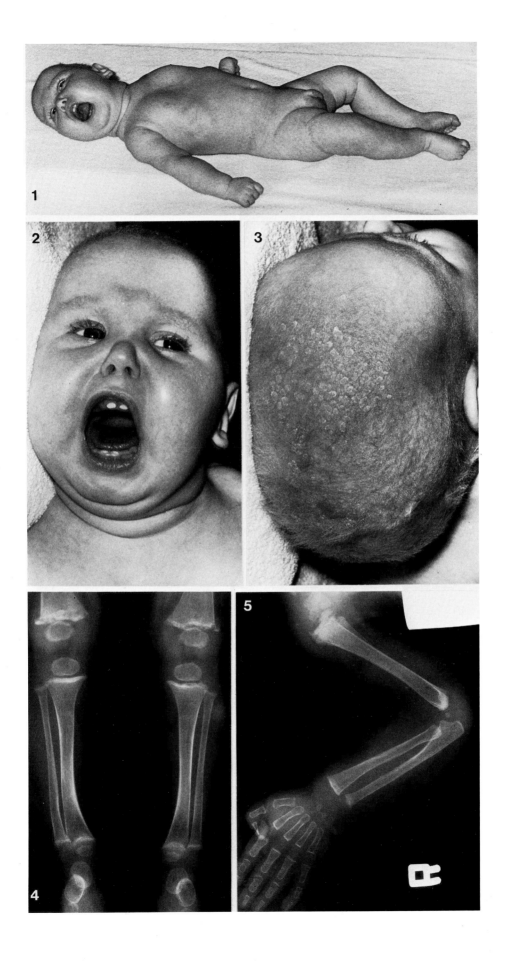

36. von Gierke Syndrome

(Glycogenosis Syndrome Type I)

A hereditary metabolic disease with typical facies, growth deficiency, and protuberant abdomen.

Main Signs:
1. Facial dysmorphism, best described as a Rubens or doll face (**1, 2, 4,** and **5**).
2. Small stature.
3. Protuberant abdomen as a result of liver enlargement (**3**).
4. Mental retardation due to hypoglycaemia and hypoglycaemic seizures.
5. Poorly developed hypotonic musculature (**3**).

Supplementary Findings: Susceptibility to infections.
Tendency to bleeding.
Enlargement of the kidneys; hepatoma.
Osteoporosis.
Xanthomas, gouty tophi and arthritis.
Fasting hypoglycaemia unresponsive to glucagon or adrenalin; elevation of lactate, pyruvate, triglycerides, phospholipids, cholesterol, and uric acid.

Manifestation: At birth. Growth retardation apparent late in infancy. Xanthomas, gouty tophi and arthritis usually not before adulthood.

Aetiology: Autosomal recessive hereditary disease. Glucose-6-phosphatase not demonstrable in liver, kidneys, or intestinal mucosa. This enzyme catalyses the last step in glycogenolysis.

Frequency; Rare (ca. 1:400 000).

Course, Prognosis: Average life expectancy somewhat limited due to lactic acidotic metabolic state and susceptibility to infections in the first years of life, later due to gouty nephritis. Progression of liver enlargement probably limited to childhood.

Treatment: Frequent carbohydrate-rich meals; at night constant feeding by means of a gastric tube. Alkalisation in stress situations during the first years of life; prompt antibiotic treatment of bacterial infections; allopurinol to lower the uric acid level.

Illustrations:
1–3 Patient 1 at age 1½ years. Delayed development; height deficit 11 cm.
4 and 5 Patient 2 at age 1½ years. Height deficit 9 cm. Hypoglycaemic seizures up to the 6th year of life. Liver at the level of the umbilicus. At follow-up at 10 years, no further enlargement of the organ determinable. Height deficit now 13 cm.

Reference:
Stanbury J.B., Wyngaarden J.B., Fredrickson D.S.: The Metabolic Basis of Inherited Disease. McGraw-Hill Book Company, 4th edn., 1978, p.143

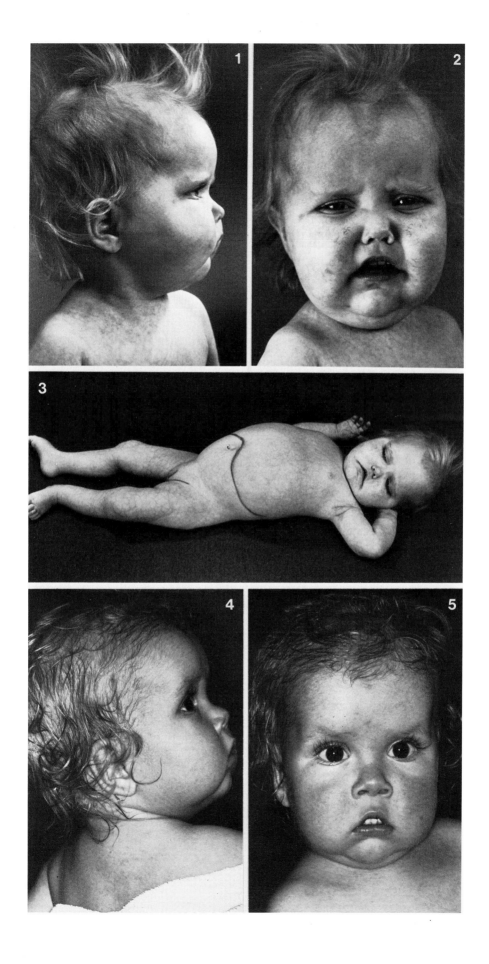

37. Hurler Syndrome

(Pfaundler–Hurler Syndrome, Mucopolysaccharidosis I-H)

An autosomal recessive inherited mucopolysaccharide storage disease, which leads to the development of a typical facial dysmorphism and to growth deficiency, dementia, corneal clouding, and hepatosplenomegaly.

Main Signs:
1. Characteristic facies with depressed, flat nasal root; broad tip of the nose and large nostrils; hypertelorism; exophthalmos; corneal clouding; thick pouting lips (1–4); large tongue; widely spaced teeth; hypertrophy of the alveolar processes and gums (8). Macrocephaly (6). Hair of the head abundant, thick, and strong (1 and 2). Increasing dementia.
2. Short stature after a period of normal growth in infancy; very short neck; thoracolumbar gibbus (4 and 6).
3. Joint contractures (3), claw hands (7), broad feet. Indurations of skin and cartilage.
4. Protuberant abdomen, diastasis recti, hernias.

Supplementary Findings: Chronic purulent rhinitis, abundant lanugo-like body hair.

Heart: Valvular defects, enlargement, insufficiency.

Progressive changes in bone structure, of a dysostosis multiplex type: Osteoporosis with coarse trabeculae, thickening of the roof of the skull, broad ribs and clavicles, crudely shaped scapulae, oval and in part hook-shaped vertebral bodies; broadening and shortening of the long bones with loss of characteristic details (5), pelvic dysplasia.

Frequently increased intracranial pressure when circulation of the cerebrospinal fluid is impaired by mucopolysaccharide infiltrates in the meninges. Increased excretion of chondroitin sulphate and heparitin sulphate in the urine; alpha-L-iduronidase not demonstrable, or demonstrable only in diminished amounts, in tissues.

Manifestation: Biochemically, after birth; radiologically, in the first months of life; clinically, in the second half-year of life.

Aetiology: Autosomal recessive hereditary disorder. Owing to absence of alpha-iduronidase, the above-mentioned mucopolysaccharides are not degraded, but stored in various organs, leading to morphological and functional anomalies of the latter.

Frequency: About 1:100 000.

Course, Prognosis: Constant progression of signs and symptoms until death in the second decade of life. Death due to infection, heart failure, or aspiration.

Differential Diagnosis: The Hunter syndrome (mucopolysaccharidosis II) affects males only. It is clinically similar, but milder (however, with relatively early impairment of hearing), more slowly manifest, and runs a more prolonged course. As a rule, no corneal clouding in Hunter syndrome.

Treatment: Symptomatic. Prevention by means of prenatal diagnosis.

Illustrations:
1–5 Patient 1 at age 5 years. Height 93 cm (50th percentile for a 2½-year-old girl), marked dementia, pronounced hepatomegaly.
6 Patient 2 at age 1¼ years. Height 85 cm (97th percentile), head circumference 52.5 cm (50th percentile for a 10-year-old boy). Hepatomegaly. Bilateral inguinal hernia.
7 and 8 Patient 3. Hand and oral cavity at age 2½ years.

References:
Spranger J.: Mucopolysaccharidosen. Hdb. inn. Med., Bd VII/I 209 Berlin, Heidelberg, New York, Springer 1974
Spranger J. W., Langer, jr L. O., Wiedemann H.-R.: Bone Dysplasias. An Atlas of Constitutional Disorders of Skeletal Development. Stuttgart and Philadelphia, G. Fischer and W. B. Saunders, 1974
McKusick V. A.: Heritable Disorders of Connective Tissue. Mosby, Saint Louis 1979

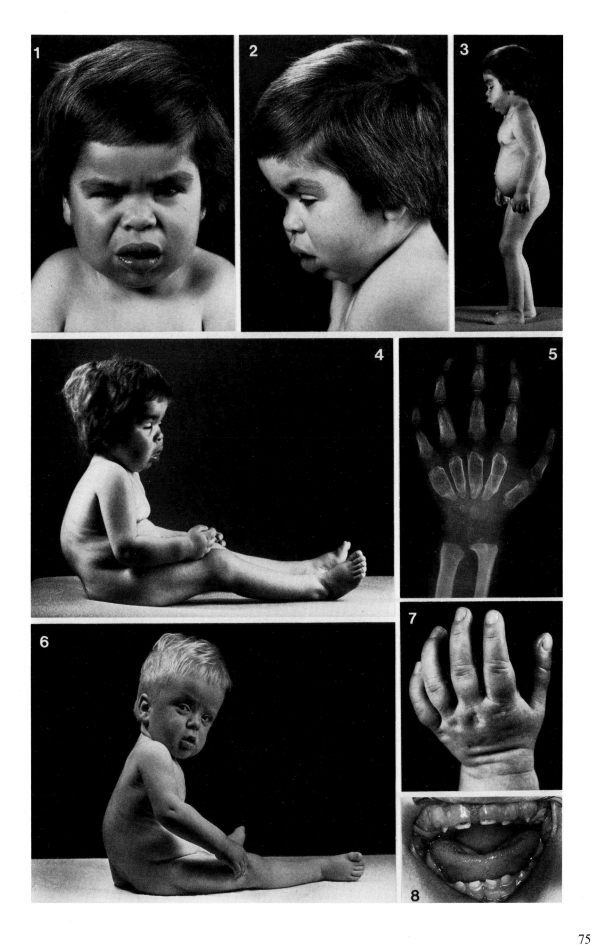

38. Hunter Syndrome

(Mucopolysaccharidosis II)

A mucopolysaccharidosis storage disease exclusively of males which leads to relatively typical facial dysmorphism, early hearing impairment, hepatosplenomegaly, small stature, and more or less severe mental retardation.

Main Signs:
1. Coarse facial features – similar to, but not as pronounced as in Hurler syndrome – with broad and low nose, hypertelorism, 'full' cheeks, thick lips, large tongue, widely spaced teeth, and macrocephaly (**4** and **5**). Impaired hearing beginning in early childhood. Usually no corneal clouding. Erethistic feeblemindedness or dementia (not with type B, see below).
2. Small stature after transiently normal growth in the first year or two of life; short neck.
3. Joint contractures (**1** and **2**), claw hands (**3**). Indurations of skin and cartilage, not infrequently nodose in character.
4. Pes cavus, hernias (**1** and **2**), diastasis recti. Protuberant abdomen (**2**). ·

Supplementary Findings: Chronic suppurative rhinitis. Hepatosplenomegaly.
   Heart: Valvular defects, enlargement, insufficiency.
   Changes of bony form and structure as in Hurler syndrome; however, less severe at a given age. Coxarthrosis (type B). Increased intracranial pressure from impaired flow of the cerebrospinal fluid, seldom progressive.
   Increased excretion of chondroitin sulphate and heparitin sulphate in the urine.

Manifestation: Biochemically, from birth on; clinically, after the end of the first year of life.

Aetiology: X-linked recessive hereditary disease. Decreased activity of the enzyme iduronate sulphatase results in storage of mucopolysaccharides in various organs and thus to anomalies of their function and morphology.

Frequency: About 1:50000.

Course, Prognosis: In the first years of life, slowly progressive. After the 4th and 5th years of life, two forms can be distinguished on the basis of their different courses: Type A, rapidly progressive, with death before the 15th year of life. Type B: slowly progressive and in particular, with only slight or no noticeable mental impairment; death – usually from cardiac failure – in adulthood. The oldest patient lived to age 60 years.

Differential Diagnosis: Hurler syndrome (p.74).

Treatment: Symptomatic. Genetic counselling. Prenatal diagnosis possible.

Illustrations:
1–5 Patient (type A) at age 5 years (**1, 2,** and **4**) and at 4 years (**3** and **5**). Psychomotor development up to 1½ years of age, normal; thereafter developmental standstill. At 111 cm, height still normal. Liver four fingerbreadths below the costal margin. At 5¾ years, a shunt operation because of increased intracranial pressure.

References:
Spranger J.: Mucopolysaccharidosen. Hdb. Inn. Med. Bd. VII/1, 209. Berlin, Heidelberg, New York, Springer 1974
Spranger J. W., Langer jr L. O., Wiedemann H.-R.: Bone Dysplasias. An Atlas of Constitutional Disorders of Skeletal Development. Stuttgart and Philadelphia, G. Fischer and W. B. Saunders, 1974
McKusick V. A.: Heritable Disorders of Connective Tissue. The C. V. Mosby Company, Saint Louis 1979

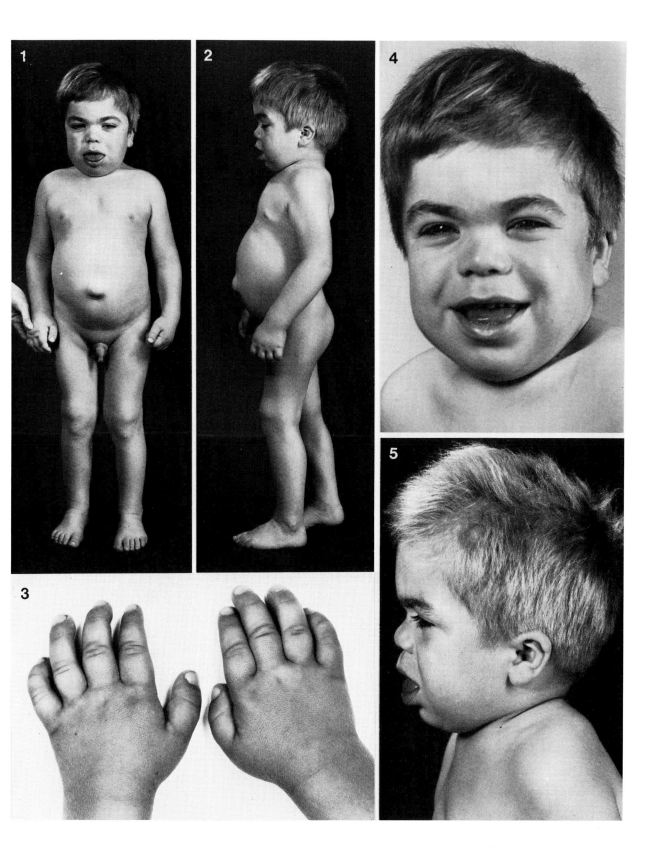

39. Sanfilippo Syndrome

(Mucopolysaccharidosis III)

A recessive hereditary mucopolysaccharide storage disease, which leads to coarsening of the facial features, to behavioural disturbances and dementia, and to hepatomegaly.

Main Signs:
1. Flat nasal root; full, pouting lips; enlarged tongue; coarsened facial features, which in older children are reminiscent of those in Hurler syndrome. Abundant bristly hair of the head; thick, bushy eyebrows and sometimes synophyrs (1–5).
2. Increasing erethistic behaviour, aggressiveness, dementia.
3. Up to the 10th year of life, above average height; thereafter, slowing of growth.
4. No corneal clouding.

Supplementary Findings: Hepatosplenomegaly. Broad dental laminae. Occasionally umbilical or inguinal hernia, decreased joint mobility. Increased susceptibility to infections.

Sleep disorders. Optic atrophy in isolated cases.

Changes of bony structure and form similar to those of Hurler syndrome, but much less severe.

Increased excretion of the mucopolysaccharide heparitin sulphate in urine.

Manifestation: Biochemically, from birth; clinically, by behavioural disturbance and mental retardation after the 3rd year and by somatic signs after about the 4th or 5th years of life.

Aetiology: Autosomal recessive hereditary disease. The seemingly uniform clinical picture is based on absence of the enzyme heparin sulphate sulphatase (Sanfilippo syndrome type A), of alpha-N-acetylglucosaminidase (type B), or of acetyl CoA: alpha-glucosaminid-N-acetyltransferase (type C).

Frequency: About 1:50000, possibly greater.

Course, Prognosis: Characterised by rapid loss of mental and motor abilities, so that meaningful communication usually becomes impossible by 6 to 10 years of age. Spastic tetraplegia with dysphagia in the terminal phase. Death, usually as the result of pneumonia, in the second decade of life.

Treatment: Symptomatic. Genetic counselling. Prenatal diagnosis possible.

Illustrations:
1 and 2 Patient 1 at age 7 years: macrocephaly (head circumference 55.5 cm). Height 138 cm (average height of a 10-year-old girl). IQ 38 (Kramer–Binet). Mild joint contractures.
3–5 Patient 2 at age 3 years. Head circumference, height, and psychomotor development still within normal limits. Hepatomegaly. Biochemically type B. Note that the facial features in the younger patient are more similar to those of Hurler syndrome than are the features of the older patient.

References:
Spranger J.: Mucopolysaccharidosen. Hdb. Inn. Med. Bd. VII/1, 209, Berlin, Heidelberg, New York, Springer 1974
Spranger J. W., Langer jr L. O., Wiedemann H.-R.: Bone Dysplasias. An Atlas of Constitutional Disorders of Skeletal Development. Stuttgart and Philadelphia, G. Fischer and W. B. Saunders 1974
McKusick V. A.: Heritable Disorders of Connective Tissue. V. Mosby, Saint Louis 1979

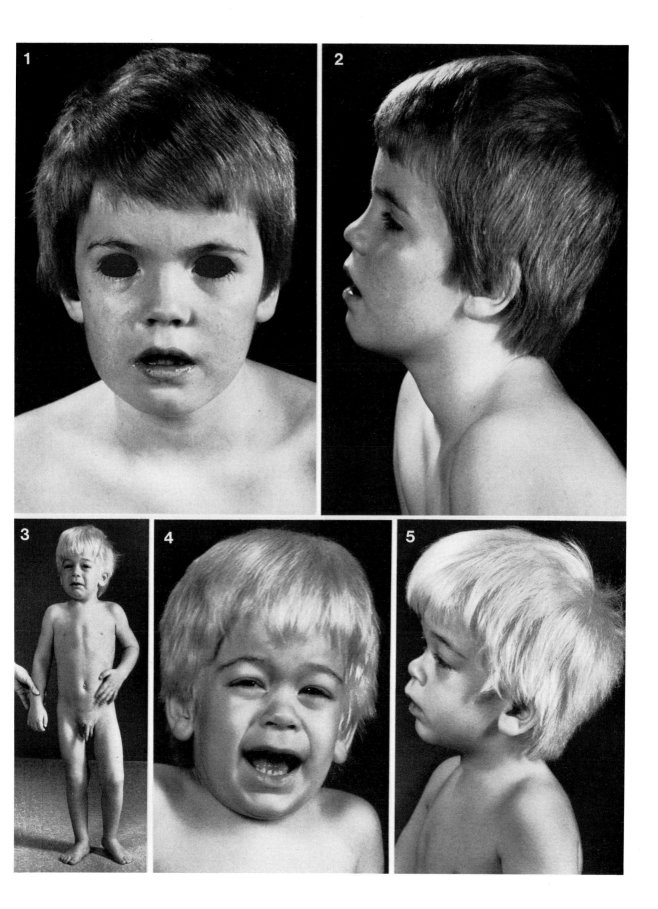

40. Morquio Syndrome

(Morquio–Brailsford Syndrome, Mucopolysaccharidosis IV)

A mucopolysaccharide storage disease with relatively typical facial dysmorphism, marked disproportional growth retardation, joint dysplasia, corneal clouding, all in all yielding a characteristic picture.

Main Signs:
1. Moderately coarse facial features with macrostomia, short nose, and accentuated jaws (**1** and **2**). Corneal clouding, dental diastemata, grey-blue discoloration of the teeth as a result of enamel hypoplasia.
2. Severe dwarfism, especially of the trunk, with a very short neck (**1** and **2**). Head held in retraction. Pectus carinatum, flaring of the lower rib cage, kyphoscoliosis.
3. Swelling and limitation of motion at the joints with malpositioning (ulnar deviation of the hands, pronounced knock knees), hyperextensibility of the finger joints, and instability of the vertebral ligaments. Hands and feet short and stubby.

Supplementary Findings: Normal intelligence. Inguinal hernias. Inelastic, indurated skin.

Onset of progressive hearing impairment in the second decade of life.

Aortic insufficiency.

Changes in bony form and structure similar to those in Hurler syndrome, but with marked involvement of the epiphyses and more severe, generalised platyspondyly.

Hypo- or aplasia of the odontoids.

Increased urinary excretion of the mucopolysaccharides keratin sulphate and chondroitin-4-sulphate; in this respect a tendency to normalisation with increasing age.

Manifestation: Biochemically, from birth; radiologically, in later infancy; clinically, from the 2nd or 3rd year of life. Corneal clouding recognisable only with a slit lamp before age 10 years.

Aetiology: Autosomal recessive hereditary disease. Deficiency of galactosamine-6-sulphate sulphatase.

Frequency: Estimated at about 1:100 000.

Course, Prognosis: Progressive signs and symptoms. Adult height usually not greater than 1m. Average life expectancy shortened by heart failure, but especially also from the results of compression of the medulla oblongata, and spinalis. Life expectancy, which in the past was about 20 years, has been definitely prolonged since the introduction of therapy.

Differential Diagnosis: Other mucopolysaccharide types, especially the Hurler syndrome (p.74), which, however, shows mental retardation or dementia, early appearance of corneal clouding, a different MPS urinary excretion pattern, etc.

Also, skeletal dysplasias in which the vertebrae are especially severely affected (see spondyloepihyseal dysplasia congenita, p.174; metatropic dysplasia, p.170; osteodysplasia type Kniest, p.176).

Treatment: Causal treatment unknown. Fusion of the upper cervical vertebrae no later than the 5th year of life. Orthopaedic measures. Replacement of the aortic valve worth considering. Hearing aids when required.

Illustrations:
1 and **2** A 14-year-old girl. Increased excretion of keratin sulphate.

References:
Spranger J. W., Langer jr L. O., Wiedemann H.-R.: Bone Dysplasias. An Atlas of Constitutional Disorders of Skeletal Development. Stuttgart and Philadelphia, G. Fischer and W. B. Saunders 1974
McKusick V. A.: Heritable Disorders of Connective Tissue. Mosby, Saint Louis 1979
Holzgreve W., Gröbe H., v. Figura K., et al: Morquio syndrome. Clinical findings in 11 patients with MPS IV A and in 2 patients with MPS IV B. Hum. Genet. 57:360 (1981)

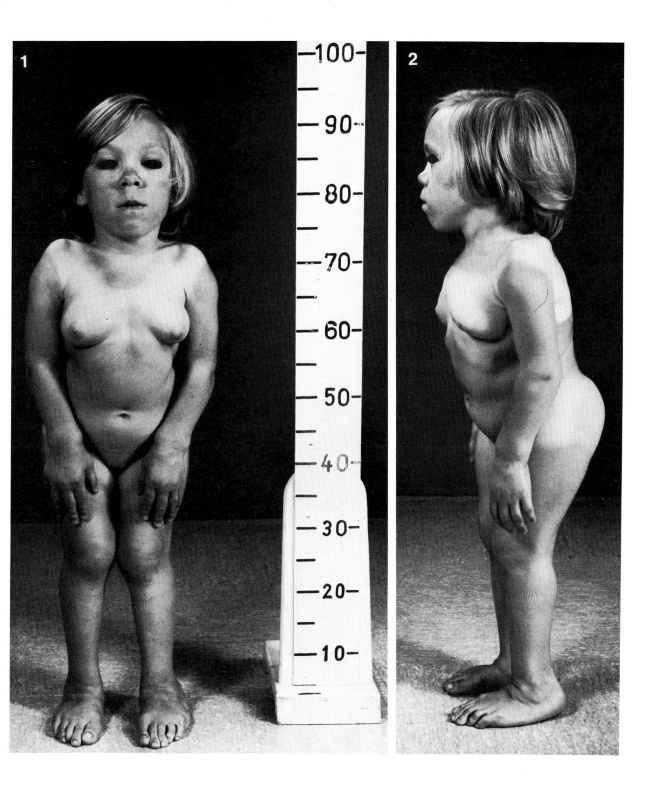

41. Exomphalos–Macroglossia–Gigantism Syndrome

(EMG Syndrome, Wiedemann–Beckwith Syndrome)

A relatively frequent and very characteristic congenital dysplasia syndrome of practical importance, consisting of characteristic facies, 'scored' ears, inborn and/or postnatal generalised 'gigantism', in some cases umbilical hernia, macroglossia, and other organomegalies as well as possible severe postnatal hypoglycaemia.

Main Signs:

1. Frequent mild exophthalmos often associated with a relatively small head and possible protruding occiput (**2 and 4–6**), as well as numerous telangiectatic naevi of the upper half of the face in infancy. Hypoplasia of the midface, possible soft tissue folds under the eyes (**5, 9, and 10**). Variously developed slit- or notch-like indentations of the external ears (**12–14**) and/or a groove on the dorsal edge of the helix in the great majority of cases. Congenital macroglossia, often with macrostomia, prognathism. Omphalocele (**1**); possibly simply the development of a large umbilical hernia (**2**). Congenital nephromegaly (ultrasonography imperative), hepato-, pancreato-, and possible cardiomegaly. Connatal macrosomia and/or postnatal 'gigantism', in connection with which the height, weight, and skeletal and dental maturity may be in advance of the norm for years.

2. Possible severe, prolonged, therapy-resistant hypoglycaemia in the newborn period and in infancy.

Supplementary Findings: Not infrequently the presence or development of hemihypertrophy (of the lower extremity alone or of the whole half of the body).

Rarely hypertrophy of the clitoris or penis.

Substantially increased tendency to blastomatosis (especially Wilms tumours and carcinoma of the adrenal cortex), especially in children with distinct hemihypertrophy.

Prediabetic metabolism possible later in childhood.

Mental development usually normal (in the absence of severe hypoglycaemic damage).

Manifestation: Birth and later (macrosomia).

Aetiology: Genetically determined syndrome often with ambiguous mode of inheritance; basic defect unknown; perhaps heterogeneity.

In apparently sporadic cases (i.e., examination of possible carriers negative), risk of recurrence low; with familial occurrence, risk of recurrence up to 50%.

Frequency: Relatively frequent; since publication of this syndrome in 1964, hundreds of cases have become known.

Course, Prognosis: After survival of possible post partum adaptive difficulties, polycythaemia, hypoglycaemia, respiratory and feeding difficulties, etc., usually good. Regression of splanchnomegaly, gradual slowing of growth (eventually normal adult height, unremarkable sexual maturation); tendency to attain normal proportions, including those of the facial features, and better tongue to mouth proportions.

Regular follow-up, especially of the abdomen for possible tumour development and with routine ultrasonography of the kidneys, absolutely mandatory.

Differential Diagnosis: Fetopathia diabetica; here, no macroglossia, no indentations of the external ears, no umbilical hernias, etc. Hypothyroidism (because of the enlarged tongue); ruled out by accelerated growth, absence of obstipation, etc., blood tests.

Treatment: Initially regular blood sugar determinations; in some cases prednisolone or diazoxide. Repair of omphalocele. Partial glossectomy may be indicated, possibly even in the small infant. Orthodontic care. Orthopaedic treatment for hemihypertrophy. Genetic counselling. In given cases, prenatal diagnosis with ultrasonography.

Illustrations:

1 Premature infant; omphalocele, macroglossia; brother of the 6-year-old patient in **10**.

2 6-month-old child; typical facies (ear shown in **12**), large umbilical hernia; probably frequent early hypoglycaemic seizures; still tendency to hypoglycaemia.

3, 7, and 11 Toddlers, post partum surgery for omphalocele, accelerated growth, normal mental development.

4–6 and 8–10 Typical facies at various ages.

13 Ear of patient in **3**.

14 Ear of patient in **5**.

References:

Wiedemann H.-R.: Exomphalos-Makroglossie-Gigantismus-Syndrom … Z. Kinderheilkd. *115*:193 (1973)

Kosseff A. L., Herrmann J., Gilbert E. F., et al: Studies of malformation syndromes of man XXIX: The Wiedemann-Beckwith syndrome. Eur. J. Pediatr. *123*:139 (1976)

Sommer A., Cutler E. A., Cohen B. L., et al: Familial occurrence of the Wiedemann-Beckwith syndrome … Am. J. Med. Genet. *1*:59 (1977)

Puissan Ch., Risbourg B., Lenaerts C., et al: Syndrome de Wiedemann et Beckwith. J. Génét. Hum. *28*:281 (1980)

Sotela-Avila C., Gonzalez-Crussi F., Fowler J. W.: Complete and incomplete forms of Beckwith-Wiedemann syndrome: Their oncogenic potential. J. Pediatr. *96*:47 (1980)

Best L. G., Hoekstra R. E.: Wiedemann-Beckwith syndrome: Autosomal dominant inheritance in a family. Am. J. Med. Genet. *9*:291 (1981)

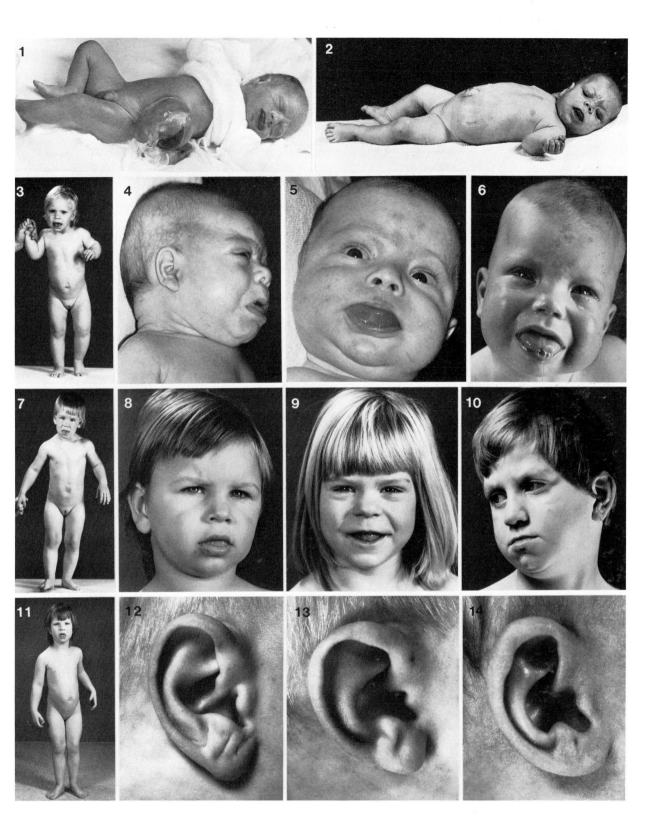

42. Sotos Syndrome

(Cerebral Gigantism Type Sotos)

A syndrome of childhood gigantism usually with above-normal size at birth, unusual facies, acromegalic changes, and signs of nonprogressive cerebral involvement.

Main Signs:
1. Inborn macrosomia and/or postnatal somatic gigantism (**3** and **4**) with accelerated osseous maturation and teething.
2. Macrocrania and abnormally large hands and feet.
3. Unusual physiognomy [high, prominent forehead with 'receding' hairline or 'frontal baldness' (**1**); hypertelorism; slightly out- and downward slanting of the lid axes]·
4. Congenital, nonprogressive cerebral impairment with retarded psychomotor development, disturbance of fine motor activity.

Supplementary Findings: Usually dolicocephalus, large ears, prognathism, high palate, and unusually long arms. Not infrequently development of kyphoscoliosis. On echoencephalography or CCT, slight to moderate enlargement of the cerebral ventricles, especially the IIIrd (no increased intracranial pressure).

No evidence of a constant endocrine or biochemical abnormality.

Manifestation: At birth and in infancy.

Aetiology: Genetically determined syndrome. Usually sporadic occurrence. Not only dominant inheritance observed, but also evidence for possible recessive transmission acknowledged. Thus, probable heterogeneity.

Frequency: Not rare (since 1964 about 170 cases have appeared in the literature).

Course, Prognosis: Accelerated growth self-limited by the end of the first, or at least the beginning of the second decade of life. Onset of puberty at the usual age or somewhat earlier. Adult height average, less than, or possibly greater than normal. The degree of mental retardation of decisive significance. Apparently an increased disposition to development of malignant tumours.

Differential Diagnosis: Other primordial gigantism syndromes (see, e.g., p.82, p.86).

Treatment: Regular follow-up examinations. All appropriate measures to further children with developmental or psychomotor retardation. Attention to scoliosis and early treatment in certain cases. Genetic counselling.

Illustrations:
1–4 A child with the Sotos syndrome. Length at birth 60 cm. At age 14 months (**1**, **3**, and **4**), average height of a 2¼-year-old, head circumference corresponding to that of an 8-year-old. Hand length of a 5-year-old, early eruption of teeth, bone age 3 years. Prominent forehead with frontal baldness, appearance of a child older than his age; large, somewhat low-set ears; large genitalia; very large feet. Statomotor retardation, clumsy motor performance; clearly enlarged IIIrd ventricle. At 2 years 4 months, height of a 4-year-old; enormous feet. At 3 years 11 months, (**2**) average height of a 6¼-year-old. 'Too old' appearing. Clumsy, restless, mentally subnormal behaviour.

References:
Jaeken J., van der Scheuren-Lodeweyck M., Eeckels R.: Cerebral gigantism syndrome. A report of 4 cases and review of the literature. Z. Kinderheilkd *112*:332 (1972)
Wiedemann H.-R.: Diencephale Syndrome des Kindesalters. Pädiatr. Prax. *11*:95 (1972)
Sotos J.F., Cutler E.A., Dodge P.: Cerebral gigantism. Am. J. Dis. Child. *131*:625 (1977)
Beman H., Nilsson D.: Sotos syndrome in two brothers. Clin. Genet. *18*:421 (1980)
Smith A., Farrar J.R., Silink M., et al: Dominant Sotos syndrome. Arch. Dis. Childh. *55*:579 (1980)

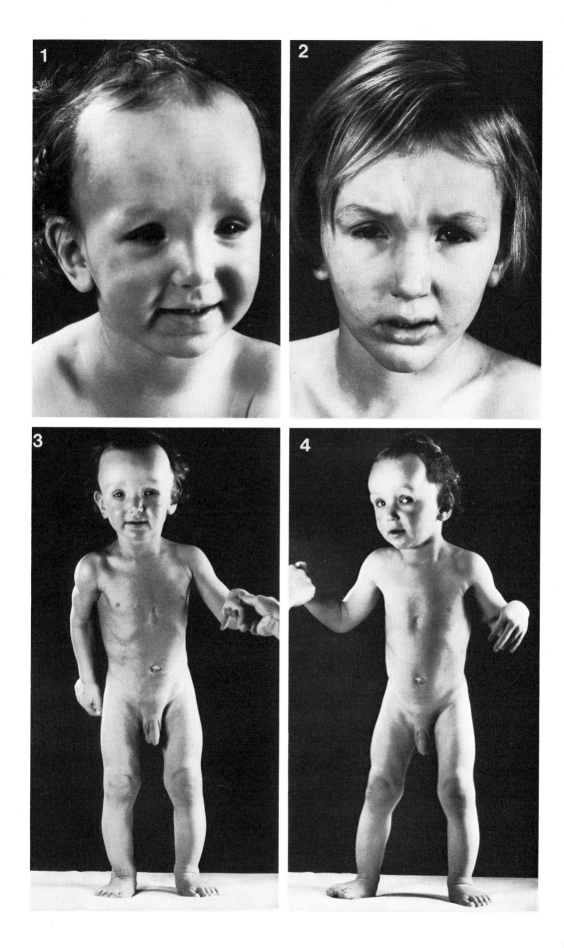

43. Weaver Syndrome

A further syndrome of 'gigantism' in childhood with congenital macrosomia, macrocrania, distinctive facies, unusual voice, muscular hypertonia, and additional anomalies.

Main Signs:
1. Congenital macrosomia and postnatal somatic gigantism (**1**).
2. Marked macrocrania (without signs of increased intracranial pressure) with broad, protruding forehead (**2**).
3. Distinctive appearance: pronounced hypertelorism; low-set, broad root of the nose; accentuated, long philtrum; receding chin; large ears (**1** and **2**).
4. Deep, hoarse voice. Muscular hypertonia.

Supplementary Findings: Possible initial limitation of motion of the elbow and knee joints. Club feet. Possible camptodactyly of the fingers, clinodactyly of the toes, broad thumbs, simian creases. Thin, deeply inserted nails; prominent fingertip pads.

Loose skin of the neck; inguinal and/or umbilical hernias.

Developmental retardation.

X-rays: Discordantly accelerated osseous maturation; upper ilial regions low and broad; widening of the distal ends of the long bones, especially the femora (**3**).

Manifestation: From birth on.

Aetiology: Unknown; to date, only sporadic cases are known (recently also the first known affected girl).

Frequency: Rare (since 1974, just half a dozen observations have been reported).

Course, Prognosis: Long-term follow-up not yet possible; however, the adult height would be expected to be normal or less than normal, rather than unusually tall. The intellectual development is key to the prognosis of the individual case.

Differential Diagnosis: Other primordial gigantism syndromes (see, e.g., p.82, p.84).

Treatment: Symptomatic. All possible aids to psychomotor development. Early measures to prevent obesity.

Illustrations:
1–3 A 15-month-old boy, the first child of healthy, young, nonconsanguineous parents. Birth at term after an unremarkable pregnancy: 57 cm, 4970 g, and head circumference 36 cm; club feet. At 15 months, 93 cm (like a 2½-year-old), about 17 kg, and head circumference 52 cm (both like those of a 4-year-old). (By kind permission of Prof. F. Majewski, Düsseldorf).

References:
Weaver D.D., Graham C.B., Thomas I.T., et al: A new overgrowth syndrome with accelerated skeletal maturation, unusual facies, and camptodactyly, J.Pediatr. *84*:547 (1974)
Fitch N.: The syndromes of Marshall and Weaver. J.Med.Genet. *17*:174 (1980)
Majewski F., Ranke M., Kemperdick H., et al: The Weaver syndrome: A rare type of primordial overgrowth. Eur.J.Pediatr. *137*:277 (1981)
Meinecke P., Hamburg: Personal communication concerning a case in a female

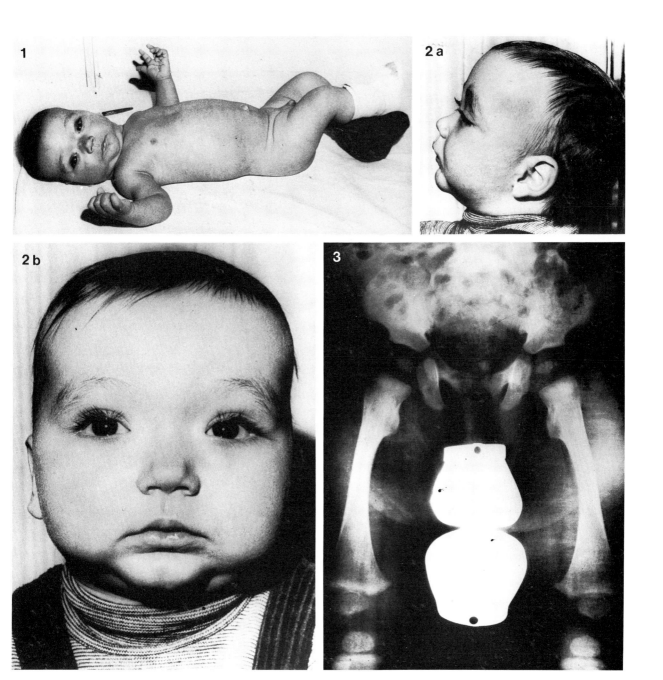

44. Marfan's Syndrome

(Arachnodactyly)

A characteristic hereditary syndrome of disproportionate tall stature, defects of the eye, and tendency to develop aortic aneurysm.

Main Signs:
1. Tall stature, especially due to excessively long extremities, particularly the distal portions, resulting in eunuchoid body proportions and arachnodactyly (**1** and **2**).
2. Marked deficit of fatty tissue. Muscular hypoplasia and hypotonia (**1**, **4**, and **6**).
3. Long, narrow face with high palate (**1** and **4**) and narrowly spaced teeth; dolichocephaly.
4. Signs of connective tissue weakness: hernias, hyperextensible joints, luxation of the joints, kyphoscoliosis, pedes plani, among others; pectus carinatum or excavatum (**1** and **4**).

Supplementary Findings: Dislocation of the lenses in about 75% of cases, usually upwards; when less pronounced, recognisable by split-lamp examination; danger of glaucoma. Usually marked myopia. Retinal detachment. Round lenses. Blue sclera.

General dilatation of the aorta (aortic valve insufficiency), dissecting aneurysm. Less frequently corresponding involvement of the pulmonary artery or the mitral and tricuspid valves.

Manifestation: In infancy. However, usually not diagnosed until childhood or later.

Aetiology: Autosomal dominant hereditary disease with variable expressivity; new mutations may be assumed for about 15% of cases, often associated with increased paternal age. A fundamental connective tissue disorder is likely, although the exact defect has not been determined.

Frequency: About 1 in 66000 of the population.

Course, Prognosis: Death as a result of cardiovascular complications possible at any age, especially after puberty. On average, patients attain 30 to 50 years. The possible occurrence of valvular endocarditis carries a very poor prognosis. Danger of going blind.

Differential Diagnosis: Homocystinuria (p.92), which must be ruled out in every case since it is basically amenable to therapy. Stickler's syndrome (p.404). (Contractural arachnodactyly see p.90.)

Treatment: Timely limitation of growth by means of hormone therapy, also as an attempt to prevent severe scoliosis. Propranolol seems to slow the development of aneurysms.

Vascular or cardiac surgery as indicated. Avoidance of marked physical exertion. Genetic counselling.

Illustrations:
1–3 Patient 1 at age 14 years: height 174 cm, weight 48 kg (normal weight of a girl 159 cm tall). Second toes operatively shortened bilaterally as they were 1.5 cm longer than the first toes. No evidence of cardiac defect at present. Myopia.
4 Patient 2 at age 9 years. No definite evidence of a cardiac defect. Myopia on the right, astigmatism on the left, round lenses. Lenses *not* dislocated. Height at 13 years, 196.5 cm.
5–7 Patient 3 (sister of patient 2) at age 6 years. Evidence of ballooning of the mitral valve. Round lenses, *no* luxation. Normal amino acid chromatogram. Height at age 10 years, 174.5 cm.

References:
Pyeritz R. E., McKusick V. A.: The Marfan syndrome: Diagnosis and management. N. Engl. J. Med. 772 (1979)
Donaldson R. M., Emanuel E. W., Olsen E. G. J., et al: Management of cardiovascular complications in Marfan syndrome. Lancet *II*:1178 (1980)
Boucek R. J., Nobel N. L., Gunja-Smith Z., et al: The Marfan syndrome: A deficiency in chemically stable collagen cross-links. N. Engl. J. Med. 988 (1981)

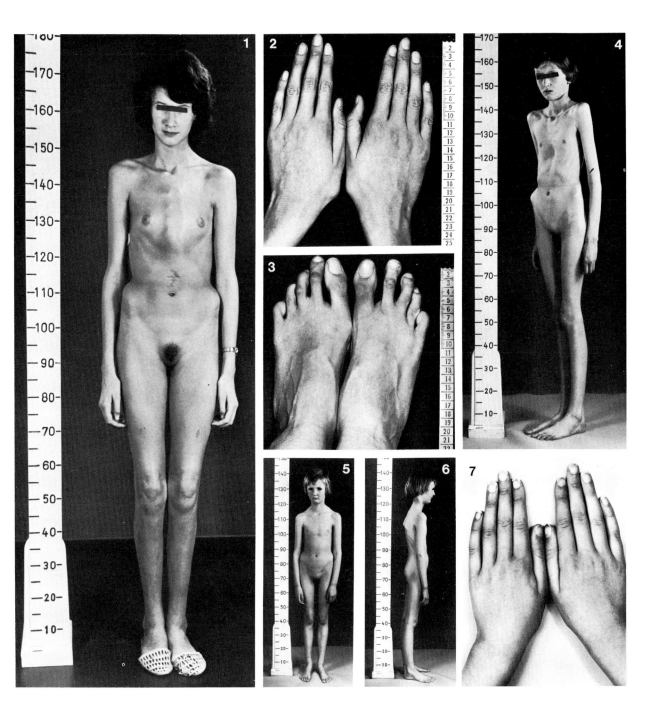

45. Syndrome of Contractural Arachnodactyly

A hereditary syndrome of arachnodactyly with multiple congenital contractures of the extremities.

Main Signs:
1. Multiple, largely symmetrical, congenital contractures of finger joints, knees, ankles, elbows, and (usually mild involvement) hips. Long, thin extremities, including hands and fingers, feet and toes, the proximal phalanges being particularly long. Flexion contractures of the fingers at the proximal interphalangeal joints, often with ulnar deviation; thumbs often adducted; toes may be slightly pronated. Pedes equino vari or calcaneo valgi (1 and 3).
2. Height normal or above average. Pectus excavatum or carinatum. Frequent development of kyphoscoliosis (1).
3. Eyes possibly somewhat deep-set; external ears may be posteriorly rotated with anomalies of the helix or antihelix and concha; retrogenia (2). Short neck (1c).

Supplementary Findings: No luxation of the lens or iridodonesis as in Marfan's syndrome (p.88) and homocystinuria (p.92); however, ocular anomalies may occur.

Cardiovascular involvement (as in Marfan's syndrome) much less frequent than in Marfan's syndrome, but may occur.

Manifestation: At birth.

Aetiology: Autosomal dominant hereditary disease with variable expressivity.

Frequency: Rare.

Course, Prognosis: Initially, possible delay in statomotor development, especially as a result of knee and ankle contractures. Normal life expectancy (however not when, as an exception, a severe cardiac defect is present). Tendency for improvement of the contractures. Tendency for progression of kyphoscoliosis when present.

Differential Diagnosis: Arthrogryposis (p.302); the total clinical picture permits the differentiation. In case of – atypical – mental subnormality and of rib and vertebral anomalies (supernumerary), a chromosome aberration (trisomy 8) must be ruled out.

Treatment: Symptomatic, with intensive physiotherapy; if necessary, surgical correction of malpositioning of the fingers. Genetic counselling.

Illustrations:
1–3 A 3½-year-old mentally normal boy, the second child of healthy parents after the birth of a healthy girl. Birth length 57 cm; subsequent height measurements above the 97th percentile. Congenital flexion contractures of the fingers and bilateral clinodactyly; long, narrow feet, initially in slight club-foot position (later, crura valga, pedes plani). Large cranium; hypertelorism; narrow, high palate with uvula fissa, slight microgenia; large ears, posteriorly rotated on the right. Bluish sclera; eyes otherwise negative at repeated follow-up examinations. Scapulae alatae; deformity of the thorax; pronounced muscular hypotonia; inguinal hernias. Kidneys normal. Chromosome analysis with banding negative. Low excretion of 5-hydroxyproline. Persistent ductus arteriosis (ligation at age 3 years). Persistence of the left superior vena cava; surgical repair of severe aortic ectasia and aortic valve replacement at age 5 years. Death due to heart failure at 5 years and 8 months.
(By kind permission of Prof. P. Heintzen and Oberärztin Dr E. Stephan, Kiel.)

References:
Beals R. K., Hecht Fr.: Congenital contractural arachnodactyly. J. Bone Jt. Surg. 53-A, 987 (1971)
Bjerkreim I., Skogland L. B., Trygstad O.: Congenital contractural arachnodactyly. Acta Orthop. Scand. 47:250 (1976)

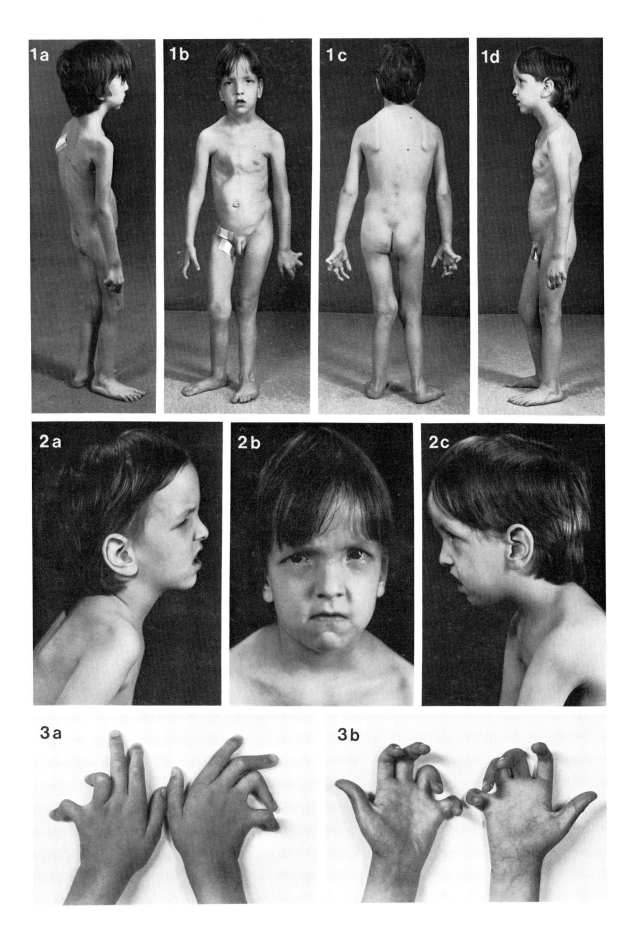

91

46. Syndrome of Homocystinuria

A metabolic disease that leads to tall stature, visual defects, and frequent mental retardation.

Main Signs:
1. A clinical picture similar to that of Marfan's syndrome, with age-dependent, in part progressive changes: tall stature often with eunuchoid proportions, conspicuous in childhood and increasing up to puberty; arachnodactyly; little subcutaneous fatty tissue. Long narrow face (see esp. patient 1, **1–3**); high palate.
2. Pectus carinatum or excavatum (**2 and 6**), scoliosis or kyphoscoliosis, knock-knees (**2**), hernias (**2**, postoperative appearance), ankylosis, 'waddling' gait.
3. Thin, sparse, dry, blond hair; flushed cheeks; translucent skin. Tendency to eczema.
4. In half to one-third of cases, mental retardation of various grades of severity. Behavioural disturbances with decreased ability to concentrate, irritability, limited social contact, etc. Possible slight microcephaly.

Supplementary Findings: Luxation of the lenses, usually inferiorly, occurring no later than the second decade of life; myopia, possible cataracts, secondary glaucoma, retinal detachment.

Tendency to form thromboemboli, even in early childhood and in every region of the body; severe premature arteriosclerosis due to homocystinuric damage to the endothelium.

Possible convulsive seizures.

Hepatomegaly.

Osteoporosis, punctate calcifications of the distal ulnar and radial epiphyses.

Evidence of homocystine in the urine or of hypermethioninaemia.

Manifestation: Biochemically, in the first weeks of life; clinically, in childhood or later.

Aetiology: Autosomal recessive hereditary disease with absence of the enzyme cystathione synthetase. Subdivided into type A and type B according to whether responsive to vitamin B6 therapy. In addition, there are further biochemically defined types of homocystinuria which, however, do not show the clinical picture described here.

Frequency: About 1:50 000 to 1:150 000 of the population.

Course, Prognosis: Life expectancy in untreated patients markedly decreased due to thromboembolic complications.

Diagnosis: By means of special tests of the urine and subsequent quantitative determination of homocystine in the blood plasma and urine. Unexplained thromboembolism in childhood should always suggest the diagnosis of homocystinuria.

Differential Diagnosis: Marfan's syndrome; here luxation of the lens is usually congenital and usually *upwards*; no flushing of the cheeks, unremarkable hair, hyperextensible joints, no mental retardation, no analogous tendency to thromboembolism, no progression of signs, and usually family history of similarly affected persons.

Treatment: About half of the cases respond to high doses of vitamin B6 (with simultaneous folic acid substitution) – type A. Long-term treatment. Type B can be favourably influenced by a methionine-poor and L-cystine-enriched diet on a long-term basis. Great restraint with operative procedures, especially with all avoidable procedures involving the vascular system (venipuncture, etc.) because of the danger of triggering thromboembolism. Genetic counselling. In appropriate cases, utilisation of prenatal diagnostic possibilities.

Illustrations:
1–4 Patient 1 at age 5½ years. Height 129 cm (average height of a 7-year-old boy). Moderate mental retardation. Blond hair, red cheeks. Subluxation of the lenses and myopia diagnosed at age 2 years.
5–7 Patient 2 at age 3¾ years. Height 109 cm (average height of a 5-year-old). No mental retardation. Blond hair. Flushed cheeks, eczema. At 2½ years slight myopia. No osteoporosis. Neither patient responded to pharmacological doses of vitamin B6.

Reference:
Pullon D.H.H.: Homocystinuria and other methioninemias. In: Neonatal Screening for Inborn Errors of Metabolism. Bickel H., et al (eds). Springer, Berlin -Heidelberg-New York 1980

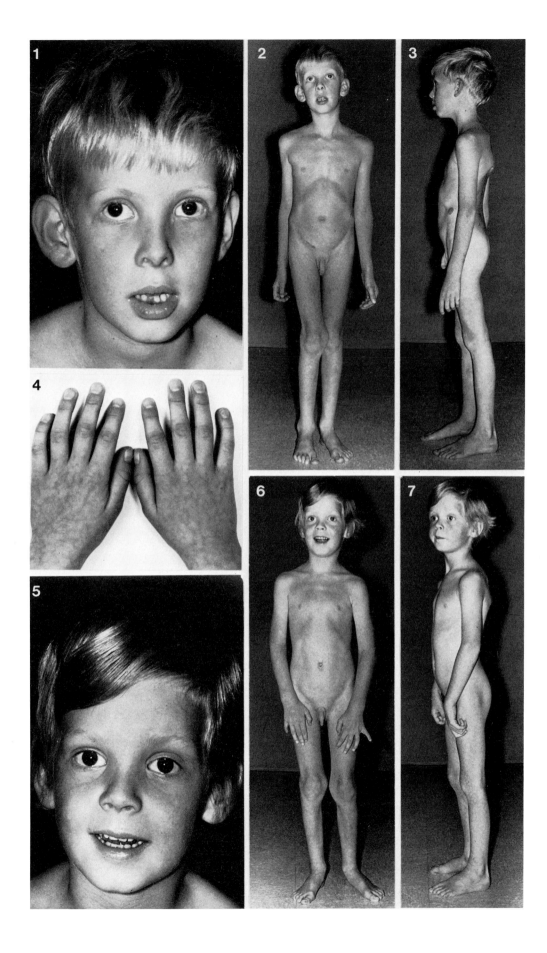

47. The XYY Syndrome

A tall stature syndrome in males with an extra Y chromosome.

Main Signs:
1. Tall stature.
2. Possible hypogenitalism.
3. Pronounced disposition to early varicosities of the lower legs and to leg ulcers.

Supplementary Findings: Intelligence as a rule below average. Frequently labile temperament; unstable patients who are easily seduced may have a history of deviant behaviour.

Evidence of a double 'Y–chromosomal sex chromatin' in simple screening tests; confirmation of the anomalous sex chromosome constitution by chromosome analysis.

Manifestation: Clinically by tall stature in childhood.

Aetiology: The syndrome, expressing the chromosomal aberration of a supernumerary Y chromosome, is caused by faulty separation of the chromosomes during spermatogenesis.

Frequency: About 1 in 1000 newborn boys.

Course, Prognosis: Average final height of about 1.85 metres; occasional patients may be much taller. Extreme tallness is a marked psychological handicap, impairing ability to cope. Possible infertility.

Differential Diagnosis: Other tall stature syndromes, especially Marfan's syndrome (p.88).

Treatment: Hormonal therapy to retard growth if excessive height is anticipated. Psychological support and in some cases adequate psychotherapy.

Illustrations:
1 and 2 A patient at age 14 years (1.82 cm) and again at 18 years (2.02 m). (By kind permission of Prof. J. Murken, Munich.)

References:
Any comprehensive textbook of paediatrics or internal medicine

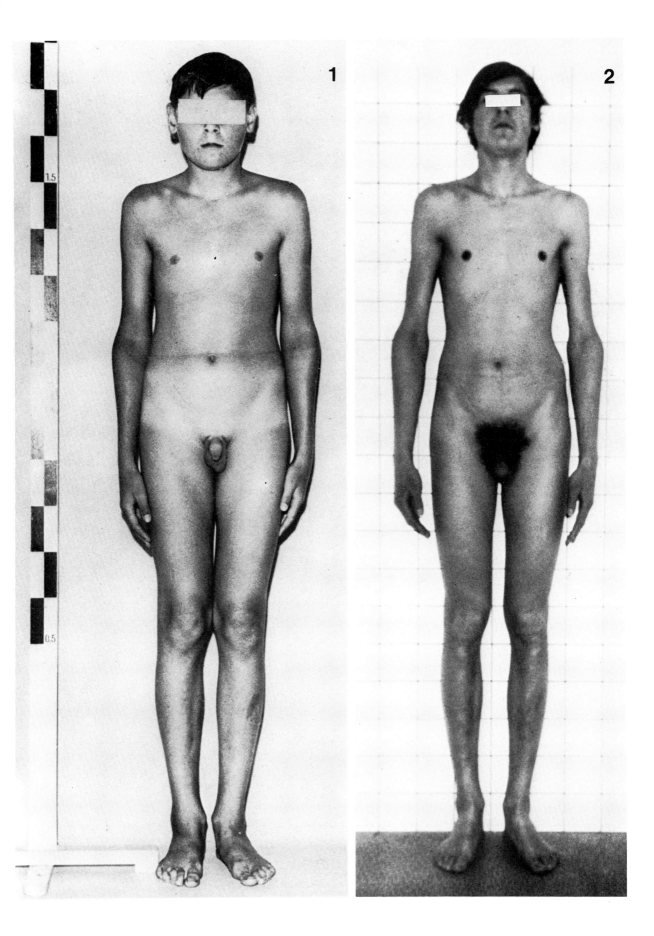

48. Russell Syndrome

(Primordial Dwarfism Type Russell)

A syndrome of pre- and postnatal slender dwarfism, relatively large cranium with correspondingly small face and microretrognathia, relatively short upper extremities, and clinobrachydactyly of the little fingers.

Main Signs:
1. Congenital small size in spite of full-term pregnancy. Disproportionately large cranium (1) with prominent frontal eminences, high hairline, and frequently very late closure of the anterior fontanelle – however, normal head circumference at birth and continuing normal growth: 'pseudohydrocephalus'. Small 'triangular' face with often finely differentiated nose, short philtrum, and large mouth with downturned corners. Microretrognathia (3).
2. Postnatal continuation of slow growth in height and especially weight (under or about the third percentile). Relatively short upper extremities (2a) with long lower extremities. Marked slenderness with narrow thorax and underdeveloped musculature (2).
3. Clino- or clinobrachydactyly of the little fingers. Delayed osseous maturation (4).

Supplementary Findings: High, squeaky voice which persists for years. Tendency to marked sweating.

Occurrence of rather minor asymmetries and of hyperlordosis, cryptorchidism, hypospadias, and other anomalies of the urogenital system.

Possible delay of motor development. Mental retardation an exception.

Manifestation: Pre- and postnatally.

Aetiology: Unknown. As a rule, sporadic occurrence. Genetic basis likely.

Frequency: Rare.

Prognosis: Dependent on the degree of development of the clinical picture and the significance of possible additional malformations and handicaps. Distinctly short adult stature to be anticipated.

Diagnosis, Differential Diagnosis: Numerous features in common with the Silver syndrome (p.98); the two syndromes may prove to be identical, as presumed by some authors ('Silver–Russell syndrome').

Treatment: See under Silver syndrome (p.98).

Illustrations:
1–4 A child born at term with birth weight 1750 g; mental development within normal limits; at 4½ months: 52 cm, 3220 g and at 3 years, 4 months: 75 cm, 5500 g (both well below the 3rd percentile). Extremely slim and delicate. Long cranium with protruding forehead, high, rather thin hairline, normal head circumference for age. Right half of face somewhat fuller than the left. Slightly low-set ears. Congenital ptosis of the left upper eyelid. Relatively large mouth with slightly down-turned corners and thin lips. Microretrognathia, overbite, narrowly spaced teeth especially of the lower jaw, dental caries. Squeaky voice. Short upper extremities. Slight clinobrachydactyly of the little fingers; zygodactyly bilaterally with double nail present on the second toe of the left foot. Exceedingly narrow, slender hand with bone age of about a 6-month-old child, pseudoepiphyses of proximal metacarpals I and II and hypoplasia of the middle phalanx of digit V. Evidence of ventricular septal defect; dilated renal pelvis of the right kidney on pyelography; hypospadias. Profuse sweats.

References:
Russell A: A syndrome of 'intrauterine' dwarfism recognisable at birth with cranio-facial dysostosis, disproportionately short arms, and other anomalies (5 examples). Proc. Roy. Soc. Med. 47:1040 (1954)
Gareis F. J., Smith D. W., Summitt L. L.: The Russell–Silver syndrome without asymmetry. J. Pediatr. 79:775 (1971). Thereto discussion: J. Pediatr. 80:1066 and 1068 (1972)
Haslam R. H. A., Berman W., Heller R. M.: Renal abnormalities in the Russell–Silver syndrome. Pediatrics 51:216 (1973)

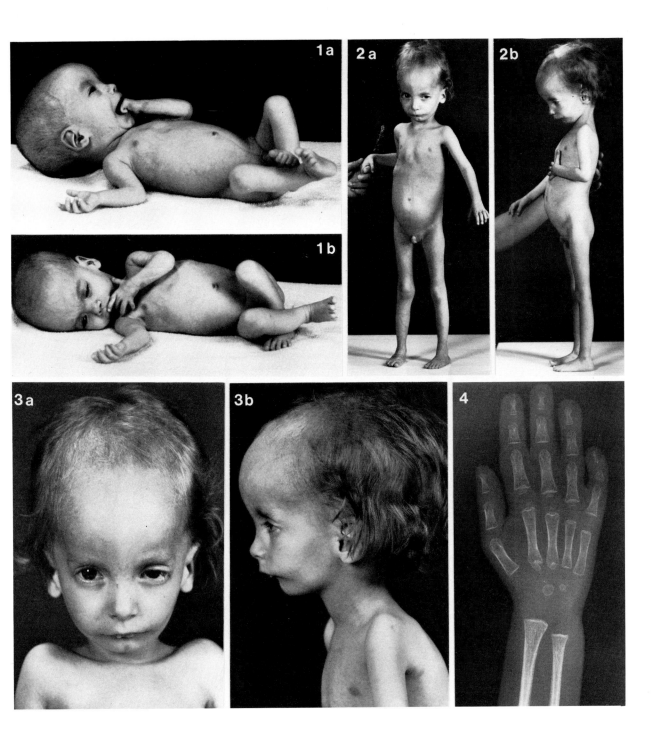

49. Silver Syndrome

A syndrome of pre- and postnatal dwarfism, asymmetry, broad forehead, clinobrachydactyly of the little fingers, and anomalies of sexual development.

Main Signs:
1. At birth, small for date; postnatal continuation of subnormal height and weight (**2**) with approximately corresponding delay of bone maturation.
2. Asymmetry due to underdevelopment of one side of the body or a part thereof (**1a, 2,** and **3**).
3. Large appearing (normal for age) cranium with wide forehead; small 'triangular' face; mouth sometimes thin-lipped with down-turned corners; micrognathia (**1**).
4. Clino- or clinobrachydactyly of the little fingers; proximal cutaneous syndactyly of the 2nd and 3rd toes (zygodactyly).
5. Signs of dissociated pubertus praecox in some cases; most frequently premature increase of urinary gonadotropins.

Supplementary Findings: Possible café-au-lait spots of the skin; hip or other skeletal dysplasias; malformations of the urogenital tract. Marked asymmetry of the lower extremities with tilting of the pelvis and secondary scoliosis.

Possible delay of statomotor development. Mental retardation rather the exception.

Manifestation: Pre- and postnatally.

Aetiology: Unknown. The – quite isolated – occurrence in siblings and reports of comparable, although milder, signs in mothers of affected children point to a genetic basis.

Frequency: Rare.

Prognosis: As a rule, probably relatively favourable; in individual cases, dependent on the severity of somatic dysplasias and on mental development.

Diagnosis, Differential Diagnosis: Overlaps with the Russell syndrome (p.96).

Treatment: Physiotherapy in some cases; orthopaedic or nephrourological care if required. Unresponsive to growth hormone, apart from exceptional cases with corresponding deficiency.

Illustrations:
1–3 A 2-year-old girl of normal psychomotor development (at term, 1800 g and 49 cm); height age, 18 months (below the 10th percentile); weight age, 9 months (below the 3rd percentile). Connatal hemihypertrophy of the right side of the body including the ear and nose (osseous hypotrophy shown in **3a**); secondary tilt of the pelvis and mild secondary scoliosis. Cranium relatively large, but normal for age (46.5 cm). Prominent, slightly bulging forehead. Small face; microretrognathia. Clinobrachydactyly of the 5th finger bilaterally; zygodactyly on the right. Rather unusually tall lumbar vertebral bodies. Ectopic ureterocele with megaureter and left hydronephrosis associated with a quiescent accessory kidney and ureter on the left. Markedly elevated gonadotropins in the urine.

References:
Silver K. H.: Asymmetry, short stature, and variations in sexual development. A syndrome of congenital malformations. Am. J. Dis. Child. *107*:495 (1964)
Tanner J. M., Ham T. J.: Low birthweight dwarfism with asymmetry (Silver's syndrome): Treatment with human growth hormone. Arch. Dis. Childh. *44*:231 (1969)
Szalay G. C.: Definition of the Russell–Silver syndrome. Pediatrics *52*:309 (1973)
Tanner J. M., Lejarraga H., Cameron N.: The natural history of the Silver–Russell syndrome: A longitudinal study of 39 cases. Pediatr. Res. 9:611 (1975)
Escobar V., Gleiser S., Weaver D. D.: Phenotypic and genetic analysis of the Silver–Russell syndrome. Clin. Genet. *13*:278 (1978)
Angehrn V., Zachmann M., Prader A.: Silver–Russell syndrome. Observations in 20 patients. Helv. Pediatr. Acta *34*:297 (1979)

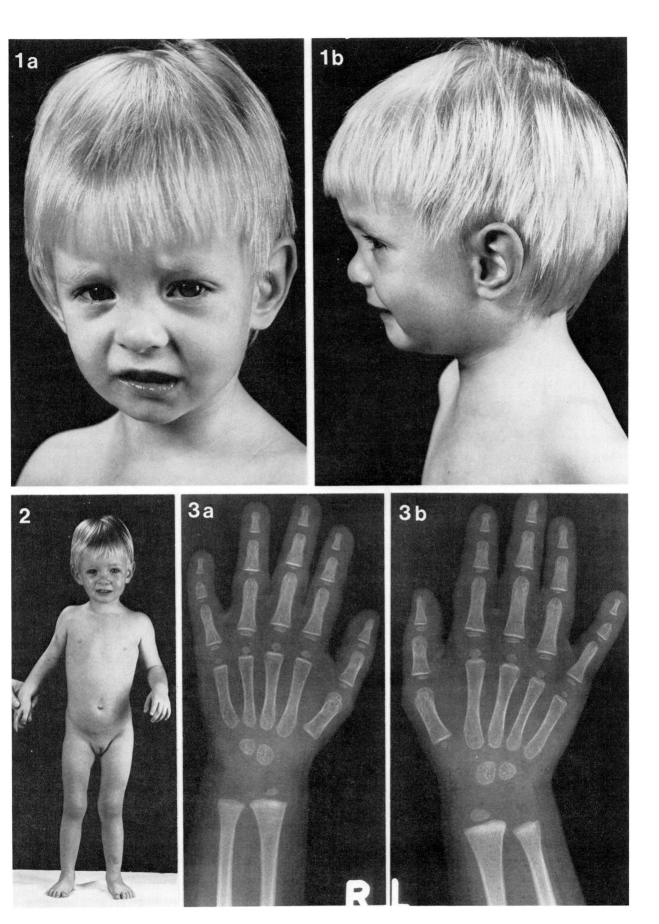

50. Primordial Dwarfism with Relative Macrocrania, Peculiar Physiognomy, Further Minor Malformations and Normal Psychomotor Development

A syndrome of primordial dwarfism, peculiar facies with blepharophimosis, large dolichocephalic head, and normal mental development.

Main Signs:
1. Primordial, for the most part proportional, gracile dwarfism, well under the 3rd percentile. Relative macrocrania with dolichocephaly (1–3).
2. Facies: Short, narrow palpebral fissures with slight antimongoloid slant under relatively striking eyebrows. Suggestion of epicanthus bilaterally. Low-set ears. Prominent nose. Small, thin-lipped, narrow mouth which appears pinched (1 and 4).

Open bite. Massive caries (? secondary to difficulty in caring for the teeth because of the small opening of the mouth).
3. Hypogonadism, bilateral cryptorchidism. Simian crease left, suggested on the right; hypoplastic-appearing distal phalanges of the fingers; clinodactyly of the 5th fingers (5).

Supplementary Findings: Slumped posture; winged scapulae; dorsal kyphosis which the child was able to compensate for. (2 and 3).

Psychomotor development normal for age.

X-rays: Dysplasia of the 1st rib on the left. Dissociated development of the ossification centres on X-ray of the hands and profoundly retarded bone age (by about 3½ years) (5).

Manifestation: At birth.

Aetiology: Unknown.

Course, Prognosis: Apart from short stature, expected to be favourable.

Differential Diagnosis: Other syndromes with dwarfism and blepharophimosis.

Treatment: Symptomatic.

Illustrations:
1–5 A 7-year-old boy, the first child of young, non-consanguineous parents of normal height. A healthy younger brother. Birth of the proband shortly before term with 2250 g and *44* cm. At 7 years, 2 months, 104 cm; head circumference at 6 years, 10 months, 52.3 cm. Large internal organs negative; thorough endocrinological examination negative; chromosome analysis negative.

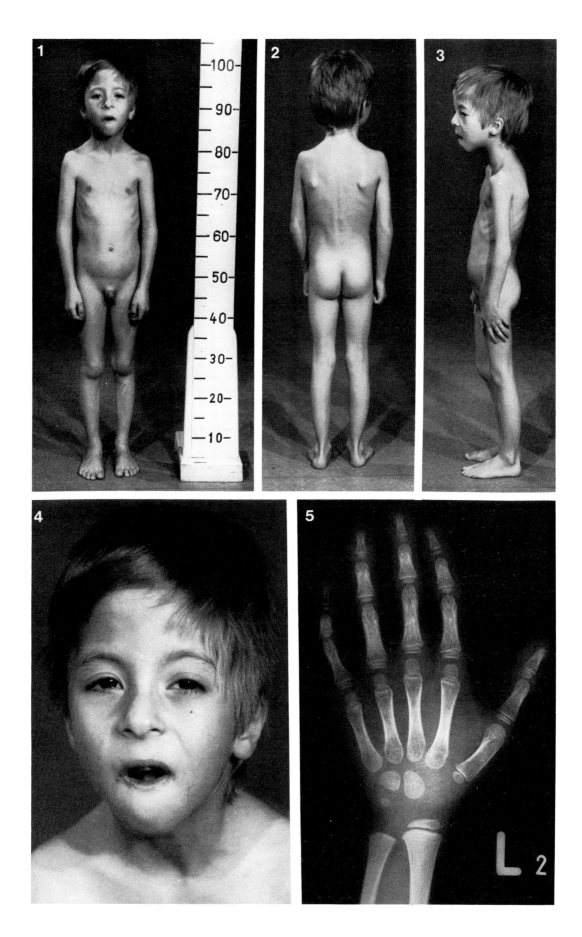

51. Syndrome of Blepharophimosis, Camptodactyly, Short Stature, Mental Retardation, and Inner Ear Hearing Impairment

A syndrome of unusual features of the face, hands, and feet in combination with growth deficiency, mental retardation, and impaired hearing.

Main Signs:
1. Facies: high forehead; short, narrow palpebral fissures; prominent eyebrows with slight synophyrs; low-set, simply formed external ears; low-set root of the nose; small mouth (with diastema, high palate, bifid uvula) (1–3).
2. Camptodactyly of fingers II–V along with clinodactyly of the little fingers (6). Hallus valgus deviation bilaterally and dysplasia of the little toes with rudimentary or absent nails.
3. Short stature (under the 3rd percentile at 5 and 13½ years) with lower extremities being somewhat too short (4 and 5).
4. Primary mental retardation (IQ at 13½ years, 44).
5. Primary inner ear hearing impairment bilaterally.

Supplementary Findings: Long narrow thorax with mild funnel chest.

Strabismus (operated); optic fundi normal.

X-rays: Cone-shaped epiphyses of the proximal phalanges of toes II–V bilaterally.

Manifestation: At birth (impaired hearing recognised in late infancy).

Aetiology: Unknown.

Course, Prognosis: Affected especially by the severe grade of mental retardation.

Differential Diagnosis: Other syndromes of short stature and blepharophimosis.

Illustrations:
1–6 The proband at age 5 years (1, 2, and 6) and 13½ years (3–5). First child of healthy, young, non-consanguineous parents; premature birth; no serious problems in rearing. Several cerebral seizures between the 3rd and 5th years of life; neurological examination negative; EEG negative; electromyelogram unremarkable. Clinical and laboratory examinations negative. Chromosome analysis negative.

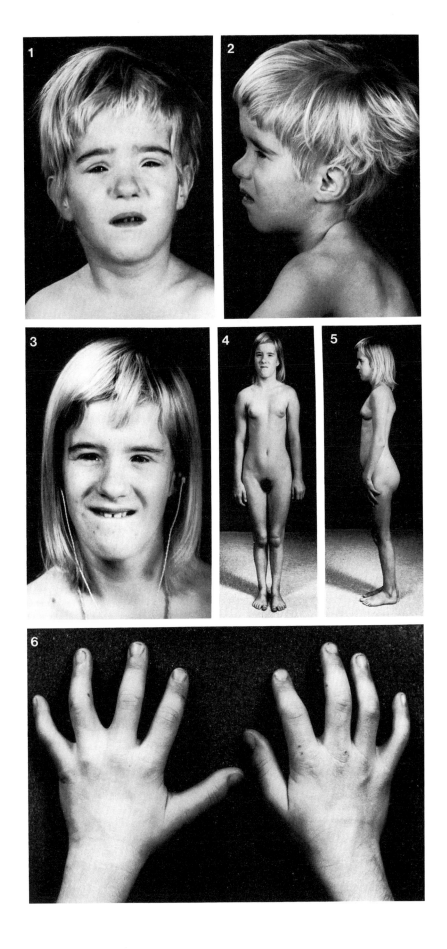

52. Rubinstein–Taybi Syndrome

A syndrome with characteristic facies, microcephalic psychomotor retardation, small stature, and anomalies of the hands and feet with broad distal phalanges, especially of the thumbs and halluces.

Main Signs:
1. Cranium and facies: Microcephaly of various grades of severity, often with protruding forehead and large anterior fontanelle. Antimongoloid slant of the palpebral fissures, broad nasal root, epicanthi, frequent strabismus, prominent eyebrows and eyelids, possible ptosis, and mild anomalies of the external ears (1 and 2). Beak-shaped nose, crooked or straight, with anterior prolongation of the nasal septum (2). High palate, slightly receding chin.
2. Broad distal phalanges of the thumbs and halluces, also often of other rays (3–5). Thumbs not infrequently radially deviated at the interphalangeal joint. Possible clinodactyly and overlapping toes.
3. Psychomotor retardation (IQ usually less than 50); frequent EEG anomalies.
4. Short stature (usually about or below the 3rd percentile).

Supplementary Findings: Frequently undescended testes. Often hirsutism. Development of kyphoscoliosis. Occurrence also of heart and kidney defects.

X-rays may show deformity of the proximal phalanges in cases with abnormal angulation of the thumbs and/or halluces; sometimes also doubling within the big toe region. Generalised delay of ossification. Possible anomalies of the pelvis, vertebrae, and/or thorax.

Manifestation: Birth and later.

Aetiology: Unclear; since there has been concordance in monozygotic twins, genetic factors must be assumed. No increased risk of recurrence in further children of parents of an affected child.

Frequency: Up to 1 in 500 mentally retarded or higher.

Course, Prognosis: For the most part dependent on the severity of mental retardation and the quality of support and education of the child. Average life expectancy probably shortened.

Differential Diagnosis: The Cornelia de Lange syndrome (p.118) should not be difficult to exclude.

Treatment: Symptomatic. All appropriate aids for the handicapped.

Illustrations:
1–5 A 6½-year-old girl, the second child of healthy, nonconsanguineous parents after a healthy sibling. Head circumference at birth with other measurements being normal, 32.5 cm; presently 47.6 cm (below the 2nd percentile). Height and weight around the tenth percentile. General developmental retardation. Hirsutism. On X-ray distinct asymmetry of the facial bones and skull; delayed ossification. Chromosome analysis negative. (By kind permission of Frau Dr U. Hillig and Prof. Dr G. G. Wendt, Marburg a.d.L.)

Reference:
Theile U., Draf U., Heldt J. P.: Das Rubinstein-Taybi-Syndrom. Dtsch. Med. Wochenschr. 1505 (1978)

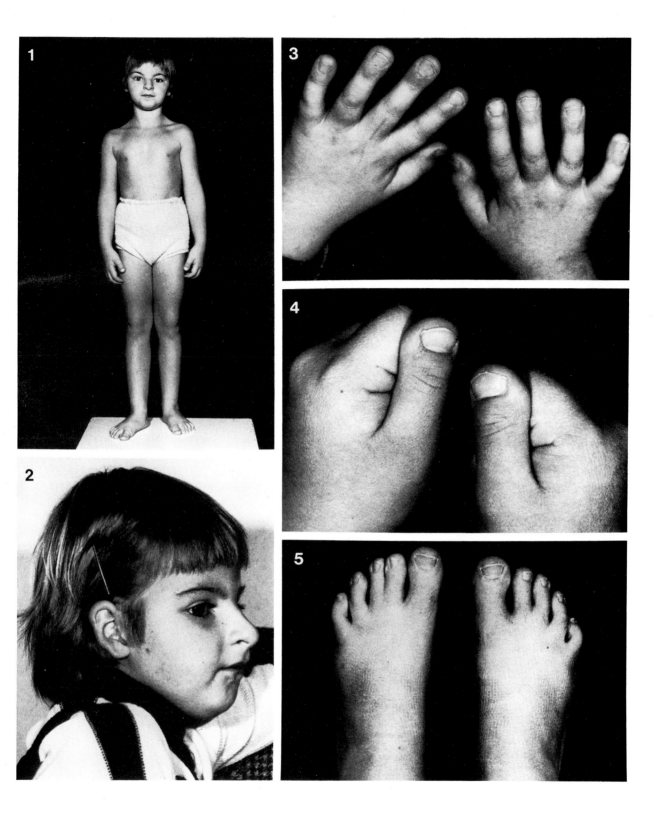

53. Syndrome of Dyscrania or Microcephaly, Psychomotor Retardation, and Short Stature with Anomalies of the Hands and Feet

A familial dyscrania–microcephaly–retardation syndrome with small stature and broad, short thumbs and big toes.

Main Signs:

1. Dyscrania with high forehead, sloping occiput (**1–3, 1a–3a**); microcephaly.
2. Facies: Slight antimongoloid slant of the palpebral fissures, low-set ears, slightly receding chin (**1–3, 1a–3a**).
3. Psychomotor retardation of various grades of severity.
4. Short stature (to below the third percentile).
5. Short hands and feet with stubby, broad thumbs and halluces (**1b–3b, 4,** and **5**).

Supplementary Findings: Unilateral undescended testes in both boys as well as inguinal hernias. Micropenis and striking scrotal hypoplasia in the child in **3**.

Manifestation: At birth and later.

Aetiology: Genetically determined syndrome.

Course, Prognosis: Essentially dependent on the degree of mental retardation.

Treatment: Symptomatic.

Illustrations:

1, 1a, and **1b**   A 9-month-old infant, the first child of young, nonconsanguineous parents. Normal measurements at birth. Head circumference at 9 months about the 2nd percentile, at 2 years well below the 2nd percentile. Initially telangiectatic naevi spread over the face. Delayed closure of a very large anterior fontanelle. No psychomotor development (CCT: dilated ventricles; EEG: increased seizure activity). Small stature on and below the 3rd percentile. Short stubby thumbs, contracted in the physiological position (**1b**), and big toes. High arched palate, pectus carinatum, club feet, cardiac defect (VSD). Ocular fundi negative; detailed clinical, laboratory, and enzymatic investigations negative; chromosome analysis negative.

2, 2a, 2b, 4, and **5**   The 26-year-old mother of the proband: craniofacial dysmorphism, retardation, abnormal thumbs and big toes (also present in the mother's father and in her two sisters). Extensive similarities of the mother's and son's palmar ridge patterns.

3, 3a, and **3b**   The 13-month-old son of a sister of the mother of the proband, the first child of young, nonconsanguineous parents. Birth 3 weeks prior to term with 2300 g, 44 cm, and 32 cm head circumference. At 14 months microcephaly; premature closure of the cranial sutures; CCT: partial dilation of the cerebral ventricles. Psychomotor retardation. Growth deficiency (at 14 months under the third percentile). Plump, paw-like hands and stubby feet, broad thumbs and big toes. Fundi negative. Chromosome analysis negative (including banded preparations).

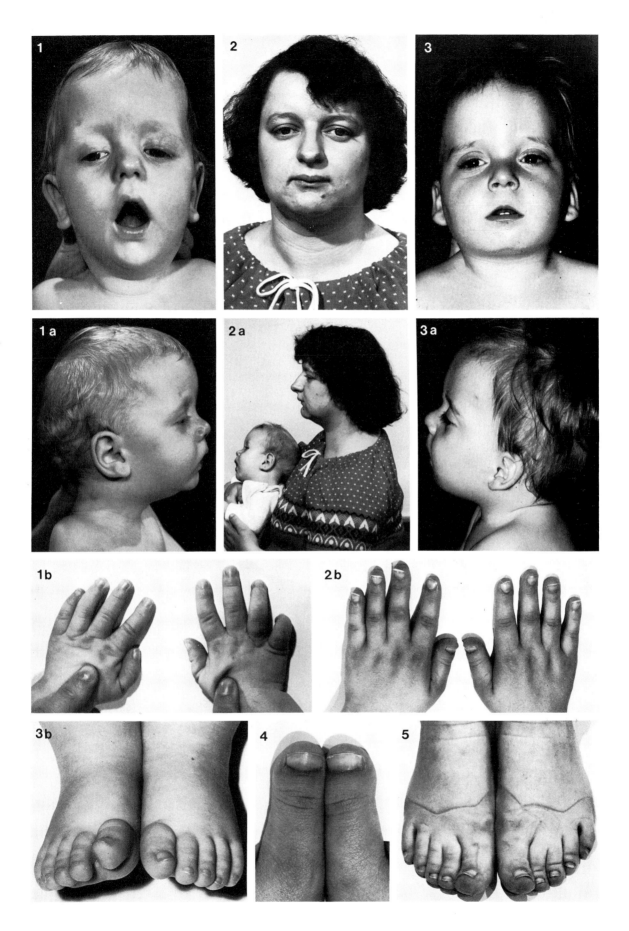

54. Cockayne Syndrome

A growth deficiency syndrome progressively manifesting from the second year of life and leading to dystrophic 'dwarfism' with typical facies, microcephaly, mental retardation, neurological and ocular defects, and other anomalies.

Main Signs:

1. Severe growth deficiency, disproportionate due to excessive length of the extremities and oversized hands and feet (1).
2. Typical facies, narrow, 'sunken in' and 'too old', with deepset eyes, thin nose, prognathism (1–3).
3. Increasingly apparent microcephaly.
4. Progressive neurological defects (ataxia, possible tremor; hearing impairment, which may progress to deafness, and decreased visual acuity – see below) as well as mental retardation.

Supplementary Findings: Development of ocular and visual defects, progressing to blindness: retinitis pigmentosa; optic atrophy; cataracts (in about one third of cases); possible corneal clouding.

Hypersensitivity to UV light with exanthemas of the skin and subsequent dyspigmentation and scarring.

Progressive development of flexion contractures of the large joints and progressive dorsal kyphosis.

Possible cryptorchidism; impaired sweating, disorder of water–salt metabolism, decreased resistance to infection.

Radiologically, calcification in the area of the cerebral basal ganglia, thickening of the calvaria, and other findings.

No evidence of a consistent endocrinological or biochemical abnormality.

Manifestation: Starting in the second year of life (after normal development for at least the initial, greater part of the first year of life).

Aetiology: Autosomal recessive inherited disease. Basic defect unknown.

Frequency: Very rare; about 60 cases have been described.

Course, Prognosis: Progressive, on to complete invalidism. Decreased life expectancy.

Differential Diagnosis: 'Seckel syndrome' (p.110), Dubowitz syndrome (p.112), progeria (p.194), and Bloom syndrome (p.270) can be readily ruled out.

Treatment: Symptomatic. Avoidance of exposure to sunlight. In some cases cataract operation, hearing aids. Genetic counselling of the parents.

Illustrations:

1–3 An 18-year-old, the only child of healthy parents. Birth measurements 3875 g and 55 cm. Quite unremarkable development until age 2 years, thereafter progressive slowing of physical and mental development. Presently, typical senile facial appearance, microcephaly (43.5 cm), dwarfism (97.5 cm) with very long extremities and large hands and feet. Ataxia, tremor, oligophrenia. Photosensitivity. Visual and hearing impairments. (By kind permission of Prof. H. Schönenberg, Aachen.)

References:
Schönenfeld H., Frohn K.: Das Cockayne-Syndrom. Monatschr. Kinderheilkd. *117*:103 (1969)
Bensman A., Brauner M., Teboul-Faure, et al: Le syndrome de Cockayne. J. Radiol. Electrol. *59*:375 (1978)
Soffer D., Grotzky H.W., Rapin I., et al: Cockayne syndrome. Unusual neuropathologic findings and review of the literature. Ann. Neurol. 6:340 (1979)

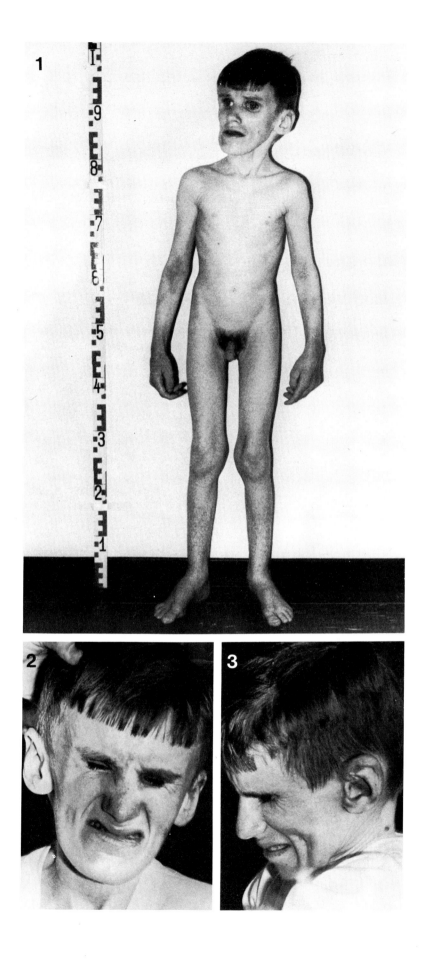

106

55. 'Seckel Syndrome'

('Bird-headed Dwarfism')

An unclassified complex of cases with hereditary pre- and postnatal stunted growth, microcephaly, 'bird face', mental retardation, and further anomalies.

Main Signs:
1. Congenital small size (relative to gestational age).
2. Microcephaly (**1–6**) with mental or psychomotor retardation.
3. 'Bird face' due to its narrowness; sloping forehead; large eyes; prominent, large, more-or-less beak-shaped nose; receding chin (**1–6**). Possibly low-set, dysplastic ears (**3**).
4. Continuation of growth deficiency postnatally.

Supplementary Findings: Frequent facial asymmetry, strabismus. Anomalies of the upper extremities (clinodactyly, simian crease, hypoplasia of the 1st ray) and of the lower limbs (hip dysplasia, club feet, or other deformities) and possibly also of the trunk (decreased number of ribs, kyphoscoliosis, etc.). Cryptorchidism.
Possible hypotrichosis.
Relatively 'too old' appearance.

Manifestation: At birth.

Aetiology: Not uniform. Autosomal recessive inheritance.

Frequency: Rare.

Course, Prognosis: Poor with respect to mental development.

Differential Diagnosis: Other more or less well-delineated primordial dwarfism–microcephaly forms.

Therapy: Symptomatic. Genetic counselling. In case of further pregnancies in the mother, prenatal diagnosis with ultrasonography.

Illustrations:
1–6 The second child of young, healthy, nonconsanguineous parents after a healthy girl. (**1–3**, the patient after birth; **4–6**, 6 months later.) Spontaneous birth 9 days after term; measurements: 1200 g, 36 cm, and 27 cm (head circumference). Facial asymmetry; strabismus. Dry scaly skin, hypotrichosis; initially limited extension of the large joints. Fingers sharply tapered distally, clinodactyly and simian crease bilaterally. Lax knee joints. Rockerbottom feet. Bilateral cryptorchidism; right hydronephrosis with ureteral stenosis. Length at age 6 months, 52 cm; head circumference 31 cm (both well under the 2nd percentile). CCT: Hydrocephalus *int. et ext. e vacuo*; evidence of bilateral hypoplasia of the frontal lobes. Severely impaired psychomotor development. Chromosome analysis from lymphocyte and fibroblast cultures, negative (including banded preparations). (By kind permission of Dr P. Meinecke, Hamburg.)

References:
McKusick V. A., Mahloudji M., Abott M., et al: Seckel's bird-headed dwarfism. New Engl. J. Med. *277*:279 (1967)
Boscherini B., Iannaccone G., La Cauza C., et al: Intrauterine growth retardation...Eur. J. Pediatr. *137*:237 (1981)

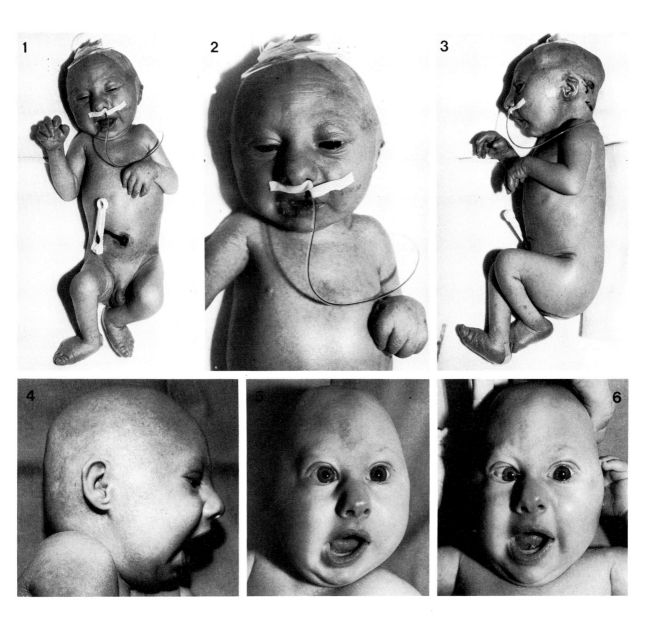

56. Dubowitz Syndrome

A malformation–retardation syndrome of primordial growth deficiency, unusual facies, marked microcephaly, moderate mental retardation, hyperactivity, and eczema.

Main Signs:
1. Typical facial dysmorphism, especially characterised by epicanthic folds superiorly, hypertelorism, relatively short palpebral fissures, occasional ptosis, low nasal bridge (most pronounced in young children). Thin hair, hypoplasia of the lateral portion of the eyebrows; micrognathia (**1** and **2**).
2. Primordial growth deficiency. Pronounced microcephaly with comparatively mild mental retardation. Hyperactivity. High-pitched voice.
3. Decreased subcutaneous fatty tissue. Eczematous skin changes, especially after exposure to sunlight, (**1–4**).

Supplementary Findings: Syndactyly of the 2nd and 3rd toes (**6**).
   Pes planus, pes planovalgus. Short, radially deviated 5th fingers (**5**).
   Cryptorchidism.
   Vomiting and diarrhoea in infancy.
   Frequent infections. Anaemia.

Manifestation: At birth.

Aetiology: Autosomal recessive hereditary disease.

Frequency: Since the first description in 1971 until 1980, somewhat over 30 cases had been reported.

Prognosis: Occasionally catch up of growth. Improvement of eczema after about the 3rd year of life. The further prognosis cannot be given since almost all known patients are still in the paediatric age grouup.

Differential Diagnosis: Bloom syndrome (p.270): here, no mental retardation; skin manifestations are of telangiectatic erythema, and not of eczema; typical chromosomal changes. Fetal alcohol syndrome (p.364): here, corresponding maternal history, cardiac defect in the child.

Treatment: Symptomatic. Genetic counselling; in case of further pregnancy, prenatal diagnosis by ultrasonography.

Illustrations:
1–6 A patient at age 8 years. Birth weight 2750 g. Eczema and vomiting during infancy. IQ 62. Hyperactivity. Pendulous testes. Measurements at age 8 years: height 106 cm (corresponding to that of a 4½-year-old boy), weight 12 kg (corresponding to that of a 21-month-old boy), head circumference 48 cm (corresponding to that of an 18-month-old boy).

References:
Grosse R., Gorlin J., Opitz J.M.: The Dubowitz syndrome. Z. Kinderheilkd. *110*:175 (1971)
Majewski F., Michaelis R., Moosmann K., Bierich J.R.: A rare type of low birthweight dwarfism: The Dubowitz syndrome. Z.Kinderheilkd. *120*:238 (1975)
Orrison W.W., Schnitzler E.R., Chun R.W.M.: The Dubowitz syndrome: Further observations. Am.J.Med.Genet. *7*:155 (1980)

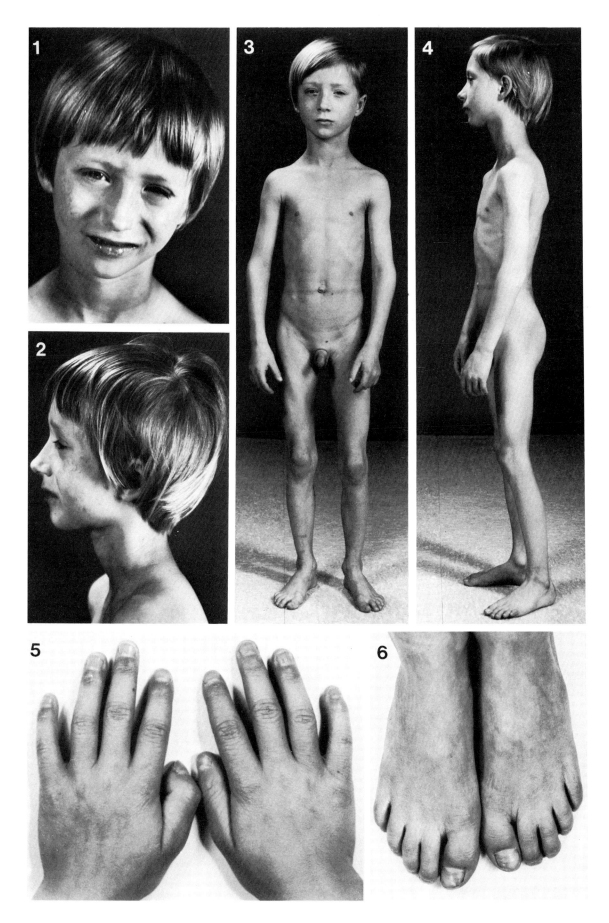

57. A Further Microcephaly–Small Stature – Retardation Syndrome

An unfamiliar syndrome of peculiar facies, microcephaly and mental retardation, growth deficiency, anal atresia, and further anomalies.

Main Signs:
1. Facies: Antimongoloid slant of the palpebral fissures, bilateral ptosis (left more marked than right; suspected IIIrd and XIIth nerve paresis); broad nasal bridge; low-set and prominent, dysplastic ears; narrow prolabium; and receding chin (**1–8**).
2. Microcephaly (around the 2nd percentile) with substantial psychomotor retardation.
3. Small stature (between the 3rd and 10th percentiles).
4. Anal atresia.

Supplementary Findings: High palate, dysodontiasis, bipartite uvula, persistent ductus arteriosis. Synostosis of the first ribs bilaterally; crudely shaped scapulae and clavicles. Narrow hands; pillar-like, poorly modelled legs (**6** and **9**).

Manifestation: At birth.

Aetiology: Unknown.

Course, Prognosis: In view of the mental retardation, poor.

Differential Diagnosis: Other microcephaly–small stature syndromes.

Treatment: Appropriate handicap aids.

Illustrations:
1–9 The 3rd child of healthy parents; numerous healthy siblings. Birth measurements 3100 g, 49 cm, and 33.5 cm (head circumference). No maternal alcoholism. Chromosome analysis normal.

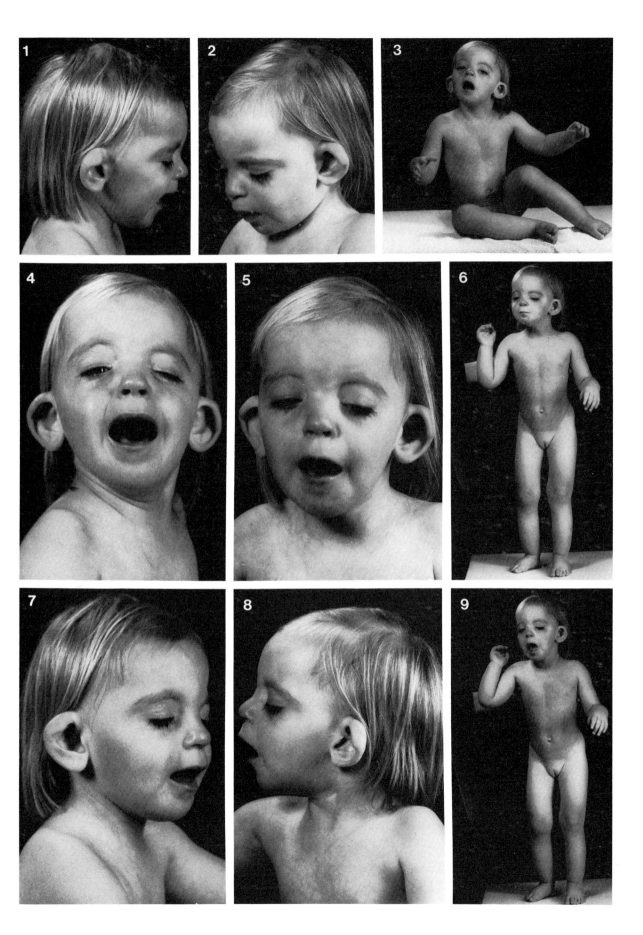

58. Mietens Syndrome

A malformation–retardation syndrome of small stature, short forearms held in flexion, unusual facies, corneal clouding, and moderate mental retardation.

Main Signs:

1. Flexion contractures of the elbows with dislocation of the head of the radius and abnormally short forearms (**1–4**).
2. Small stature and mental retardation (IQ about 70–80).
3. Unusual facies with bilateral corneal clouding, nystagmus, strabismus, narrow pointy nose with hypoplastic alae nasi (**1** and **2**).

Supplementary Findings: Pedes plani et valgi, moderately severe flexion contractures of the knees (**2**), hip dysplasia; pectus excavatum as well as clinodactyly may also be present.

Manifestation: Pre- and postnatally.

Aetiology: Genetically determined syndrome; mode of inheritance not completely clear, most likely autosomal recessive.

Frequency: Very rare.

Course, Prognosis: Intelligence may be difficult to evaluate due to defective vision and limited arm function. *If* vascular anomalies (see below, text of Illustrations) prove to be part of the syndrome, the prognosis must be guarded.

Differential Diagnosis: Other forms of congenital shortening of the forearm must be considered.

Treatment: Ophthalmological and orthopaedic care. All appropriate measures to promote the developmentally retarded child.

Illustrations:

1 and 2 Two of four affected siblings. Small stature; mental retardation. Corneal clouding; strabismus. Narrow nose with hypoplasia of the alae nasi. Abnormally short forearms with flexion contractures of the dislocated elbows. Flexion contractures of the knees; pedes valgi et plani. The girl has a history of a ruptured aneurysm of the right anterior cerebral artery.
3 X-ray of a 5-month-old sibling.
4 X-ray of the boy shown in **1**.
(By kind permission of Prof. C. Mietens, Bochum.)

References:
Mietens C., Weber H.: A syndrome characterised by corneal opacity, nystagmus, flexion contracture of the elbows, growth failure, and mental retardation. J. Pediatr. 62:624 (1966)
Warring III G. O., Rodrigues M. M.: Ultrastructure and successful keratoplasty of sclerocornea in Mietens' syndrome. Am. J. Ophthalmol. 90:469 (1980)

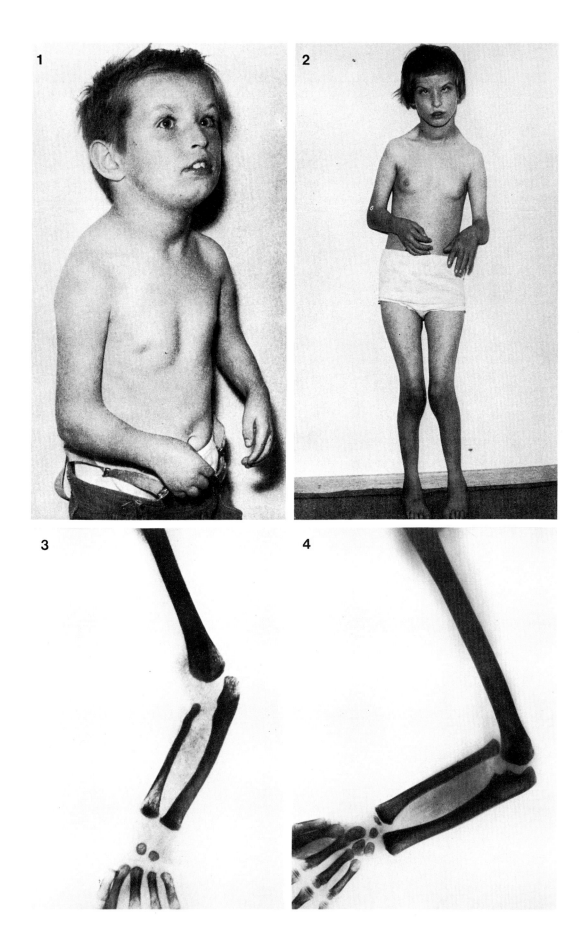

59. Cornelia de Lange Syndrome

(Brachmann–de Lange Syndrome, Typus Degenerativus Amstelodamensis)

A malformation–mental retardation syndrome of unknown aetiology with characteristic facial dysmorphism, primordial growth deficiency, and reduction anomalies of the extremities.

Main Signs:
1. Pathognomonic facies with bushy eyebrows meeting over the root of the nose, hypertelorism, antimongoloid slant of the palpebral fissures, anteverted nostrils, increased naso-labial distance or protruding philtrum, narrow lips, and down-turned corners of the mouth. Low anterior and posterior hair lines. Microbrachycephaly. Deep, coarse, expressionless voice.
2. Severe psychomotor retardation. Prominent musculature, sometimes with hypertonia severe enough to interfere with feeding.
3. Hirsutism.
4. Small stature.
5. Short hands and feet, thumbs displaced proximally, short 5th finger, simian crease. In cases with marked reduction, retrogression of the rays from the ulnar side, with monodactyly or arm stumps in extreme cases; lower extremities generally not as severely affected.

Supplementary Findings: Cylindrical trunk, small nipples. Cutis marmorata. Myopia, nystagmus, strabismus. Cardiac defects. Undescended testes, hypoplastic genitalia.

Manifestation: At birth.

Aetiology: Unknown. the vast majority of cases are sporadic. The nonuniform chromosome anomalies reported on several occasions are considered optional manifestations.

Frequency: Not rare; up to 1971, about 250 cases had been published.

Course, Prognosis: No progression. Infections pose a threat to severely retarded and markedly hypertonic children, especially in infancy.

Treatment: Symptomatic.

Illustrations:
1–4 Patient 1 at age 10½ years. Birth weight 2450 g, length 39 cm. Subsequently, height just below the 3rd percentile. In infancy, frequent infections. At 12 years, onset of grand mal epilepsy. Mental retardation. Head circumference, 49 cm, corresponds to that of a 3-year-old girl.
5–7 Patient 2 at age 7 months; weight 5000 g, length 58 cm, head circumference 36.5 cm (birth weight 1770 g, length 41 cm, head circumference 28.5 cm). Marked muscular hypertonia, severe psychomotor retardation; feeding possible only with stomach tube; seizures.

References:
Grosse F. R., Opitz J. M.: The Brachmann–de Lange syndrome, editorial comments. In: Gellis S., (ed) Year Book of Pediatrics 1971, Year Book Medical Publishers, Chicago
Beck B.: Epidemiology of Cornelia de Lange's syndrome. Acta paediatr. Scand. 65:631 (1976)
Johnson H. G., Ekman P., Friesen W.: A behavioral phenotype in the de Lange syndrome. Pediatr. Res. *10*:843 (1976)
Beck B., Mikkelsen M.: Chromosomes in the Cornelia de Lange syndrome. Hum. Genet. *59*:271 (1981)

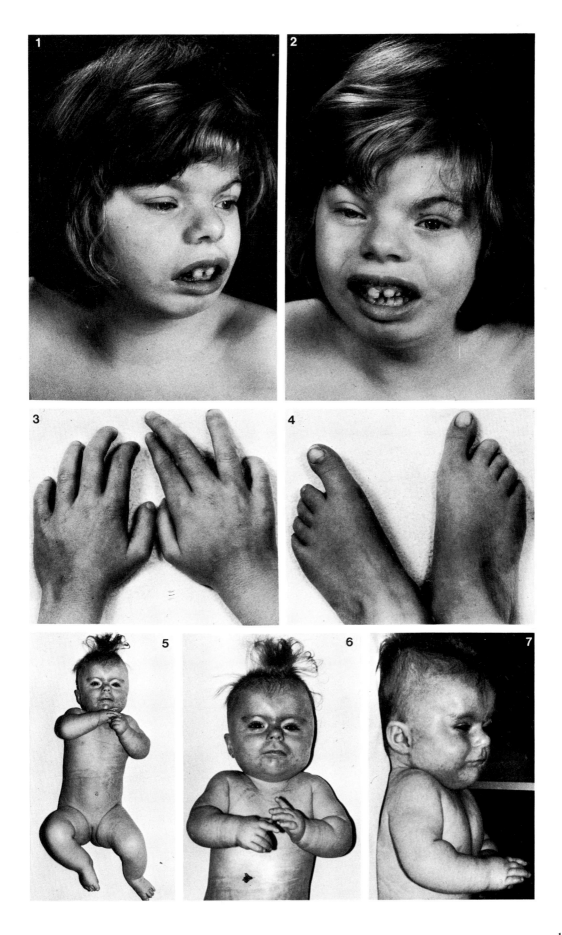

119

60. Syndrome of Oligosymptomatic Hypothyroidism

A form of hypothyroidism of delayed onset, with mainly osseous manifestations and with growth deficiency as the presenting complaint.

Main Signs:
1. More or less severe, for the most part proportional, growth deficiency with a thick-set appearance; thorax often broad and bell-shaped; frequent dorsal kyphosis and lumbar lordosis; and quite pronounced muscle contours, especially of the thighs (**1, 3,** and **4**).
2. As a rule, definite waddling gait.
3. Radiologically, general delay of ossification and epiphyseal dysgenesis, the latter usually most pronounced in the hip joints as a multicentric crumbly appearance of the capital femoral epiphysis. Also flattening of the vertebral bodies. All in all, a picture similar to that of polyepiphyseal dysplasia (**5–7**).
4. Mental development may seem normal; skin and hair may be quite unremarkable; obesity, obstipation, etc., may be completely absent and the conventional laboratory diagnostic laboratory tests (e.g., T_4 determination) may not yield clearly abnormal results.

Supplementary Findings: Delayed dentition.
Unequivocal identification via TSH determination (including TRH test). Ectopic thyroid tissue frequently demonstrable.

Comment: This mild form of hypothyroidism with ectopic thyroid glands is apparently not always picked up by TSH- newborn screening.

Manifestation: Clinical diagnosis is practically impossible before the third year of life.

Aetiology: Unclear. As a rule, sporadic occurrence. Girls more frequently affected (ratio 70:30).

Frequency: Not so rare.

Course, Prognosis: With timely recognition and prompt initiation of specific substitution therapy, favourable.

Differential Diagnosis: This disorder should no longer be confused with epiphyseal and spondylo-epiphyseal osteodysplasias.

Treatment: Immediate initiation of substitution therapy with L-thyroxin leads to rapid normalisation of the pathological laboratory values, rapid advancement of ossification, catch-up of growth, and possibly also definite improvement of intellectual performance.

Illustrations:
1–3 and **5–7**   An 11½-year-old girl; height 117.5 cm – below the 3rd percentile.
4   A 4½-year-old girl; height 94 cm – below the 3rd percentile.
8   Pelvic X-ray of a 6-year-old girl.
9   X-ray of the same girl as in **8**, 6 months after initiation of substitution therapy.

Reference:
Oldigs H.-D., Schnakenburg K. L., Wiedemann H.-R.: Zum Krankheitsbild der oligosymptomatischen Hypothyreose. Med. Welt 32:885 (1981)

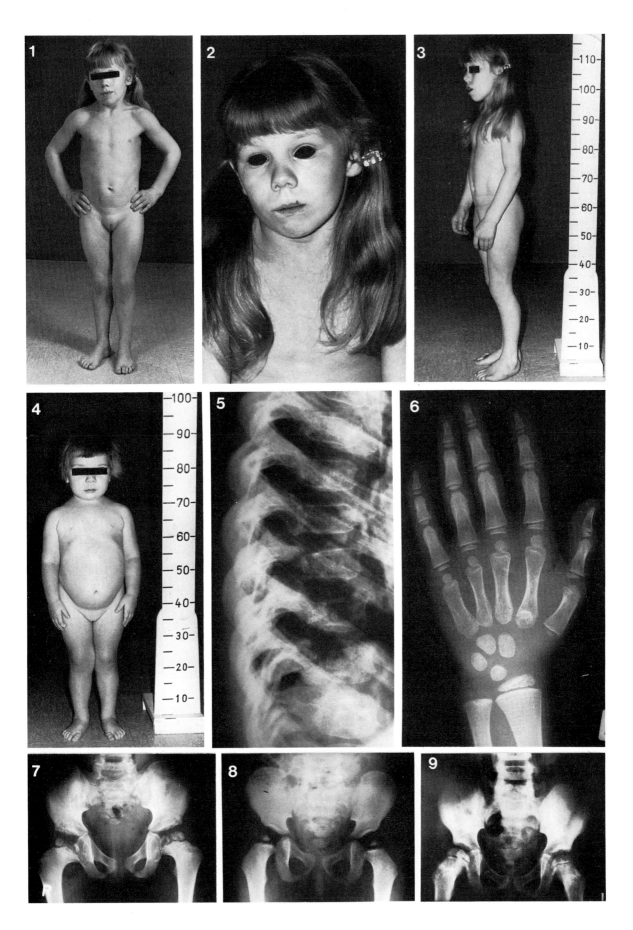

121

61. Short Stature Associated with Vitiligo, and – in One Case – Chronic Hypoparathyroidism.

Small stature associated with vitiligo in three siblings, one of whom in addition has chronic 'idiopathic' hypoparathyroidism.

Main Signs:
1. Small stature: Height of the 16-year-old girl (2) on the 15th percentile for her age; of her 12-year-old brother (1), below the 3rd percentile; and of her 10-year-old sister, on the 3rd percentile.
2. Vitiligo: Typical focuses below the knee caps in the 16-year-old (5), also symmetrically on the iliac crests (2), below the larynx, and on the lower back. The same affecting her brother on the eyelids, chin, inner surfaces of the upper arms, penis, distal lower legs, the backs of the feet, and other locations (1, 4, 6, and 7). The same on the trunk of her younger sister.
3. Chronic idiopathic hypoparathyroidism (established biochemically and endocrinologically and controlled therapeutically with dihydrotachysterol) solely in the – mentally retarded, erethistic – boy; pseudohypoparathyroidism ruled out; to date no evidence of autoimmune disease. Both girls of normal intelligence, normocalcaemic, and euparathyroid.

Supplementary Findings: Additional anomalies in the boy: Asymmetric brachycephaly, dysplastic auricles, hypertelorism, epicanthi, and broad nasal root (3).

Manifestation: Small stature in the first decade of life. Vitiligo appearing in the 11th, 9th, and 10th years of life respectively. First seizure in the boy at 3 months; years later, the first medical records of characteristic tetanic paroxysms.

Aetiology: Uncertain.

Course, Prognosis: Regarding hypoparathyroidism: with adequate treatment, favourable for life expectancy.

Comment: In these cases, the small stature is familial (father, 1.67; mother, 1.52 m; in the mother's sibship, further cases of small stature). Generalised vitiligo, as present in these siblings, is considered an autosomal dominant hereditary defect with variable penetrance. Primary idiopathic hypoparathyroidism manifested in early childhood occurs in an X-chromosomal recessive and in an autosomal dominant form, among others. Combinations of vitiligo with diverse endocrinopathies, including chronic idiopathic hypoparathyroidism, are known. The association of small stature and generalised vitiligo in the siblings shown here, one of whom has chronic hypoparathyroidism, will be viewed for the present as a chance combination.

Illustrations:
1, 3, 4, 6, and 7 A 12-year-old boy with early manifested, chronic idiopathic hypoparathyroidism, generalised vitiligo, and (familial) short stature.
2 and 5 One of his two euparathyroid sisters with short stature at age 16 years; generalised vitiligo.

References:
Lerner A. B., Nordlund J. J.: Vitiligo. What is it? Is it important? JAMA 239: 1183 (1978)
McBurney E. I.: Vitiligo. Clinical picture and pathogenesis. Arch. Int. Med. 139:1295 (1979)

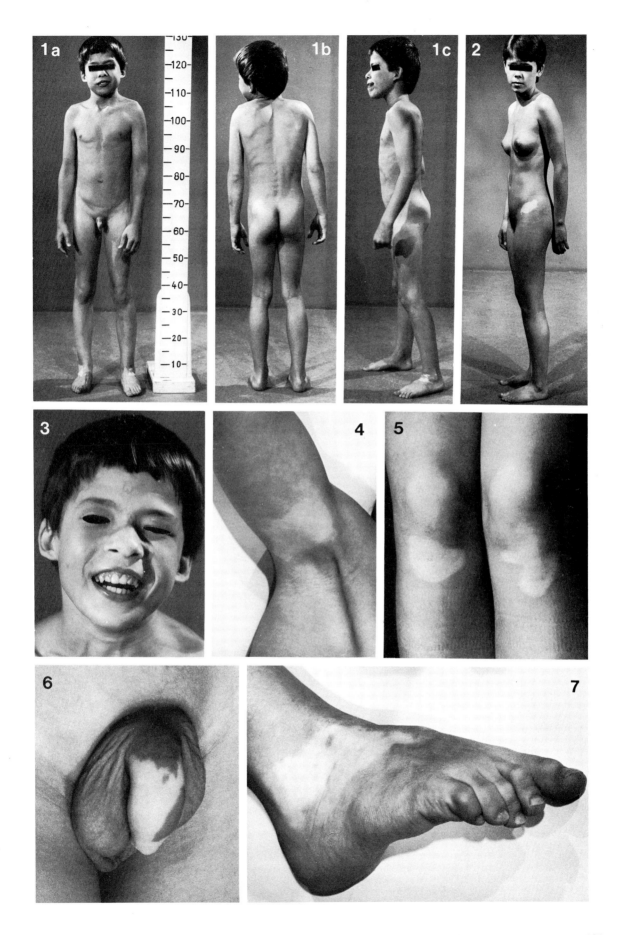

123

62. Pseudohypoparathyroidism

(Syndrome of Albright Hereditary Osteodystrophy)

A hereditary syndrome of small stature, obesity, round face, brachydactyly due to abnormally short metacarpal or metatarsal bones, mental retardation, and possible seizures.

Main Signs:
1. Short, stocky physique with short neck, short extremities, and round face (1). Adult height between about 1.38 and 1.52 metres, occasionally greater.
2. Obesity – usually of moderate severity.
3. Short hands and/or feet as a result of abnormal shortness of one or more metacarpal and metatarsal bones – especially IV or V, III, and I (2 and 3).
4. Mental retardation of quite varied severity, occasionally not present.

Supplementary Findings: Manifestations of abnormal mineral metabolism, including tetanic seizures or convulsions, delayed eruption of the teeth, enamel defects, and ectopic calcifications (in: subcutaneous tissues, especially in the extremities and around the joints; lenses of the eyes; the basal ganglia of the brain). Biochemically, typical findings of hypocalcaemia/hyperphosphataemia, high serum level of immunoreactive parathormone, and parathormone resistance (diminished response of the kidneys to parathormone as determined by cAMP and phosphate excretion). A normocalcaemic variant may also occur.

Manifestation: Early childhood, but also frequently not until later in childhood. (Subcutaneous calcification, 'osteomata cutis', may occur as early as the first months of life.)

Aetiology: The clinical and biochemical variability reflects the differences of the presumed modes of inheritance (X-chromosomal dominant, sex-limited autosomal dominant, and other modes); apparent heterogeneity. After detailed biochemical clarification, genetic counselling should be procured.

Frequency: Rare. Girls affected predominantly.

Course, Prognosis: Normal life expectancy. The occurrence of mental retardation cannot be predicted.

Differential Diagnosis: Shortening of the 4th and 5th metacarpal bones may also occur, for instance, in Turner syndrome (p.128), which from the total clinical picture should not be difficult to exclude.

Treatment: Symptomatic (vitamin D medication, if indicated, as determined by experienced specialists). Genetic counselling.

Illustrations:
1 The 'round face' of a typically affected boy.
2 X-ray of the hands of an 11-year-old girl.
3 X-ray of the hands of the 29-year-old mother of the girl in 2.
(Figure 1 reproduced with kind permission of Dr P. Maroteaux, Hôpital des Enfants Malades, and 2 and 3, with kind permission of Prof. Dr Cl. Fauré, Hôpital Trousseau; both of Paris.)

References:
Maroteaux P.: Les maladies osseuses de l'enfant. Flammarion, Paris 1974
Spranger J. W., Langer L. O., jr, Wiedemann H.-R.: Bone Dysplasias. An Atlas of Constitutional Disorders of Skeletal Development. Stuttgart and Philadelphia, G. Fischer and W. B. Saunders 1974
Boscherini B., Coen G., Bianchi G., et al: Albright's hereditary osteodystrophy. Acta Pediatr. Scand. 69:305 (1980)

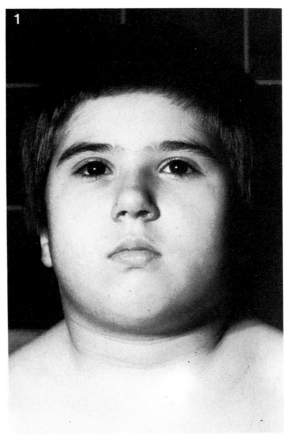

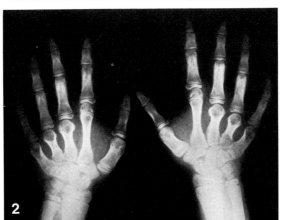

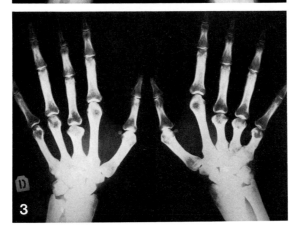

63. Syndrome of Acrodysostosis

A syndrome of peripheral dysostosis, growth deficiency, hypoplasia of the nose, and mental retardation.

Main Signs:
1. Markedly shortened hands and feet with short, stubby fingers and toes; loose, wrinkled soft tissue on the dorsal surfaces; and short broad nails (1).
2. Often small size at birth; postnatal growth deficiency increasingly apparent. Relatively short forearms held in flexion; restricted extension at the elbows (1).
3. Characteristic facies: Nasal hypoplasia with low insertion of nasal root, nose usually short and flat with a broad tip, possibly indented medially; anteverted nares and long philtrum (1). In some cases hypoplasia of the upper jaw, hypertelorism, epicanthi, prognathism, dysodontiasis, wide mandibular angle.
4. Mental retardation of different grades of severity, which as an exception may not be a feature.

Supplementary Findings: Radiologically, markedly shortened metacarpals and metatarsals with deformity of the epiphyses, shortened phalanges with cone-shaped epiphyses, and frequent bowing and other deformity of the bones of the distal forearm (2).

Occasionally defective hearing.

Manifestation: At birth or thereafter, with increasingly apparent signs.

Aetiology: Although occurring sporadically to date almost without exception – predominantly in girls – there is little doubt of a genetic basis, and among others, dominant new mutations should be considered.

Frequency: Rare.

Course, Prognosis: Influenced by mental retardation, growth deficiency, increasingly impaired function of the hands, feet, and elbow joints, and increasingly distorted facial features. Apparently normal life expectancy.

Comment: Pseudohypoparathyroidism (p.124) and acrodysostosis are considered by some as different forms of the same fundamental clinical entity.

Treatment: Symptomatic. Plastic or cosmetic surgery may be considered in cases of severe facial deformity.

Illustrations:
1 and 2 A 1.17 m tall, 15-year-old girl with psychomotor retardation, the first child of nonconsanguineous parents. Patient shows the full clinical picture.
(By kind permission of Dr P. Maroteaux, Paris.)

References:
Robinow M., Pfeiffer R. A., Gorlin R. J., et al: Acrodysostosis. Am. J. Dis. Child. *121*:195 (1971)
Ablow R. C., Hsia Y E., Brandt I. K.: Acrodysostosis coinciding with pseudohypoparathyroidism and pseudopseudohypoparathyroidism. Am. J. Roentgenol. *128*:95 (1977)

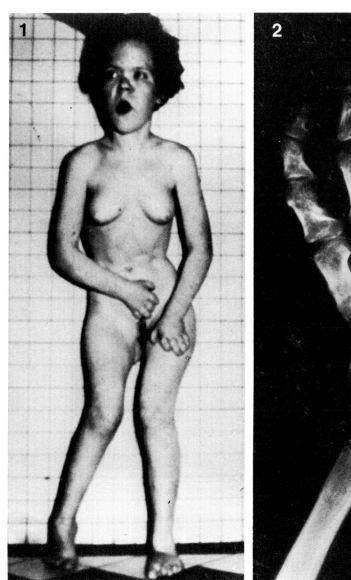

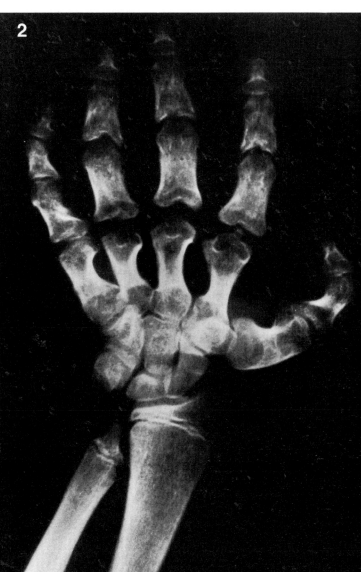

64. Turner Syndrome

(Ullrich–Turner Syndrome)

A malformation syndrome characterised especially by small stature, failure of puberty to occur, pterygium, lymphoedema of the hands and feet, and characteristic facies, all of which can be attributed to complete or partial absence of the X chromosome in phenotypic females.

Main Signs:
1. Small stature, usually from birth on, adult height usually less than 144 cm; failure of puberty to occur; pterygium, cutis laxa, or in some cases oedema of the neck region; broad thorax (**1** and **7**).
2. Cubitus valgus; at birth lymphoedema of the dorsum of the hands and feet, which usually regresses by late infancy (**9**); shortening of the 4th and 5th metacarpals; narrow, dysplastic, sometimes spoon-shaped or short nails (**9** and **10**).
3. Ptosis of the eyelids, epicanthic folds (**1, 2,** and **4**); micrognathia (**1**), high and narrow hard palate with malpositioned teeth; low posterior hairline (**6**).

Supplementary Findings: Anomalies of the kidneys (for the most part horseshoe kidneys, unilateral agenesis); cardiac abnormality (mostly stenosis of the aortic isthmus); below-average intelligence; increased number of pigmented naevi and fibroma of the skin (**4** and **5**); prominent veins, especially on the arms; osteoporosis; possible hearing defect. Low oestrogen, high gonadotropin levels. Decisive chromosomal abnormality.

Manifestation: At birth; however, the child may not come to attention until later in childhood.

Aetiology: Complete (majority of the cases) or partial absence of the X chromosome – more exactly: complete or partial monosomy for the short arm of the X chromosome – in all or some somatic cells.

Frequency: About 1:3000 female births. No increased risk of recurrence for the affected family.

Prognosis: Dependent on heart and kidney malformations. Increased tendency to thyroid dysfunction and diabetes.

Differential Diagnosis: Noonan syndrome (p.132).

Treatment: Androgen administration may effect an increase in adult height. Under oestrogen therapy a pubertal growth spurt is not to be expected; thus, oestrogen treatment to develop the secondary sexual characteristics and to induce vaginal bleeding should be started as late as feasible. If needed, cardiac or renal surgery. Possibly plastic surgery and psychotherapy.

Illustrations:
1–4 Typical 'sphinx-like' facial expressions in children 3 months and 2½, 9, and 13 years old.
4 and **5** Child with very marked pterygium colli, pigmented naevi.
6 Same child as in **3**: low posterior hairline.
7 and **8** 7-year-old girl with shield chest, increased intermamillary distance; somewhat masculine habitus; height corresponding approximately to that of a 4½-year-old.
9 9-day-old baby; marked lymphoedema; short, dysplastic nails.
10 1-day-old baby; narrow, hyperconvex nails.

References:
Palmer C. C., Reichmann A.: Chromosomal and clinical findings in 100 females with Turner syndrome. Hum. Genet. *35*:35 (1976)
Urban M. D., Lee P. A., Dorst J. P., et al: Oxandrolone therapy in patients with Turner syndrome. J. Pediatr. *94*:823 (1979)

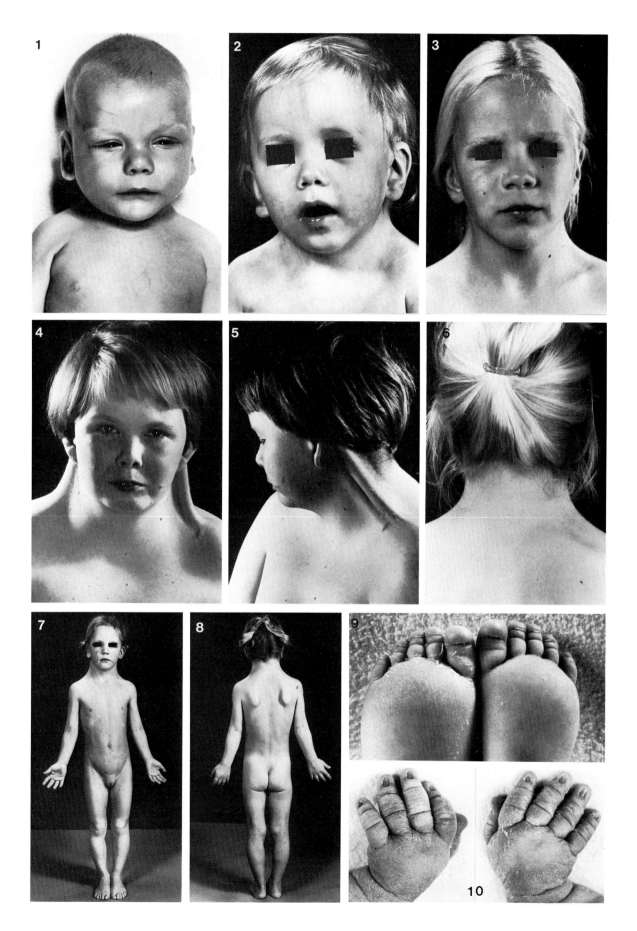

65. Aarskog Syndrome

A malformation syndrome occurring in males with growth deficiency, unusual facies, typical genital peculiarities, and other anomalies.

Main Signs:
1. Small stature, frequently with a long trunk.
2. Face characterised by a prominent forehead with wedge-shaped hairline; hypertelorism; possible slight antimongoloid slant of the palpebral fissures; uni- or bilateral ptosis; hypoplasia of the midface; short, broad nose with anteverted nares and long wide philtrum; anomalies of the pinnae; horizontal groove directly below the lower lip; prognathism (1 and 3).
3. Shawl-like formation of the scrotal folds above the root of the penis, cryptorchidism (2 and 4).
4. Short and broad hands with simian creases and short, broad feet (metatarsi adducti; stubby toes). Short fingers frequently with mild cutaneous syndactyly and especially short 5th fingers, often with only one flexion crease. Unusual hyperextensibility of the proximal interphalangeal joints when the hands are extended at the metacarpophalangeal joints and the distal interphalangeal joints are flexed.

Supplementary Findings: Pectus excavatum. Inguinal hernias.

Possible anomalies of the cervical vertebral bodies, craniosynostoses.

Occasionally mild mental retardation.

Manifestation: At birth; delayed growth (usually normal birth measurements) noted during the first year of life.

Aetiology: Apparently an X-chromosomal recessive characteristic since the mothers and other female relatives of affected boys not infrequently show mild signs of the syndrome (especially the hands and face, possibly also somewhat small stature). However, autosomal dominance – see captions to the illustrations – as well as X-chromosomal semi-dominance have also been considered. Possible heterogeneity.

Frequency: Apparently not rare; between the time of the first description in 1970 until 1980, about 100 cases were reported.

Prognosis: Good. Although initial growth is around or below the 3rd percentile, satisfactory adult height is usually attained after a normal puberty.

Differential Diagnosis: Noonan syndrome (p.132), which does not show the penoscrotal anomaly, but includes pulmonary stenosis, pterygium, mental retardation. Robinow syndrome (p.146).

Treatment: Symptomatic. Genetic counselling.

Illustrations:
1 and 2 Case 1 at age 9 months (length 66 cm, corresponding to that of a 5-month-old boy). Stubby broad hands, undescended testes. Bilateral simian creases. Premature closure of the sagittal suture (also present in his similarly affected sister). The father of both children shows mild signs of the syndrome.
3 and 4 Case 2 at age 3¾ years. Height 95 cm, corresponding to that of a 3-year-old boy. Postherniorraphy; seizure disorder.

References:
Hoo J.: The Aarskog (facio-digito-genital) syndrome. Clin. Genet. *16*:269 (1979)
Berry C., Cree J., Mann Tr.: Aarskog's syndrome. Arch. Dis. Childh. *55*:706 (1980)

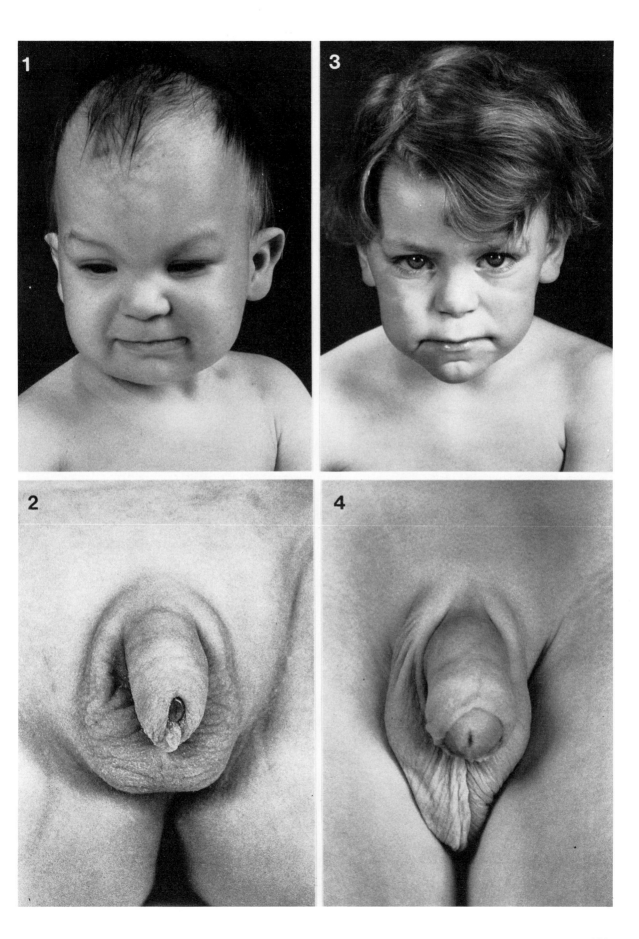

131

66. Noonan Syndrome

('Male Turner Syndrome' or XY-Turner Phenotype, 'Female Pseudo-Turner Syndrome', XX-Turner Phenotype, Ullrich Syndrome, Ullrich–Noonan Syndrome)

A probably heterogeneous malformation–retardation syndrome occurring in both sexes (without chromosomal aberration) with characteristic facies, short stature, cardiac defect, and multiple other, usually less severe anomalies.

Main Signs:
1. Usually mild proportional growth deficiency.
2. Frequent mild mental retardation; occasionally defective hearing.
3. Typical facies (**1, 2, 4,** and **6**), mainly characterised by hypertelorism, antimongoloid slant of the palpebral fissures, epicanthus, ptosis, down-turned corners of the mouth, and micrognathia.
4. Low posterior hairline, pterygium or cutis laxa of the lateral neck (**1** and **7**); low-set ears with unusual edges; high palate.
5. Broad thorax with pectus carinatum and/or excavatum.
6. Pulmonary stenosis (valvular, supravalvular, peripheral), less frequently atrial septal defect, or other.

Supplementary Findings: Cryptorchidism; possibly small testes (postpubertally). In some cases delayed puberty; fertility in both sexes possible.

Cubitus valgus; short, radially deviated 5th fingers; broad, short fingernails (**5**); possibly lymphoedema of the dorsum of the hands and feet.

Hypertrophic cardiomyopathy and, much less frequently, pulmonary lymphangiectasia may be present; exceptionally, chylothorax has been observed.

Manifestation: At birth; however, the child may not come to attention until later in childhood.

Aetiology: Genetically determined syndrome; probably heterogeneity. Occurrence of autosomal dominant transmission.

Frequency: Considerable (exact figures still not available); estimation: 1 in 1000 liveborn children.

Course, Prognosis: Essentially dependent on the cardiac defect and on mental development.

Treatment: In some cases cardiac surgery, operation for cryptorchidism, removal of pterygium; hormone substitution. Genetic counselling.

Differential Diagnosis:
1. Turner syndrome (p.128): pronounced growth deficiency, usually normal mental development, failure of puberty to occur, frequent renal anomalies, and stenosis of the aortic isthmus as the usual cardiac defect. Chromosome anomaly.
2. Syndrome of multiple lentigines (LEOPARD syndrome; p.240): Usually normal intelligence, skin covered by freckles, abnormal ventricular conduction on ECG, possible hearing defect, autosomal dominant transmission.
3. Aarskog syndrome (p.130).

Illustrations:
1 and 2 Patient 1 with quite typical facies at age 16¾ years. Height 151 cm (average height of a 12½-year-old). Menarche at 14 years. Intelligence in the normal range.
3–5 Patient 2 at age 6 years. Height 111 cm (3rd percentile). Birth measurements and heights at ages 11 months and 2¼ years within the norm. Testes not descended until after the 2nd year of life. Infundibular and valvular pulmonary stenosis. Debility.
6–7 Patient 3 at age 3 weeks. Definite psychomotor retardation at 6 months. Mild supravalvular pulmonary stenosis, marked septation of the left ventricle. Malrotation II.

References:
Wilroy R.S., jr, Summit R.L., Tipton R.E., et al: Phenotypic heterogeneity in the Noonan syndrome. Birth Defects 15/5B:305 (1979)
Duncan W.J., Fowler R.S., Farkas L.G., et al: A comprehensive scoring system for evaluating Noonan syndrome. Am J. Med. Genet. 10:37 (1981)

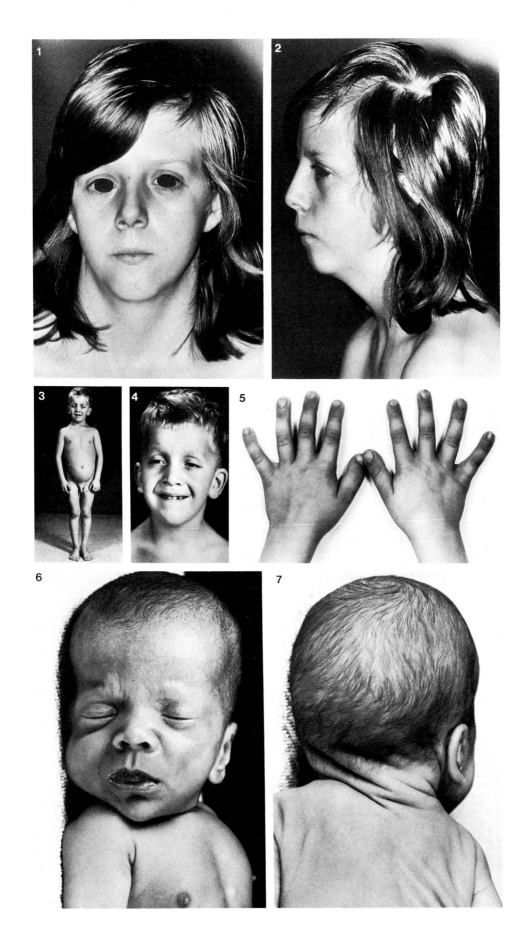

67. Syndrome of Abnormal Facies, Growth Deficiency, and Psychomotor Retardation

A syndrome of facial dysmorphism, short stature with thickset physique, and considerable mental retardation.

Main Signs:
1. Facies: Flat and broad with wide, low-set root of the nose, hypertelorism, short 'pug' nose, and high philtrum. Short, narrow palpebral fissures, epicanthi (left more pronounced than right). High narrow palate. Low-set, dysplastic ears (1–6). Similarity of the boy's facial features with those of his father (7) and his father's father.
2. Primordial short stature, well below the 3rd percentile. Short neck, thickset trunk, stubby hands and feet. Unusual pudgy physique during infancy and early childhood with extremities at first relatively too short, but later rather too long (3 and 4).
3. Primary, moderately severe mental retardation.

Supplementary Findings: Strabismus convergans alternans. Left lower extremity shorter (2½ cm) and thinner than the right. Mild clinodactyly of the little fingers (8).

Manifestation: At birth.

Aetiology: Unknown.

Course, Prognosis: Influenced by the marked mental retardation.

Comment: The clinical picture brought to mind several well-known syndromes, but could not be classified under any of them. Maternal alcoholism *non aderat*.

Treatment: Symptomatic.

Illustrations:
1, 3 and 5 The affected child aged 3½ years.
2, 4, 6–8 The same child at 6 years, 10 months.
7 Together with his father.
The third child of young, nonconsanguineous, healthy, but small (father 1.64 cm; mother 1.52 cm), parents. Two older siblings healthy and of normal height. Proband born 10 days before term after a normal pregnancy, birth measurements 2.6 kg and *44* cm. At 6¾ years 104.5 cm. Large internal organs negative (blunted renal pelves on IVP). Ocular fundi, EEG negative. Cysterna interventricularis et cavum septi pellucidi communicans on pneumoencephalogram. Clinical, blood chemistry, and endocrinological investigations negative. Chromosome analysis (banding technique) negative.

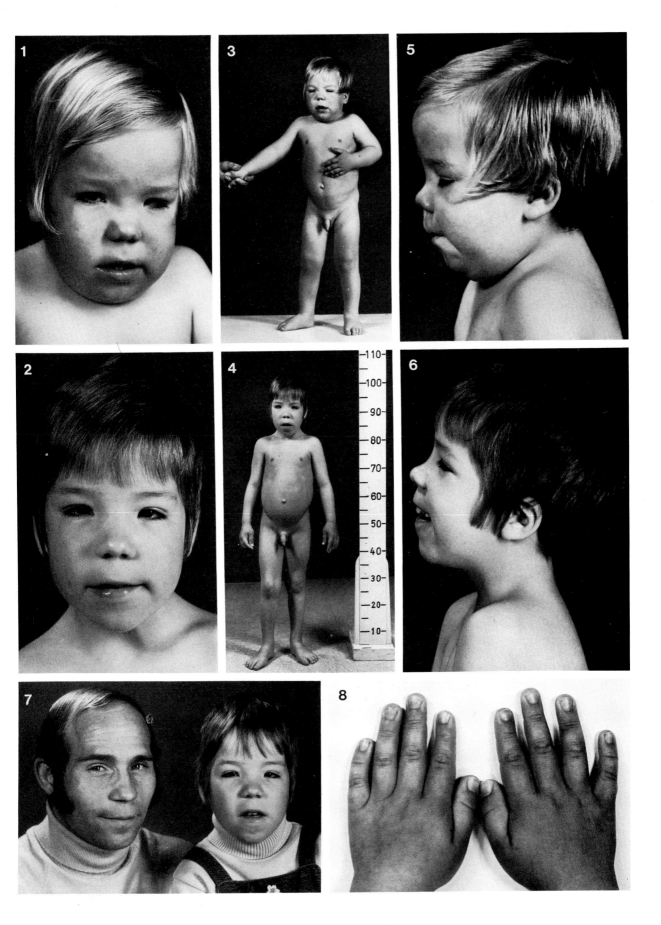

68. Syndrome of Pyknodysostosis

(Maroteaux, Lamy)

A characteristic hereditary syndrome of the skeleton with typical facial dysmorphism, small stature, and osteosclerosis.

Main Signs:
1. Small stature from early infancy, mainly due to shortness of the extremities. Adult height between 1.30 and 1.55 m.
2. Large, long, and narrow cranium with prominent forehead 4 and 5), delayed closure of the fontanelles and sutures (7), in part until adulthood; relatively small facial part of the cranium with prominent nose, hypoplasia of the lower jaw, microgenia, and marked flattening or even extension of the submaxillary angle (7). Possible mild exophthalmos; bluish sclera.
3. Short, stubby hands (8) and feet, especially the fingers and toes, with abnormal, very brittle nails (8).
4. Frequently increased tendency to fractures.

Supplementary Findings: Dysodontiasis (anomalies of eruption, malocclusion, and others). Radiologically, generalised osteosclerosis. Hypoplasia of the clavicles. Dysplasia or acro-osteolysis of the distal phalanges of the fingers and toes (9), especially in the index finger.

Manifestation: From infancy.

Aetiology: Monogenic hereditary disorder, autosomal recessive.

Frequency: Rare. Up to now, about 130 cases described in the literature.

Course, Prognosis: Life expectancy not or hardly affected. Severity of the tendency to fractures varies from case to case; fractures heal well.

Differential Diagnosis: Cleidocranial dysplasia (p.22) and, readily excluded, osteopetrosis.

Treatment: Early qualified orthodontic supervision.

Illustrations:
1–9   The same child at 2½, 5, and 10 years (1–3 and 4–6); growth deficiency respectively of about 4.5, 9.5, and 16 cm from the median for age. Skull X-ray at age 3½ years (7): thickening of the base of the skull; thickening and outward bulging of the os frontale and occipitale; anterior fontanelle and lambdoid sutures wide open; hypoplasia of the mandible with absence of the angle. X-ray of the hand at age 8 years (9): osteosclerosis; acro-osteolysis of the distal phalanges.

References:
Wiedemann H.-R.: Pyknodysostose. Fortschr. Röntgenstr. *103*:590 (1965)
Spranger J. W., Langer L. O., jr, Wiedemann H.-R.: Bone Dysplasias. An Atlas of Constitutional Disorders of Skeletal Development, Stuttgart and Philadelphia, G. Fischer and W. B. Saunders, 1974
Srivastava K. K., Bhattacharya A. K., Galatius-Jensen F., et al: Pycnodysostosis (Report of four cases). Aust. Radiol. *22*:70 (1978)

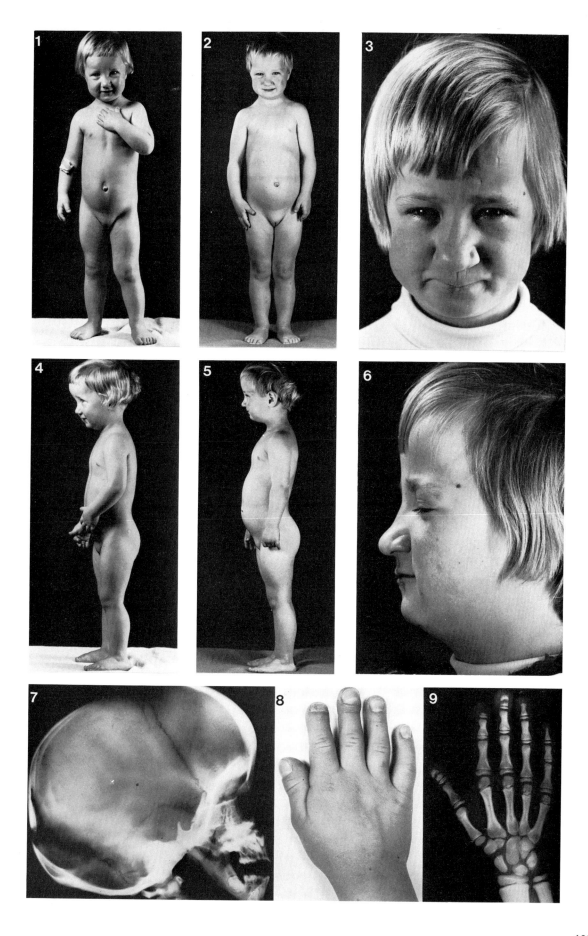

69. Syndrome of Dyschondrosteosis

(Léri–Weill Syndrome)

A hereditary syndrome of short forearms with Madelung deformity and varying degrees of shortening of the lower legs resulting in disproportionate ('mesomelic') dwarfism.

Main Signs:
1. Reducible dorsal subluxation of the distal end of the ulna (Madelung deformity; **1, 2**) bilaterally, with limited mobility.
2. More or less distinct dwarfism, disproportionate due to conspicuous relative shortness of the – slightly bowed – forearms and possibly also lower legs.

Supplementary Findings: Occasionally short hands and feet, exostoses of the proximal tibiae and fibulae, hyperlordosis, legs bowed or knock-kneed.

Radiologically, shortening, bowing, broadening, and increased separation of the bones of the forearm, dorsal subluxation of the head of the ulna, pyramid-like compression of the carpal ossification centres at the wrist.

Manifestation: From infancy, but more frequently later in childhood, with small stature and wrist deformities; development of the complete X-ray picture of the Madelung deformity by the age of puberty.

Aetiology: Autosomal dominant hereditary disorder with more severe expression in females.

Frequency: Relatively rare.

Course, Prognosis: Normal life expectancy. Adult height between about 135 and somewhat over 150 cm.

Treatment: Orthopaedic measures in cases of increased fatigability and painfulness of the wrists (e.g., leather supports; exceptionally, surgery). Genetic counselling.

Illustrations:
A 15-year-old girl with dyschondrosteosis.
1 Reducible dorsal subluxation of the distal end of the ulna and bayonet-like volar displacement of the hand ('Madelung deformity').
2 Shortening, bowing, and broadening of the radii, increased ulnar deviation of the distal radial epiphyses, ulnae slender distally, angulation of the carpal bones.

References:
Spranger J.W., Wiedemann H-R.: Dyschondrosteose. Hdb., Kinderheilkd. H. Optiz and F. Schmid, eds. Bd. VI, 204; Berlin, Heidelberg, New York, Springer 1967
Spranger J.W., Langer L.O., jr, Wiedemann H.-R.: Bone Dysplasias. An Atlas of Constitutional Disorders of Skeletal Development, Stuttgart and Philadelphia, G. Fischer and W.B. Saunders, 1974
Lichtenstein J.R., Sundaram M., Burdge R.: Sex-influenced expression of Madelung's deformity in a family with dyschondrosteosis. J. Med. Genet. *17*:41 (1980)

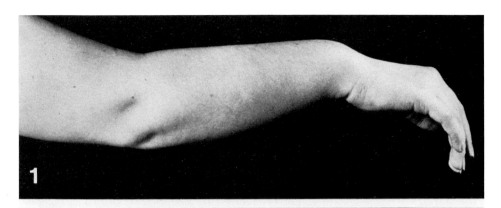

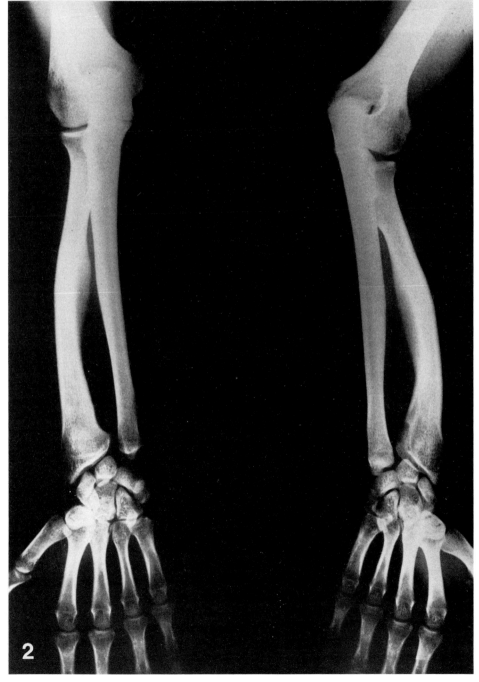

70. Mesomelic Dysplasia Type Langer

A hereditary disproportionate dwarfism from severe shortening of the forearms and lower legs with characteristic radiological findings.

Main Signs:
1. 'Mesomelic dwarfism' from shortening (and bowing) of the forearms and lower legs with distinct ulnar deviation of the hands, possibly also malpositioning of the feet, and limited motion at the elbow, wrist, and possibly ankle joints (1).
2. Radiologically, symmetrical, profound shortening, bowing, and broadening of the bones of the forearms and lower legs (2 and 3) with unusual hypoplasia of the distal ulnae (3) and proximal fibulae (2).

Supplementary Findings: Not infrequently hypoplasia of the mandible. Increased lumbar lordosis. Normal mental development.

Manifestation: At birth.

Aetiology: Hereditary disorder. In an increasing number of cases, both parents have been shown to be carriers of dyschondrosteosis (see p.138); the proband would be regarded as homozygous for the dyschondrosteosis gene.

Frequency: Rare.

Course, Prognosis: Normal life expectancy. Adult height of about 1.30 m.

Differential Diagnosis: Other types of mesomelic dysplasia (p.142, p.146, p.188) as well as dyschondrosteosis (p.138); acrodysostosis (p.126).

Treatment: Physiotherapy and in some cases orthopaedic treatment. Genetic counselling.

Illustrations:
1–3 A toddler, the first living child of nonconsanguineous parents after three spontaneous abortions and two interrupted pregnancies (indications not clear). Both parents: dyschondrosteosis. Height of the proband around the third percentile.
(By kind permission of Prof. H. Helge and Priv. Doz. J. Kunze, Berlin.)

References:
Spranger J. W., Langer L. O., jr, Wiedemann H.-R.: Bone Dysplasias. An Atlas of Constitutional Disorders of Skeletal Development. Stuttgart and Philadelphia, G. Fischer and W. B. Saunders, 1974
Esperitu C., Chen H., Wooley P. V.: Mesomelic dwarfism as the homozygous expression of dyschondrosteosis. Am. J. Dis. Child. 129:375 (1975)
Kunze J., Klemm T.: Mesomelic dysplasia, type Langer – a homozygous state for dyschondrosteosis. Eur. J. Pediatr. 134:269 (1980)

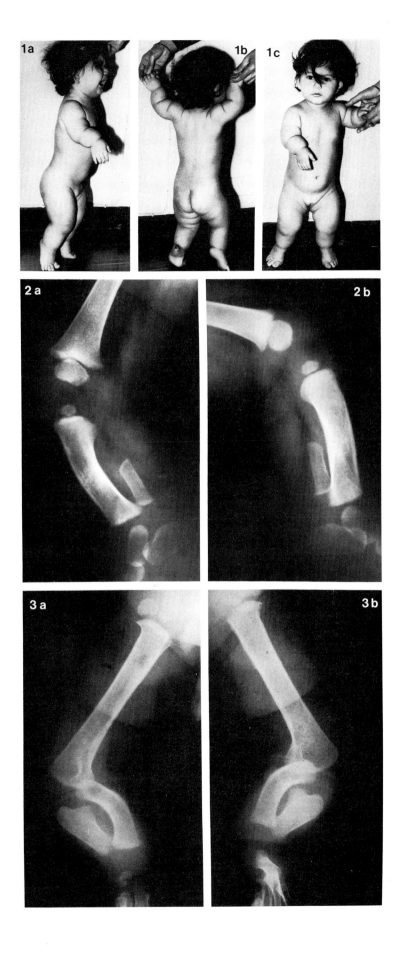

71. Nievergelt Syndrome

(Syndrome of Mesomelic Dysplasia Type Nievergelt)

An autosomal dominant hereditary syndrome of extreme shortening and deformity of the lower legs, occasionally also of the forearms, with characteristic radiological findings of the lower extremities.

Main Signs:
1. 'Lower-leg dwarfism' (**1** and **2**) with optional shortening of the forearms; sometimes atypical club feet. Optional limitation of motion of the elbow joints as a result of radioulnar synostosis, subluxation of the head of the radius.
2. On X-ray (**3** and **4**), nearly triangular or rhomboidal configuration of the short, broad tibiae (sometimes also the radii), to a lesser degree of the fibulae (possibly also the ulnae). Development of synostoses of the tarsal bones. In some cases radioulnar synostoses (see above).

Manifestation: At birth.

Aetiology: Autosomal dominant hereditary disorder with quite variable expressivity.

Frequency: Very rare; since the first description (1944), only about 15 reported cases.

Course, Prognosis: As a rule, general health otherwise unimpaired.

Differential Diagnosis: Other forms of congenital shortening of the lower legs/forearms can be excluded radiologically.

Treatment: In some cases operative correction of club feet. Further operative–conservative orthopaedic care and general care and aids for the physically handicapped. Genetic counselling.

Illustrations:
1 and 2 A 7-year-old boy; standing height 1.05 cm, with walking prostheses 1.23 m; length of lower leg about 11 cm (upper leg 36 cm); genua et crura valga, malpositioning of the feet, deformities of the toes. Arms normal.
3 and 4 X-rays of the same patient as in **1** and **2**; massive shortening and somewhat rhomboidal broadening of the bones of the lower legs, oblique course of the terminal metaphyseal plates; synostoses of the tarsal bones.
(By kind permission of Prof. W. Blauth, Kiel.)

References:
Solonen K. A., Sulamaa M.: Nievergelt syndrome and its treatment. Ann. Chir. Gynaec. Fenn. *47*:142 (1958)
Spranger J. W., Langer L. O., jr, Wiedemann H.-R.: Bone Dysplasias. An Atlas of Constitutional Disorders of Skeletal Development, G. Fischer and W. B. Saunders, Stuttgart and Philadelphia, 1974
Young L. W., Wood B. P.: Nievergelt syndrome. Birth Defects *11*:/5:81 (1975)
Hess O. M., Goebel N. H., Streuli R.: Familärer mesomeler Kleinwuchs (Nievergelt syndrome). Schweiz. Med. Wochenschrft. *108*:1202 (1978)

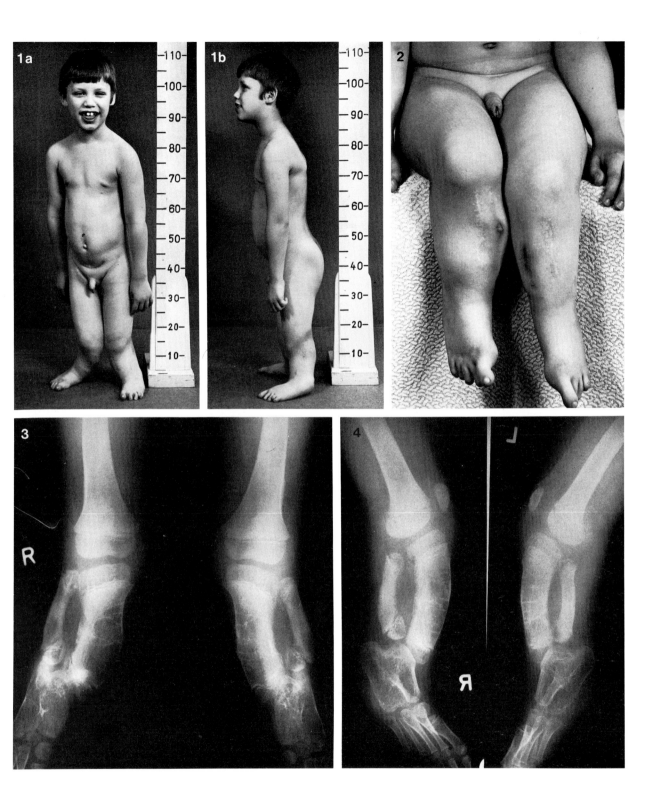

143

72. A 'New' Syndrome of Mesomelic Dysplasia

A syndrome of mesomelic dysplasia with delayed ossification of the vault of the cranium, unusual facies, short neck, and symmetrical flexion contractures of the fingers.

Main Signs:

1. Short forearms, slightly bowed. Lower extremities not short by appearance, although also bowed (**1, 8** and **10**).

2. Bilateral, for the most part symmetrical flexion contractures of fingers II–V; bilateral clinodactyly V. Pedes valgi et plani with slight malpositioning of the toes (**4** and **5**).

3. Large, round cranium with alopecia except for a cockscomb-like abundant growth of hair over the region of the sagittal suture (**1–3**). Frontal and sagittal sutures still completely open at age 9 months, wide open anterior fontanelle.

4. Unusual facies: Broad, slightly prominent forehead; slightly low-set ears; very broad, low nasal root; blue sclera; high narrow palate; microretrognathia (**1–3**). Short neck; loose skin at the neck, sometimes giving the impression of pterygium.

5. Hypospadias, glandular; cryptorchidism.

Supplementary Findings: Normal mental development.

To date, normal growth in length.

Radiologically: Subluxation of the elbow joints, the bones of the forearm being too short and slightly bowed and the right ulna showing a thorn-like ex-crescence (**9** and **11**). Tibiae somewhat too short, bowed slightly anteriorly; fibulae relatively too long, thin, with marked anterior bowing and elevation of their distal ends (**8** and **10**). Increased curvature and slight coarsening of the shape of the clavicles.

Manifestation: At birth.

Aetiology: A genetic basis certain; mode of inheritance unsettled.

Frequency: Rare.

Course, Prognosis: Apparently favourable.

Differential Diagnosis: The Robinow syndrome (p.146) shows similarities; however, it is easily ruled out.

Treatment: Symptomatic.

Illustrations:

1–11 The 1st child of young, healthy, nonconsanguineous parents after two abortions. Birth measurements 3000 g and 51 cm. Child developing well.

Reference:
Löhr H., Wiedemann H.-R.: Mesomelic dysplasia – associated with other abnormalities. Eur. J. Ped. *137*:313 (1981)

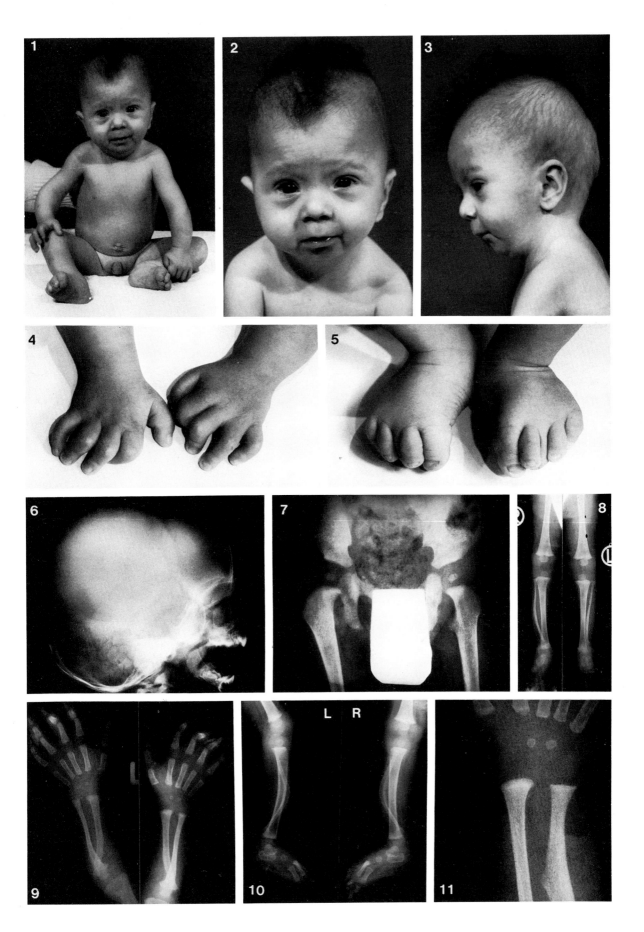

145

73. Robinow Syndrome

(Fetal Face Syndrome; Mesomelic Dysplasia Type Robinow)

A hereditary syndrome of peculiar facies, short forearms, genital hypoplasia, and growth deficiency.

Main Signs:
1. 'Fetal facial features': A disproportionately large cranium with large anterior fontanelle and protruding forehead; a relatively small face with hypertelorism, wide palpebral fissures, and correspondingly large-appearing eyes; mid-face hypoplasia; short nose with anteverted nostrils, relatively large triangular mouth with down-turned corners.
2. Mesomelic dysplasia of the upper extremities – forearms too short. Brachydactyly with clinodactyly V. Lower legs comparatively less, or not at all, remarkable (**1**).
3. Micropenis, with testicles and scrotum unremarkable as a rule (**1**). Hypoplasia of clitoris and labia minora.
4. Growth deficiency.

Supplementary Findings: Mental development normal as a rule.

Radiologically, bowing of the radius with (sub-)luxation of the head; definite shortening of the ulna. In some cases clefts of the distal phalanges of the fingers.

Frequent anomalies of the vertebral column and/or ribs (hemi- and block vertebrae, fusions) sometimes resulting in scoliosis; frequent malocclusion.

Occasional cryptorchidism, inguinal hernias.

Manifestation: At birth; delay of growth in height (birth measurements usually in the low normal range) apparent in the first years of life (under the 3rd percentile).

Aetiology: Genetically determined syndrome. Autosomal dominant transmission demonstrated repeatedly. Occurrence of an autosomal recessive form that cannot be differentiated clinically very likely. Thus, presumably heterogeneity.

Frequency: Rare; from 1969 to 1980, not many more than 20 cases described.

Course, Prognosis: With respect to general health, good. Less favourable for development of the penis. Adult height may be essentially normal. Data concerning reproduction, etc., still insufficient.

Differential Diagnosis: Other forms of mesomelic dysplasia should not be difficult to rule out. A disquieting, striking overlap of the signs with those of the Aarskog syndrome (p.130), but here the peculiar type of scrotal dysplasia as opposed to genital hypoplasia (in both sexes).

Treatment: Symptomatic. In some cases orthopaedic measures may be indicated. Possible attempt to modify the micropenis with early trials of testosterone; otherwise, constructive plastic surgery of the penis. Psychological guidance. Genetic counselling.

Illustrations:
1 A mentally normal 8-year-old boy, the 3rd child of healthy nonconsanguineous parents after two healthy children. Birth measurements 3200 g, 49 cm, cranium 39 cm. Present height below the 3rd percentile, cranial circumference with relation to his height, 98th percentile; bulging forehead. Micropenis, max. 3 cm long (post-plastic surgery!) Brachydactyly, clinodactyly; radiologically slight cleft of the distal phalanx of the thumb.
(By kind permission of Prof. F. Majewski, Düsseldorf.)

References:
Giedion A., Battaglia G. F., Bellini F., et al: The radiological diagnosis of the fetal face (= Robinow) syndrome (mesomelic dwarfism and small genitalia). Helv. Paediatr. Acta *30*:409 (1975)
Vogt J., Reinwein H., Fink M., et al: Das Robinow-Syndrom. Pädiatr. Prax. *21*:103 (1979)
Lee P. A., Migeon Cl. J., Brown T. R., et al: Robinow's syndrome. Partial primary hypogonadism in pubertal boys, with persistence of micropenis. Am. J. Dis. Child. *136*:327 (1982)

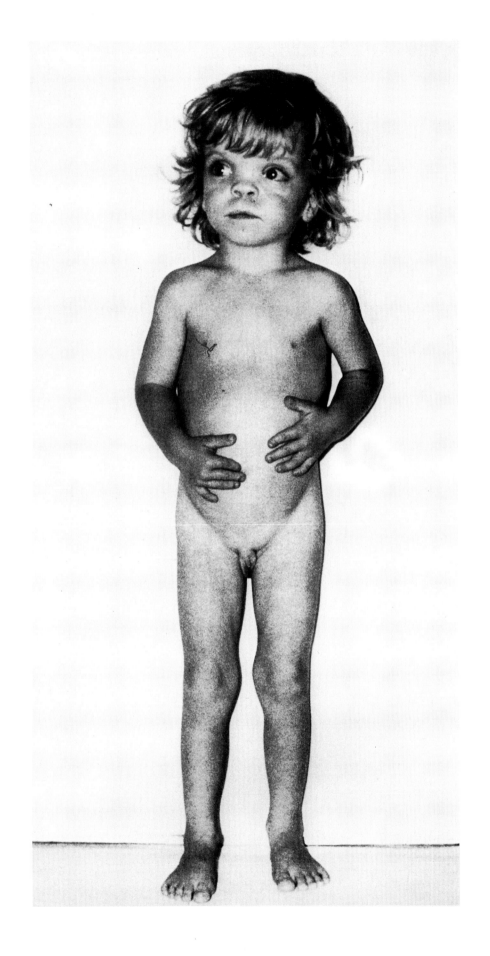

74. Syndrome of Achondrogenesis

A very severe congenital skeletal dysplasia with macrocephaly, extreme micromelia, and more or less universal hydrops.

Main Signs:
1. Macrocephaly, 'no neck'. Short trunk with distended abdomen. Extremely short extremities, generally varus positioning of the lower extremities.
2. Hydropic appearance (**1a**).

Supplementary Findings: Normal number of fingers and toes. Radiologically more or less absence of ossification of vertebral bodies, sacrum, pubic bones, and ischia (**1b**). Comparatively well-developed cranial bones, in any case the basilar.

Usually premature birth. Imminent death postnatally.

Manifestation: At birth.

Aetiology: Hereditary defect. Here too, several forms which can be differentiated clinically–radiologically and osteohistologically. Autosomal recessive mode of inheritance.

Frequency: Rare; altogether, about 85 cases described (1981).

Course, Prognosis: If not stillborn, death shortly after delivery.

Differential Diagnosis: Thanatophoric dysplasia (p.150), and a few others.

Treatment: At most, symptomatic. Genetic counselling. With subsequent pregnancies, prenatal diagnosis (X-ray, ultrasound).

Illustrations:
1a and b Child born 6 weeks prematurely (hydramnion). Length 28 cm.

References:
Wiedemann H.-R., Remagen W., Heinz H. A., Gorlin R. J., Maroteaux P.: Achondrogenesis within the scope of connately manifested generalised skeletal dysplasias. Z. Kinderheilkd. *116*:223 (1974)
Spranger J. W., Langer L. O., jr, Wiedemann H.-R.: Bone Dysplasias. An Atlas of Constitutional Disorders of Skeletal Development. Stuttgart and Philadelphia, G. Fischer and W. B. Saunders, 1974
Kozlowski K., Masel J., Morris L., et al: Neonatal death dwarfism. Aust. Radiol. *21*:164 (1977)
Schulte M. J., Lenz W., Vogel M.: Letale Achondrogenesis: Eine Übersicht über 56 Fälle. Klin. Pädiatr. *191*:327 (1978)
Andersen P. E., jr: Achondrogenesis type II in twins. Br. J. Radiol. *54*:61 (1981)
Chen H., Lin T., Yang S. S.: Achondrogenesis: A review… Am. J. Med. Genet. *10*:379 (1981)
Smith W. L., Breitweiser Th. D., Dinno N.: In utero diagnosis of achondrogenesis, type I. Clin. Genet. *19*:51 (1981)

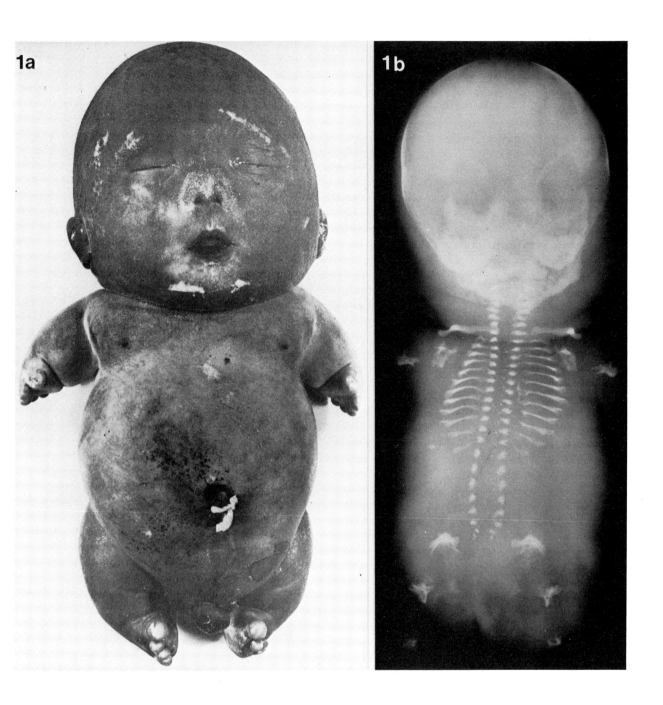

75. Syndrome of Thanatophoric Dysplasia

(Maroteaux, Lamy, Robert)

A severe congenital skeletal dysplasia with incongruously large cranium, narrow thorax, and striking micromelia.

Main Signs:
1. Macrocephaly with depressed nasal root and protruding eyes.
2. Relatively normal length of the trunk with narrow thorax.
3. Micromelia (**1a**).

Supplementary Findings: Radiologically: short ribs with narrow thorax; marked platyspondylisis with abnormal configuration of the vertebral bodies; tubular bones broad, short, and in part bowed (**1b**). Prompt development of a respiratory distress syndrome.

Manifestation: At birth; (frequent hydramnion).

Aetiology: Sporadic occurrence; genetic cause unquestioned; mode of transmission not yet established.

Frequency: Rare (up to 1980, about 100 cases described).

Course, Prognosis: As a rule, death shortly after delivery. In case of subsequent pregnancy in the mother, early diagnostic ultrasound.

Differential Diagnosis: The appearance very much resembles that of the Parrot syndrome (achondroplasia) in older individuals. However, the changes in aspect and on X-rays in newborns with the usual heterozygous (and less frequently, homozygous) achondroplasia are much less severe.

Illustrations:
1a and b A child (8-month gestation) who died on the 2nd day of life.

Reference:
Spranger J. W., Langer L. O., jr, Wiedemann H.-R.: Bone Dysplasias. An Atlas of Constitutional Disorders of Skeletal Development, Stuttgart and Philadelphia, G. Fischer and W. B. Saunders, 1974

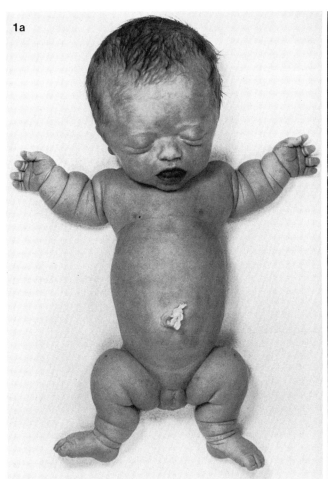

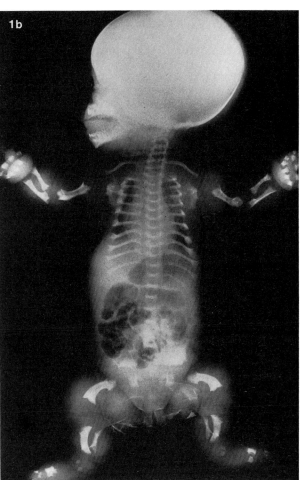

76. Short Rib–Polydactyly Syndrome of Type Saldino–Noonan

(Saldino–Noonan Syndrome)

A perinatal hereditary syndrome leading to early death and comprising narrow thorax with very short ribs, brachymelia, polydactyly, anogenital anomalies, and characteristic changes on X-ray.

Main Signs:

1. Severe narrowing of the thorax (with hypoplasia of the lungs) and distended abdomen (1). Respiratory insufficiency.
2. Brachymelia and usually postaxial polydactyly (1).
3. Anal atresia and/or genital hypoplasia.
4. Congenital hydrops as a rule.
5. Radiologically: Short, horizontal ribs; anomalies of the scapulae and pelvis; marked metaphyseal irregularities of the tubular bones, which are considerably shortened; and other findings (1b).

Supplementary Findings: Roundish, flat face. Absence of the nails. In many cases heart, kidney, pancreatic, and other anomalies at autopsy.

Manifestation: At birth.

Aetiology: Autosomal recessive hereditary disorder.

Frequency: Rare; somewhat more than 30 observations reported to date.

Course, Prognosis: Very poor. If not stillborn, the infant dies shortly after birth from respiratory insufficiency.

Differential Diagnosis: There are further rare short rib–polydactyly syndromes. In addition, Ellis–van Creveld syndrome (p.172) and D₁ trisomy syndrome (p.56) should be considered.

Treatment: Symptomatic. Genetic counselling; radiological–ultrasound prenatal diagnosis with subsequent pregnancies.

Illustrations:

1a and b A typical immature newborn (35.5 cm; 1300 g), the 1st child of young parents after an interrupted pregnancy and a spontaneous abortion. Death immediately post partum. Postaxial polydactyly of the hands and feet. (Unusual additional finding: multiple adhesions between the upper lip and the alveolar process – as in Ellis–van Creveld syndrome, p.172.)
(By kind permission of Dr Chr. v. Klinggräff, Kiel.)

References:
Spranger J. W., Langer L. O., jr, Wiedemann H.-R.: Bone Dysplasias. An Atlas of Constitutional Disorders of Skeletal Development. Stuttgart and Philadelphia, G. Fischer and W. B. Saunders, 1974
Krepler R., Weissenbacher G., Leodolter S., et al: Nicht lebensfähiger, mikromeler Zwergwuchs…Monatschr. Kinderheilkd. *124*:167 (1976)
Richardson M. M., Beaudet A. L., Wagner M. L., et al: Prenatal diagnosis of recurrence of Saldino–Noonan dwarfism. J. Pediatr. *91*:467 (1977)
Rupprecht E., Gurski A.: Kurzrippen-Polydactylie-Syndrom Typ Saldino–Noonan bei zwei Geschwistern. Helv. Paediatr. Acta *37*:161 (1982)

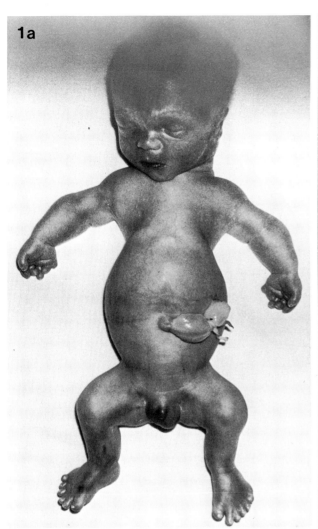 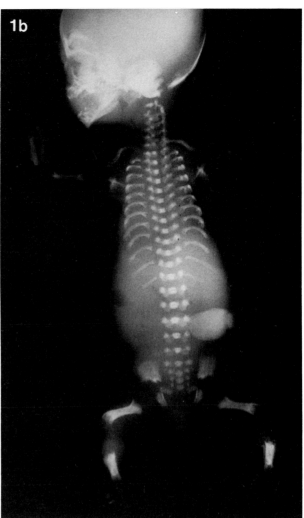

77. Chondrodysplasia Punctata, Recessive Type

(Chondrodysplasia Punctata, Rhizomelic Type)

A dysplasia syndrome with primordial dwarfism, unusual facies, psychomotor retardation, and occasionally ichthyosiform skin changes.

Main Signs:
1. Disproportionate dwarfism with symmetrical shortening of the arms and upper legs and multiple joint contractures (**1**).
2. Face flat; very full cheeks; broad, sunken nasal root – a somewhat mongoloid appearance (**1**).
3. Not infrequently ichthyosiform skin changes, alopecia.
4. Marked psychomotor retardation, tetraspasticity, generally microcephaly.

Supplementary Findings: Bilateral cataracts almost always present; optic atrophy occasionally.

Radiologically more or less severe symmetrical shortening, metaphyseal splaying, and punctate calcification of the ends of the humerus and/or femur (**2**). Pelvic dysplasia. Little or no punctate calcification ('stippling') in the vertebral column; ventral and dorsal ossification centres of the vertebral bodies (on lateral view) not joined! (Disappearance of calcium flecks usually in the course of the first year of life; fusion of the vertebral ossification centres).

Manifestation: At birth.

Aetiology: Autosomal recessive hereditary disorder.

Frequency: Very rare (up to 1971 there were 36 cases described).

Course, Prognosis: Poor. The great majority of these children do not survive infancy, usually succumbing to infection.

Differential Diagnosis: Other types of chondrodysplasia punctata (pp.156 and 158) as well as further conditions that show, or may show 'stippled epiphyses' on X-ray in the newborn period. Down's and trisomy 18 syndromes (pp.58 and 60), CHILD, Smith–Lemi–Opitz, and Zellweger syndromes (pp.160, 374, and 384), and coumarin (warfarin) embryopathy (see p.156 under Differential Diagnosis).

Treatment: Symptomatic. Genetic counselling. In appropriate cases prenatal diagnosis by ultrasound.

Illustrations:
1 and 2 A newborn infant. Early death due to pneumonia and hypoplastic lungs. Club foot on the right.

References:
Spranger J. W., Langer L. O., jr, Wiedemann H.-R.: Bone Dysplasias. An Atlas of Constitutional Disorders of Skeletal Development, Stuttgart and Philadelphia, G. Fischer and W. B. Saunders, 1974
Gilbert E. F., Opitz J. M., Spranger J. W., et al: Chondrodysplasia punctata–rhizomelic form. Eur. J. Pediatr. *123*:89 (1976)

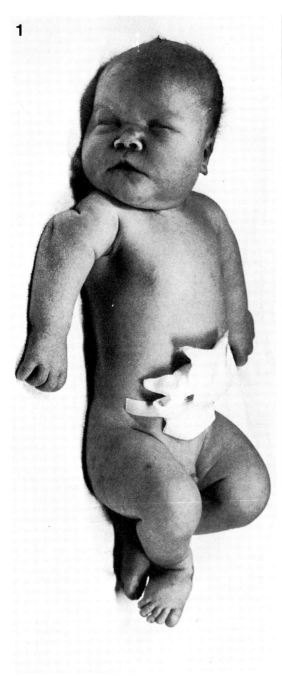

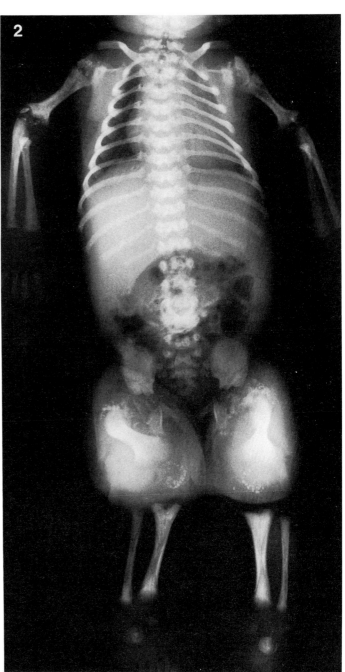

78. Chondrodysplasia Punctata, Autosomal Dominant Type

(Chondrodysplasia Punctata Type Conradi–Hünermann, Syndrome of Chondrodystrophia Calcificans, Conradi–Hünermann Syndrome)

A dysplasia syndrome with peculiar facies, shortening of the extremities, frequent curvature of the spine, and dwarfism.

Main Signs:
1. Facial dysmorphism with depressed broad nasal root, possible slight mongoloid slant of the palpebral fissures, hypoplasia of the midface, and frequent bilateral grooves on the tip of the nose (**1, 2, 4,** and **5**).
2. Short stature with symmetrical or slightly asymmetrical shortening of the extremities; frequent development of scoliosis, kyphosis; dysplasia and contracture of joints (**4** and **5**).

Supplementary Findings: No cataract; no obvious dermatoses.

Radiologically, punctate or spraylike areas of calcification at the ends of the long bones, the vertebral processes, the carpal or tarsal bones, or the ischia and pubic bones; eventual disappearance of these calcifications (**2** and **5**).

Manifestation: At birth. Scoliosis may not develop until later.

Aetiology: Autosomal dominant inheritance; sporadic cases suggest new mutations. It is possible that this is not a single uniform type.

Frequency: Rare.

Course, Prognosis: Good, after the hazardous first months of life.

Differential Diagnosis: See p.154. The use of vitamin-K antagonists during early pregnancy may lead to a more or less extensive phenocopy of a hereditary chondrodysplasia punctata (coumarin embryopathy). Medications history during pregnancy.

Treatment: Symptomatic–orthopaedic. Genetic counselling.

Illustrations:
1 and 3–5 A boy at ages 2 months (**1** and **5**, left half), 8 years (**3** and **4**), and 13 months (**5**, right half). At birth 'stippling' of the vertebral column, most of the epiphyses of the arm and leg bones, and most of the carpal and tarsal bones on X-rays. Skin and eyes normal. Height at 8½ years, 105 cm; right extremities somewhat shorter than the left; no more calcium spots. Normal intelligence.
2 Calcifications in the vertebral column and pelvis of an 8-week-old boy.

Sporadic cases; family histories unremarkable.

Reference:
Happle R.: Cataracts as a marker of genetic heterogeneity in chondrodysplasia punctata. Clin. Genet. *19*:64 (1981)

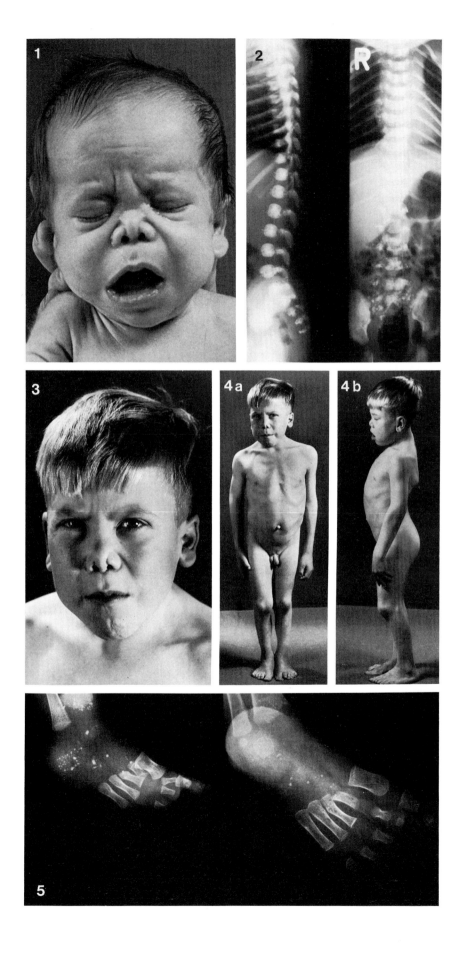

157

79. Chondrodysplasia Punctata, Sex-Linked Dominant Type

A dysplasia syndrome affecting only females as a mosaic-like distribution of skin changes and anomalies of the skeleton and eyes, all occurring asymmetrically.

Main Signs:
1. Asymmetrical skeletal anomalies with congenital shortening of the long bones (most frequently of the thigh, then of the upper arm – 2); dysplasia and contracture of joints (hips, knees, ankles, and others) as well as possible dysplastic involvement of the vertebral column, with secondary scoliosis. Unusual facies with depressed, broad nasal root, slight antimongoloid slant of the palpebral fissures, possible marked asymmetry of the facial skeleton. Possible hexadactyly (3).
2. Congenital ichthyosiform erythroderma (4 and 7) with patchy and stripe-like areas of hyperkeratosis. Later, patchy and stripe-like atrophy of the skin especially affecting the hair follicles (particularly of the forearm); localised, in part stripe-like alopecia of the head (6 and 8) and in part brittle, bristly, irregularly convoluted, lustreless hair (6); eyebrows and eyelashes sparse, growing in various directions (6). Older children often affected with ichthyosis (5).
3. Congenital or early developing cataracts, uni- or bilateral, in about two-thirds of cases; when 'bilateral', usually of unequal severity (1).

Supplementary Findings: Possible systemic stripe-like anomalies of pigmentation; in some cases flat nails with tendency to horizontal splintering (3).

Frequent short stature, in part secondary to scoliosis. Normal intellect.

Radiologically, stippling (punctate calcifications) in various parts of the skeleton, especially in the epiphyses of the long bones. Disappearance of the stippling in early years; diagnosis possible also in their absence.

Manifestation: At birth.

Aetiology: Presumptive X-chromosomal dominant hereditary disease with lethal effect of the gene on male embryos. Demonstration of mild cutaneous signs in some mothers of probands (9) suggests the possibility also of an incompletely manifested form of this hereditary type. Most cases are sporadic and should represent new mutations.

Frequency: Rare. Up to 1980, 40 cases were identified, exclusively in females.

Course, Prognosis: Good on the whole (patients handicapped by growth deficiency, scoliosis, and in some cases by ocular defects). Spontaneous regression of the congenital ichthyosiform erythroderma in infancy with development of systemic atrophoderma.

Differential Diagnosis: See p.154. The systemic anomalies of pigmentation may suggest a Bloch–Sulzburger syndrome (p.254) (transmitted by the same mode of inheritance), which should not be difficult to rule out by careful observation.

Treatment: Symptomatic (ophthalmological, orthopaedic, etc.). Careful examination of the mother for mild signs of the disorder. Genetic counselling. Prenatal diagnosis.

Illustrations:
1–6 An affected girl at birth (4), at age 6 months (1 and 3), at 6 years (2), and as an adolescent. Asymmetrical thorax and asymmetrical shortening of the extremities; postaxial hexadactyly of the left hand. At birth, multiple foci of calcium in the epiphyses of the left leg as well as in the costal cartilages. Foci of alopecia and typical changes of the hair of the head.
7 and 8 An affected girl as a newborn (also 'stippling' on X-ray, skeletal asymmetry, and unilateral cataract) and as adolescent.
9 Foci of alopecia on the head of the proband's mother.
(In part, by kind permission of E. Christophers, Kiel.)

References:
Manzke H., Christophers E., Wiedemann H.-R.: Dominant sex-linked inherited chondrodysplasia punctata: a distinct type of chondrodysplasia punctata. Clin. Genet. *17*:107 (1980)
Happle R.: X-gekoppelt dominante Chondrodysplasia punctata. Monatschr. Kinderheilkd. *128*:203 (1980)

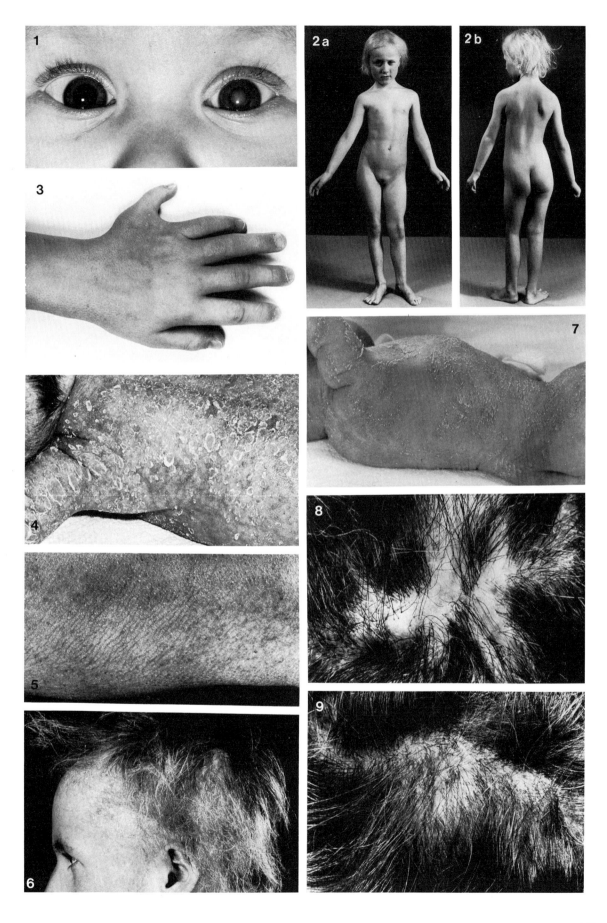

159

80. CHILD Syndrome

(syndrome of Congenital Hemidysplasia with Ichthyosiform erythroderma and Limb Defects)

A hereditary syndrome of unilateral ichthyosiform erythroderma and ipsilateral limb or skeletal defects of various grades of severity.

Main Signs:
1. Ichthyosiform erythroderma, which – more or less completely – affects one half of the body and is sharply outlined along the midline of the trunk (1, 7). Variable development – the extent possibly paralleling the severity of the skeletal and visceral defects. The face is usually spared. The nails may develop severe hyperkeratoses (3 and 4).
2. Ipsilateral skeletal hypoplasias (2 and 2a). Practically any part of the skeleton may be affected, in most cases predominantly the long bones – from mere hypoplasia of phalanges on to absence of a whole extremity. Hands and/or feet may be severely deformed.

Supplementary Findings: The right side has been affected in the vast majority of the cases observed to date; (smaller anomalies may also occur contralaterally).

In some cases secondary scoliosis (2a).

Ipsilateral anomalies of the internal organs (heart, lungs, kidneys, or other) or of the nervous system may occur.

Radiologically, in a few cases examined in the early postnatal period, epiphyseal calcium spots were demonstrated ipsilaterally in the limbs, the pelvic area, or elsewhere.

Manifestation: At birth. The dermatosis may develop later, during the first months of life.

Aetiology: Apparently a genetic syndrome. Almost exclusively girls affected. Possibly based on an X-chromosomal dominant gene with a lethal effect in males.

Frequency: Rare (up to 1980 there had been 23 reported observations).

Course, Prognosis: The dermatosis may remain constant in severity, may transiently vary somewhat, may affect new areas of skin, but also may regress spontaneously and permanently. Otherwise the prognosis depends on the presence and severity of internal and skeletal defects.

Differential Diagnosis: With chondrodysplasia punctata of the X-chromosomal type (p.158), the dermatosis occurs on both sides of the body in a different kind of pattern and (in older children) with signs of dermal atrophy. The Schimmelpennig–Feuerstein–Mims syndrome involves (p.230) a different type of skin problem.

Treatment: An effective treatment of the dermatosis is not known. Orthopaedic remedial measures, in some cases prosthetic or plastic surgery. Treatment of internal organ defects in some patients. Aids for the handicapped. Genetic counselling.

Illustrations:
1–6   An affected girl at ages 4 months (1, 2, and 2a), 1 year (3–5), and 3 years (6). Hypoplasia of the right extremities (2) with flexion contracture of the elbow joint. Hypoplasia of the right side of the mandible; the right scapula, ribs, vertebral body halves (see also spina bifida) with consequent scoliosis, and right side of the pelvis (2 and 2a). Dermatosis manifest at 2 months; sharply outlined along the midline of the trunk (1), the only areas spared being part of the face and head and the palmar and plantar surfaces. Right-sided renal aplasia. Dermatosis for the most part resistant to therapy, but eventual spontaneous regression (5 and 6). Development of severe hyperkeratosis of the nails (3 and 4).
7 and 8   A 4-year-old girl with comparable skeletal involvement and corresponding localised, medially outlined dermatosis in the right lumbar region (7) and an affected area on the left hand (8).
(By kind permission of Prof. R. Happle, Münster i. W.)

Reference:
Happle R., Koch H., Lenz W.: The CHILD syndrome. Eur. J. Pediatr. *134*:27 (1980)

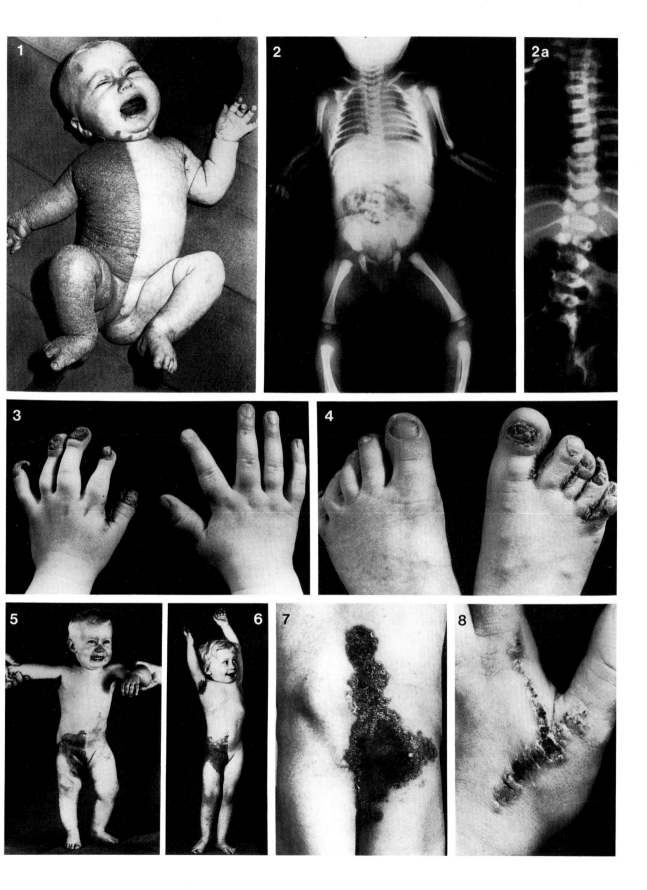

81. Syndrome of Camptomelic Dysplasia

(Camptomelic Syndrome)

An apparently uniform disorder comprising congenital symmetrical bowing and shortening of the lower extremities (with club feet), characteristic facies, and generally early death of the child from respiratory impairment – to be distinguished from other conditions with congenital deformity of the long bones.

Main Signs:
1. Disproportionate body, primarily because of shortness of the lower extremities, which show symmetrical anterior bowing (1), pretibial dimpling of the skin, and club feet. Arms possibly slightly shortened, bowed only as an exception.
2. Characteristic facies: Low root of the nose, hypertelorism, narrow palpebral fissures, long philtrum, Robin anomaly (micrognathia and cleft palate, p.52), usually relatively small mouth, anomalies of the external ears. Frequent macrodolichocephaly; wide open fontanelles (1).
3. Narrow thorax; usually a respiratory disorder.
4. Radiologically broad, short, bowed tibiae; bowed femora of normal width. Absence of the distal femoral and proximal tibial epiphyses. Severe hypoplasia of the shoulder blades, the fibulae, and other bones.

Supplementary Findings: Birth usually at term with moderate underweight; relatively frequent hydramnion.

Muscular hypotonia. Possible dislocation of the hips, elbows, halluces, fingers (with mild brachydactyly of the hands).

Phenotypic females often show a male karyotype.

At autopsy, frequent hydronephrosis, cardiac anomalies, and anomalies involving the olfactory tract and trachea.

Manifestation: At birth.

Aetiology: Mostly sporadic occurrence; definite prevalence of female cases; among these, frequently individuals with male karyotypes and absence of the HY antigen. Currently, autosomal recessive inheritance is the most prevalent assumption.

Frequency: Rare; somewhat more than 50 cases were reported up to 1980/81.

Course, Prognosis: Unfavourable; patients usually die within a few weeks of birth due to respiratory and feeding difficulties.

Differential Diagnosis: Other skeletal dysplasias with congenital bowing of the long bones.

Treatment: Symptomatic. Genetic counselling; prenatal diagnosis by X-ray for subsequent pregnancies.

Illustrations:
1 and 2   A child with typical signs of the syndrome. (By kind permission of Dr P. Maroteaux, Paris.)

References:
Hall Br.D., Spranger J.: Campomelic dysplasia. Am.J.Dis.Child. *134*:285 (1980)
Bricarelli Fr.D., Fraccaro M., Lindsten J., et al: Sex-reversed XY females with campomelic dysplasia are XY negative. Hum.Genet. *57*:15 (1981)

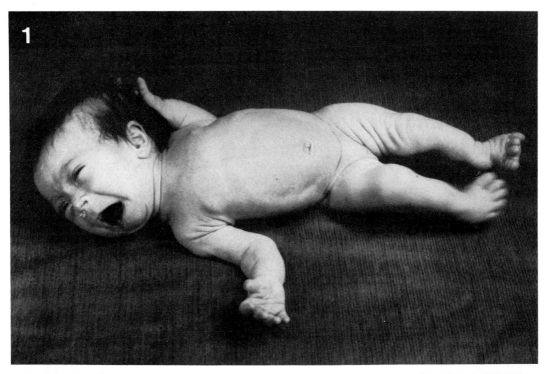

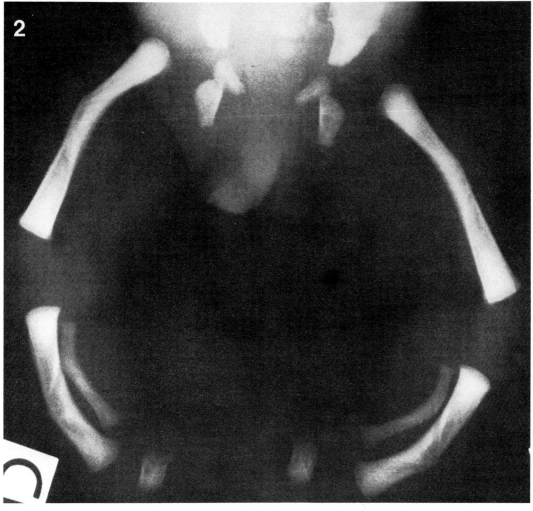

163

82. Achondroplasia

(Chondrodystrophia Fetalis, Parrot Syndrome)

A 'classic' generalised skeletal dysplasia with disproportionate, micromelic dwarfism; large head; typical facial dysmorphism; and characteristic X-ray findings.

Main Signs:
1. Primordial disproportionate growth deficiency; extremities, especially their proximal parts (arm, thigh), relatively more severely shortened than the trunk (3–7). Average adult height 124 cm for women and 131 cm for men. Ulnar deviation of the hands, splay position of the fingers ('trident hand' – 8). Limited extension at the elbow joints, genua vara, less frequently valga (3, 5, and 6).
2. Head too large for the body and rarely also for age, especially the cranial part. Coarse features, recessed nasal root, prognathism with hypoplasia of the midface region (1, 3 – 7).
3. Thorax flat, frequently bell-shaped. Thoracolumbar kyphosis, lumbosacral lordosis with protuberant abdomen (4, 5, and 7).
4. Delayed motor, but normal mental development. Occasionally (conductive or inner ear) hearing impairment.

Supplementary Findings: Large cranium with frontoparietal bossing and relatively short base. Small foramen magnum, progressive narrowing of the lumbar spinal canal caudally (which together with the progressive lumbosacral lordosis may lead to signs of compression).

Pelvis flat and broad, pelvic inlet narrow (generally dystocia), flat acetabula (9). Long bones shortened, with normal width (2), fibula relatively too long.

Manifestation: At birth.

Aetiology: Autosomal dominant hereditary disorder. The majority of cases are due to new mutations (often associated with advanced paternal age).

Frequency: About 1:25 000.

Prognosis: Apart from possible complications from compression, good as regards life expectancy. Striking rapid growth of the cranium during the first 3 years of life is the rule, and (in the absence of signs of increased intracranial pressure) no reason to worry or operate.

Differential Diagnosis: Thanatophoric dysplasia (p.150), hypochondroplasia (p.184), pseudoachondroplasia (p.192), among others.

Treatment: Symptomatic. Possible corrective osteotomy as well as specific operative measures for signs of neurological compression. Orthopaedic care; handicap aids. Genetic counselling. Early prenatal recognition with ultrasound is apparently unreliable.

Illustrations:
1 A 7-month-old infant.
2 X-ray of the left hand of a toddler.
3–5 An 8-year-old boy.
6–9 A 15-year-old boy.

References:
Silverman F. N.: Achondroplasia, Progr. Pediatr. Radiol., vol 4, Intrinsic Diseases of Bones, p.94. Karger, Basel 1973
Spranger J. W., Langer L. O., jr, Wiedemann H.-R.: Bone Dysplasias. An Atlas of Constitutional Disorders of Skeletal Development, Stuttgart and Philadelphia, G. Fischer and W. B. Saunders, 1974
Lutter L. D., Paul St., Langer L. O.: Neurological symptoms in achondroplastic dwarfs – surgical treatment. J. Bone Jt. Surg. 59-A: 87 (1977)
Hall J. G., Golbus M. S., Graham C. B., et al: Failure of early prenatal diagnosis in classic achondroplasia. Am. J. Med. Genet. 3:371 (1979)

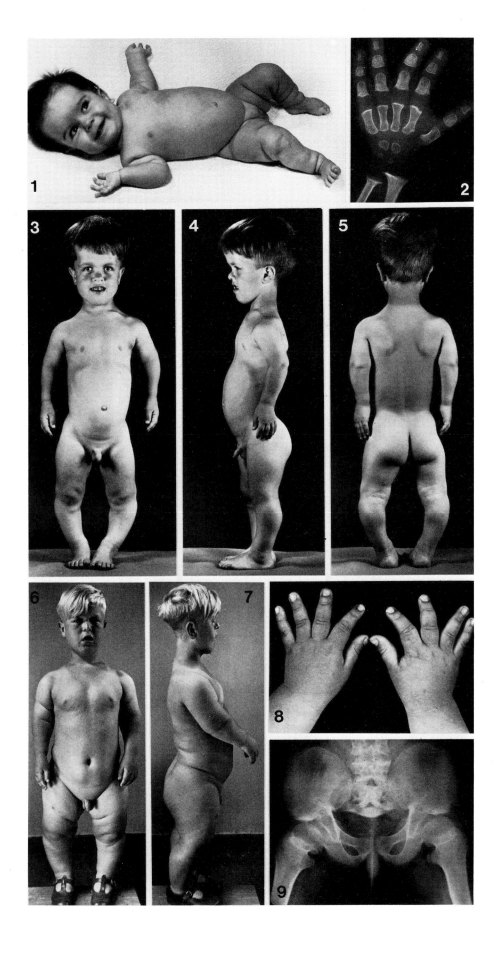

83. Syndrome of Diastrophic Dysplasia

A characteristic hereditary syndrome of severe dwarfism, club feet, joint contractures, position anomalies of the thumbs and big toes, anomalies of the auricles, and cleft palate.

Main Signs:
1. Micromelic dwarfism with club feet, joint contractures (especially of the shoulder, elbow, hip, and interphalangeal joints), and abduction of the proximally displaced, hyperextensible thumbs and halluces (1–3 and 6).
2. Anomaly of the auricles (development of cystic masses in early infancy; later, thickening and deformity) (5). Frequent cleft palate.
3. In most cases progressive thoracolumbar kyphoscoliosis and cervical kyphoses (2b and 4).

Supplementary Findings: Tendency to subluxation and luxation of the joints, promoted by laxity of the joints and ligaments.

Radiologically, severe epimetaphyseal changes of the – shortened – long bones with broadening of the metaphyses, delayed ossification and deformity especially of the proximal femoral epiphyses, more or less distinct fork-shaped deformity of the distal femoral and distal radial epiphyses, uncinate changes of the lateral ends of the clavicles, and ovoid deformity of metacarpal I in the young child, among other findings (7).

Manifestation: At birth. (Development of external ear anomalies usually between birth and the end of the first quarter year of life. Development of kyphoscoliosis usually after infancy.)

Aetiology: Autosomal recessive hereditary condition with very variable expression.

Frequency: Rare (over 70 cases are known).

Course, Prognosis: Increased incidence of early death. Later, danger of the effects of severe kyphoscoliotic changes. Adult heights range from less than 1 m to around 1.40 m. Normal mental development.

Differential Diagnosis: Pseudodiastrophic dysplasia (p.168), arthrogryposis (p.302).

Treatment: Symptomatic. Intensive orthopaedic care mandatory. All appropriate aids for the physically handicapped. Genetic counselling. Prenatal diagnosis by ultrasound in subsequent pregnancies.

Illustrations:
1, 3, 5 and 6   A 4½-year-old boy.
2, 4, and 7   A 1½-year-old girl. Note micromelia, club feet, hypermobility or abduction (up to and including subluxation) of the thumbs and halluces, early thoracolumbar kyphosis (2b) and marked cervical kyphosis (4), coarsening and deformity of the hand bones (7).

References:
Walter H.: Der diastrophische Zwergwuchs. Advances Human Genetics 2:31, Stuttgart, Thieme 1970
Spranger J. W., Langer L. O., jr, Wiedemann H.-R.: Bone Dysplasias. An Atlas of Constitutional Disorders of Skeletal Development, Stuttgart and Philadelphia, G. Fischer and W. B., Saunders, 1974
Horton W. A., Rimion D. L., Lachman R. S., et al: The phenotypic variability of diastrophic dysplasia. J. Pediatr. 93:609 (1978)
Bethem D., Winter R. B., Lutter L.: Disorders of the spine in diastrophic dwarfism. J. Bone Jt Surg. 62-A 529 (1980)
Lachman R., Sillence D., Rimion D., et al: Diastrophic dysplasia... Radiology 140:79 (1981)
Horton W. A., Hall J. G., Scott Ch. I., et al: Growth curves for height for diastrophic dysplasia... Am. J. Dis. Child. 136:316 (1982)

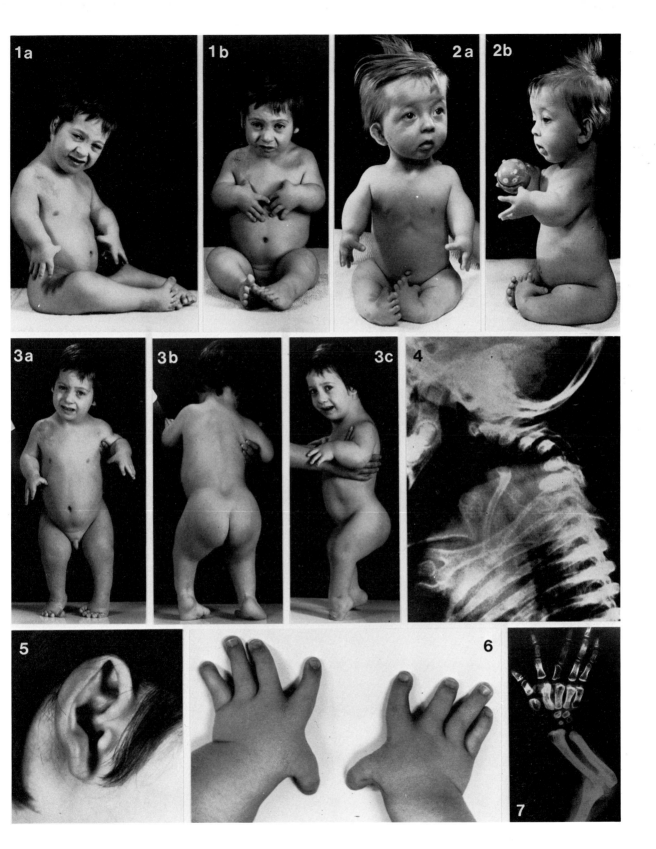

84. Syndrome of Pseudodiastrophic Dysplasia Type Burgio

A syndrome of micromelic dwarfism with characteristic facies, short neck, club feet, joint contractures and luxations, large auricles, and cleft palate.

Main Signs:
1. Congenital micromelic growth deficiency. Short neck. Bell-shaped (wider above) thorax. Almost angular, dorsolumbar kyphosis (**1, 2,** and **4**).
2. Peculiar facies with flat nose, hypertelorism, micrognathia, and abnormally full cheeks. Complete cleft palate. Large auricles (**1** and **2**).
3. Club feet. Limited motion of the metacarpal and metatarsal joints, the spine, and to a lesser degree, the knees and shoulders. Luxation of both hips, both elbows, and several finger joints (**3**).

Supplementary Findings: On X-ray, shortening and broadening of all bones of the extremities (**3**). Hypoplasia of the scapulae with dysplasia of the joint fossae; broad, square deformed ilia. Hypoplasia of the cervical vertebrae; platyspondylisis of the lower vertebrae with narrowing of the interpediculate, widening of the intersomatic spaces.

Manifestation: Birth

Aetiology: No doubt of a genetic basis. Autosomal recessive inheritance may be assumed.

Frequency: Rare.

Course, Prognosis: Increased early mortality. In case of longer survival, danger from the effects of severe kyphoscoliotic changes.

Differential Diagnosis: Diastrophic dysplasia (p.166), arthrogryposis (p.302).

Comment: Although designated pseudodiastrophic dwarfism because of signs overlapping with those of diastrophic dysplasia, this syndrome is osteochondro-histologically and -histochemically and especially radiologically an independent clinical entity, the similarities being limited to appearance.

Treatment: Symptomatic. Genetic counselling. Prenatal diagnosis by ultrasonography in case of subsequent pregnancies.

Illustrations:
1–4 The 1st child of healthy, young, nonconsanguineous parents. Birth measurements: 3120 g, 44 cm. Progression of the kyphoscoliosis. The peculiar facies persisted unchanged. Chromosomal analysis negative. Frequent episodes of fever of unknown aetiology (normal immune globulins). Sudden death at age 8 months. A female sibling born subsequently showing the same clinical picture died at age 4 days with unexplained hyperthermia.
(By kind permission of Prof. R. Burgio and Dr G. Beluffi, both of Pavia.)

References:
Burgio G. R., Belloni C., Belluﬁ G.: Nanisme pseudiastrophique. Etude de deux soers nouveaunées. Arch. Franc. Péd. *31*:681 (1974)
Gorlin R. J., Pindborg J. J., Cohen M. M., Jr.: Syndromes of the Head and Neck. 2nd Ed. McGraw-Hill Book Co., New York 1976
Kozlowski K., Masel J., Morris L., Kunze D.: Neonatal death dwarfism (a further report). Fortschr. Röntgenstr. *129*:626 (1978)
Stanescu V., Maroteaux P.: Etude morphologique et biochemique du cartilage de croissance dans les osteochondroplasies. Arch. Franc. Péd. Suppl. *1*:34 (1977)

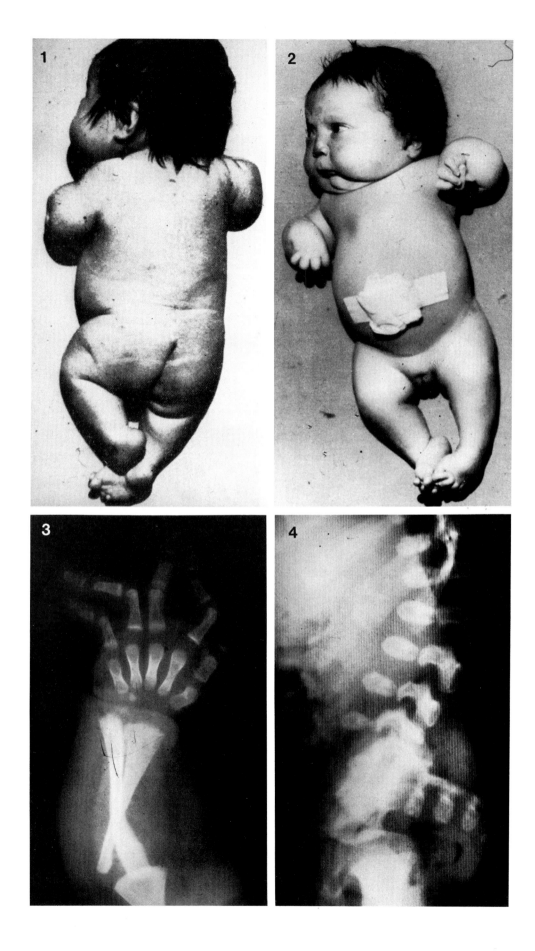

85. Metatropic Dysplasia

(Metatropic Dwarfism)

A hereditary syndrome leading to severe dwarfism with 'turnabout of proportions' during the course of childhood (initially, relatively short extremities; subsequently, more conspicuous shortening of the trunk) combined with limitation of motion of the large joints and frequently with a tail-like formation in the sacral area.

Main Signs:
1. In the newborn and young child, a disproportionately long trunk with narrow thorax and short extremities (**1–3**).
2. In the older child (and adults), 'spinal column-dwarfism' as a result of platyspondylisis (**8**) and usually also severe kyphoscoliosis; extremities now appearing abnormally long (**5** and **7**).
3. Frequent tail-like appendage formed medially over the sacral area (**3c, 5b,** and **7b**).
4. Restricted motion at the more or less prominent large joints (**1, 5,** and **7**).

Supplementary Findings: Secondary deformities of the thorax.

Hyperextensibility of the finger joints.

Radiologically aniso- and platyspondylisis (**8**), remarkable anomalies of size and form of the pelvic bones and proximal femora (**4**), severe epimetaphyseal abnormalities of the – shortened – tubular bones with broadening of the metaphyses and marked irregularities of the epiphyseal ossification centres (**2** and **6**).

Manifestation: Birth and thereafter by the change of proportions.

Aetiology: Monogenic hereditary disorder; heterogeneity; occurrence of autosomal recessive as well as autosomal dominant inheritance.

Frequency: Relatively rare.

Course, Prognosis: Increased infant mortality due to the effects of congenitally narrowed thorax. Patients eventually endangered by the effects of severe kyphoscoliosis. The adult height in severe cases may be around 1.10 or 1.20 m. Normal mental development.

Differential Diagnosis: Particularly the Kniest syndrome (p.176) and Morquio syndrome (p.80).

Treatment: Symptomatic. Intensive orthopaedic supervision and in some cases, therapy. All appropriate aids for the physically handicapped. Genetic counselling.

Illustrations:
1 A child at ages 1¼ years, 3 years (**1c**), and 4 years (**1b**).
2 and 4 X-rays of a newborn.
3 and 5 A girl at 10 months and at 7 years ('turnabout proportions').
6–8 A 7-year-old child; X-ray of a hand (**6**) and of the spinal column (**8**).

One can observe the early onset of manifest kyphosis in **3a** and the severe progression in **5**. 'Tail formations' seen in **3c, 5b,** and **7**.

References:
Maroteaux P., Spranger J., Wiedemann H.-R.: Der metatropische Zwergwuchs. Arch. Kinderheilkd. *173*:211 (1966)
Spranger J. W., Langer L. O., jr, Wiedemann H.-R.: Bone Dysplasias. An Atlas of Constitutional Disorders of Skeletal Development, Stuttgart and Philadelphia, G. Fischer and W. B. Saunders 1974
Miething R., Stöver B., Noeske H.: Metatroper Zwergwuchs. Monatschr. Kinderheilkd. *128*:153 (1980)

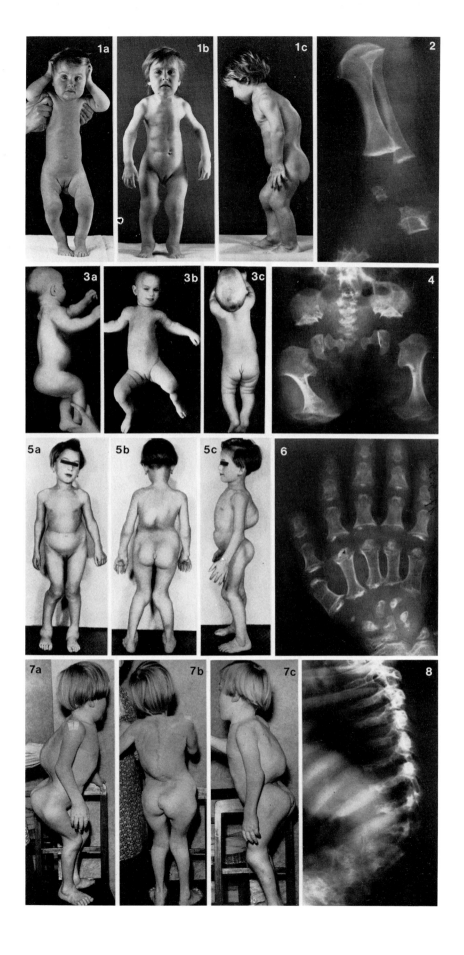

171

86. Chondroectodermal Dysplasia

(Ellis–van Creveld Syndrome)

A hereditary syndrome of congenital short-limbed dwarfism with hexadactyly on the little-finger side, hypoplasia of the nails, and abnormal bridges of mucous membrane between the upper lip and the alveolar process.

Main Signs:
1. Disproportionate, short-limbed dwarfism with progressive shortening of the extremities distally (**1**).
2. Hexadactyly of the hands, postaxial (i.e., on the little-finger side), occasionally also of the feet (**1**, **3**, and **4**).
3. Hypo- and dysplasia of the nails (**3** and **4**).
4. Short upper lip, joined to the aveolar ridge by more or less numerous additional frenula (**2**).
5. Dysodontiasis (possible congenital teeth, partial anodontia, small or late-erupting teeth, malpositioning of teeth).
6. In well over half of the cases, congenital cardiac defect (usually large atrial septal defects).

Supplementary Findings: Possible narrow thorax; later, genua valga.

Radiologically, distinctly increasing hypoplasia of the fingers distally; possible bony fusion of metacarpal bones or phalanges, or of the capitate and hamate; and many other anomalies.

Manifestation: At birth.

Aetiology: Autosomal recessive hereditary disorder with rather variable expressivity.

Frequency: Rare.

Course, Prognosis: In infancy, substantially increased mortality as a consequence of pulmonary complications or cardiac defect. Adult heights varied, between about 1.05 and 1.60 m.

Differential Diagnosis: The fully expressed syndrome can hardly cause diagnostic difficulties.

Treatment: Symptomatic. Orthopaedic treatment of polydactyly and genua valga. Early dental care. In some cases, operative correction of a cardiac defect. Genetic counselling.

Illustrations:
1–4 A 9-month-old boy, the 1st child of young, healthy, nonconsanguineous parents. The characteristic disproportion is more marked on the left side (**1**, **3**, and **4**); ulnar deviation of the left hand; clinodactyly of the 5th and 6th fingers bilaterally. Marked hypoplasia of the upper part of the left ilium with hip dysplasia and sublaxatio coxae. Bilateral pes valgus. Delayed dentition. Small penis.
(By kind permission of Frau Dr U. Hillig and Prof. G. Wendt, Marburg a. d. L.)

References:
Spranger J. W., Langer L. O., jr, Wiedemann H.-R.: Bone Dysplasias. An Atlas of Constitutional Disorders of Skeletal Development, Stuttgart and Philadelphia, G. Fischer and W. B. Saunders, 1974
Milgram J. W., Bailey J. A.: Orthopaedic aspects of the Ellis–van Creveld syndrome. Bull Hosp. Joint Dis. *36*:11 (1975)
Oliveira E., Silva D., Janovito D. et al: Ellis–van Creveld syndrome: Report of 15 cases…J. Med. Genet. *17*:349 (1980)

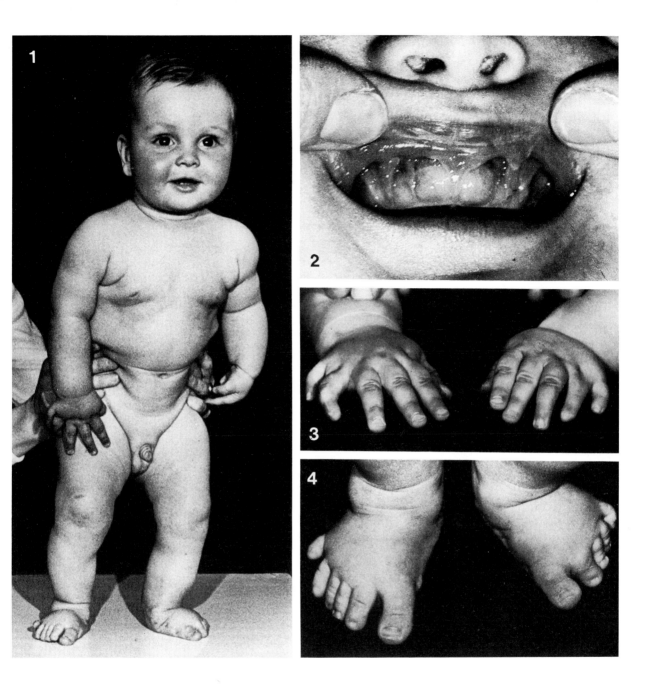

87. Syndrome of Spondyloepiphyseal Dysplasia Congenita

A hereditary syndrome of disproportionate dwarfism with severe shortening of the spinal column; barrel-shaped chest; low lumbar lordosis; severe dysplasia of the epiphyses, especially those near the trunk; essentially unremarkable cranium, hands, and feet; frequent myopia; and possible retinal detachment.

Main Signs:
1. Disproportionate dwarfism with marked shortening of the vertebral column. Short neck, compressed-appearing trunk with barrel-shaped thorax and pectus carinatum, lumbar hyperlordosis, possible kyphoscoliosis of the thoracic part of the spine (**1a-d**).
2. Relatively long extremities. Frequent waddling gait with severe hip dysplasia and marked coxa vara. Frequent genua valga (less frequently vara). Normal-sized hands and feet (**1**).
3. Impaired vision due to myopia and/or retinal detachment in about half of the cases.

Supplementary Findings: Flat face (occasionally with hypertelorism) (**1a** and **d**).

Occasional cleft palate.

Unobstructed movement at the joints, in part hyperextensibility (with possible exception of the hip, shoulder, and elbow joints). Lax ligaments.

Muscular hypotonia in infancy.

Occasionally club feet.

Delayed motor, normal mental development.

Inner ear hearing impairment not rare.

Radiologically, delayed ossification (see also **3**), especially in the pelvic bones and at the hip joints (with severe coxa vara), flattening and diverse irregularities of the vertebral bodies with hypoplasia of the odontoid process, epimetaphyseal dysplasia of the long bones, relatively normal skeletons of the hands and feet.

Manifestation: At birth.

Aetiology: Autosomal dominant hereditary disorder with quite variable expressivity. Probable heterogeneity.

Frequency: Not so rare.

Course, Prognosis: Retinal detachment may occur relatively early; thus, regular check-ups by an ophthalmologist are mandatory. There is danger of compression of the cervical part of the medulla in connection with hypoplasia of the odontoid and laxity of the ligaments, which requires orthopaedic care. The adult heights vary between about 90 and 130 cm. Increasing arthroses and corresponding handicaps related to the large joints in adulthood.

Differential Diagnosis: Especially the Morquio syndrome (later manifestation, among other differences), see p.80; also Stickler syndrome (p.404).

Treatment: Symptomatic. Early treatment of club feet when present; closure of cleft palate as required; careful neurological supervision as well as orthopaedic meaures to allay the danger of spinal cord compression; coagulation treatment for retinal detachment in some cases. All necessary aids for the physically handicapped. Genetic counselling.

Illustrations:
1a–d   A child at 6 months (height 14 cm below average for age) and 7¼ years (height deficit about 40 cm). Early kyphoscoliosis. Hypoplasia of the odontoid, at that time without abnormal mobility at the atlanto-occipital joint. Cleft palate.
2   X-ray of a hand of a 4-year-old female patient (father similarly affected).
3   A hand X-ray of the child in **1** at age 5 years.

References:
Spranger J. W., Langer L. O. jr, Wiedemann H.-R.: Bone Dysplasias. An Atlas of Constitutional Disorders of Skeletal Development, Stuttgart and Philadelphia, G. Fischer and W. B. Saunders 1974
Luthardt Th., Reinwein H., Schönenberg H., Spranger J., Wiedemann H.-R.: Dysplasia spondyloepiphysaria congenita. Klin. Pädiatr. 187:538 (1975)
Kozlowski K., Masel J., Nolte K.: Dysplasia spondyloepiphysealis congenita Spranger-Wiedemann. Aust. Radiol. 21:260 (1977)
Horton W. A., Hall J. G., Scott Ch. I., et al: Growth curves for height for diastrophic dysplasia, spondyloepiphyseal dysplasia congenita…Am. J. Dis. Child. 136:316 (1982)

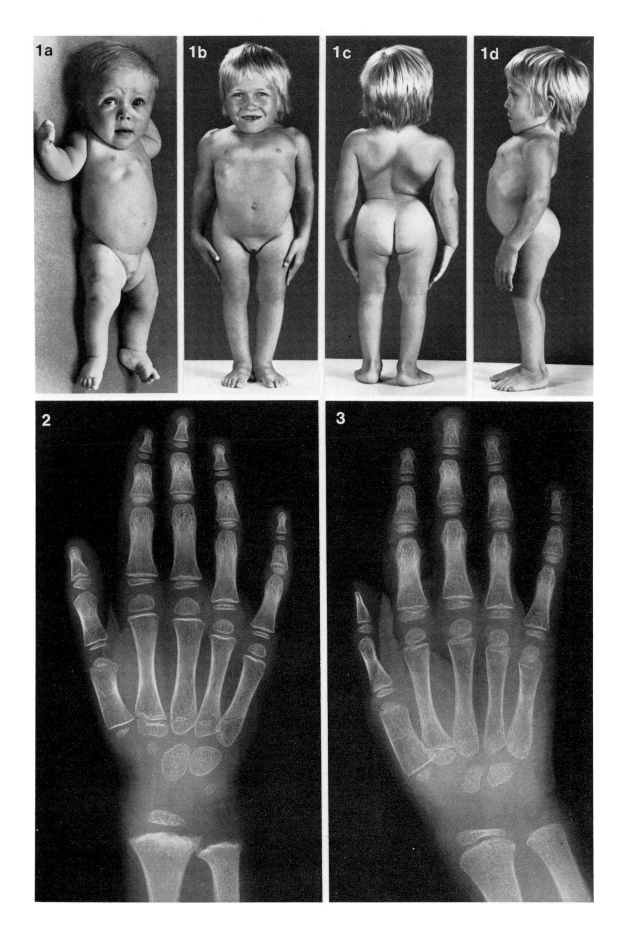

175

88. Osteodysplasia Type Kniest

(Kniest Syndrome)

A hereditary disease of disproportionate dwarfism with kyphoscoliosis, flat facies, frequent hearing and visual impairments, and characteristic X-ray findings.

Main Signs:
1. Disproportionate dwarfism with short trunk, broad thorax, marked lumbar lordosis, thoracic kyphoscoliosis, and short extremities, which appear swollen at the joints and too long relative to the trunk (**1**). Adult height between 100 and 145 cm.
2. Flat facies with possible hypertelorism and possible flat orbits with exophthalmos, flat nasal root, and (in about half of the cases) cleft palate.
3. Frequent limitation of motion at the joints (especially at the hip joints); long fingers.
4. Frequent hearing impairment (conductive and/or inner ear damage) as well as frequent severe myopia with retinal degeneration and danger of glaucoma, cataract, and retinal detachment with loss of sight.

Supplementary Findings: Frequent umbilical and inguinal hernias. Radiologically, conspicuous anomalies of size and form of the pelvic and thigh bones. Platyspondyly, marked epimetaphyseal alterations of the long bones with broadened metaphyses and marked irregularity of the epimetaphyses in the form of honeycombed, porous translucencies and delayed ossification (especially of the heads of the femora).

Manifestation: Birth (shortened, deformed extremities; restricted joint mobility); and thereafter. Delayed motor development.

Aetiology: Hereditary disease. Mode of transmission not settled beyond doubt, probably autosomal dominant. Perhaps heterogeneity.

Frequency: Rare.

Course, Prognosis: Probably approximately normal life expectancy, however with considerable to severe physical handicaps – articular and possibly ocular and acoustic.

Differential Diagnosis: Above all, metatropic dysplasia (p.170) and spondyloepiphyseal dysplasia congenita (p.174). The Morquio syndrome (p.80) as well as diastrophic and pseudodiastrophic dysplasia (pp.166 and 168) should be comparatively easy to rule out.

Treatment: Starting at an early age, regular qualified follow-up with ophthalmological and audiometric examinations. Closure of possible cleft palate and eventual speech therapy as required. Orthopaedic care for joint contractures and kyphoscoliosis. All appropriate aids for the physically handicapped. Genetic counselling.

Illustrations:
1 A 7-year-old with Kniest syndrome and his healthy twin brother.
(By kind permission of Prof. Dr O. Butenandt, Munich.)

References:
Spranger J. W., Langer L. O., jr, Wiedemann H.-R.: Bone Dysplasias. An Atlas of Constitutional Disorders of Skeletal Development, Stuttgart and Philadelphia, G. Fischer and W. B. Saunders 1974
Lachman R. S., Rimoin D. L., Hollister D. W., et al: The Kniest syndrome. Am. J. Roentgenol. *123*:805 (1975)
Kniest W., Leiber B.: Kniest-Syndrom. Monatschr. Kinderheilkd. *125*:970 (1977)

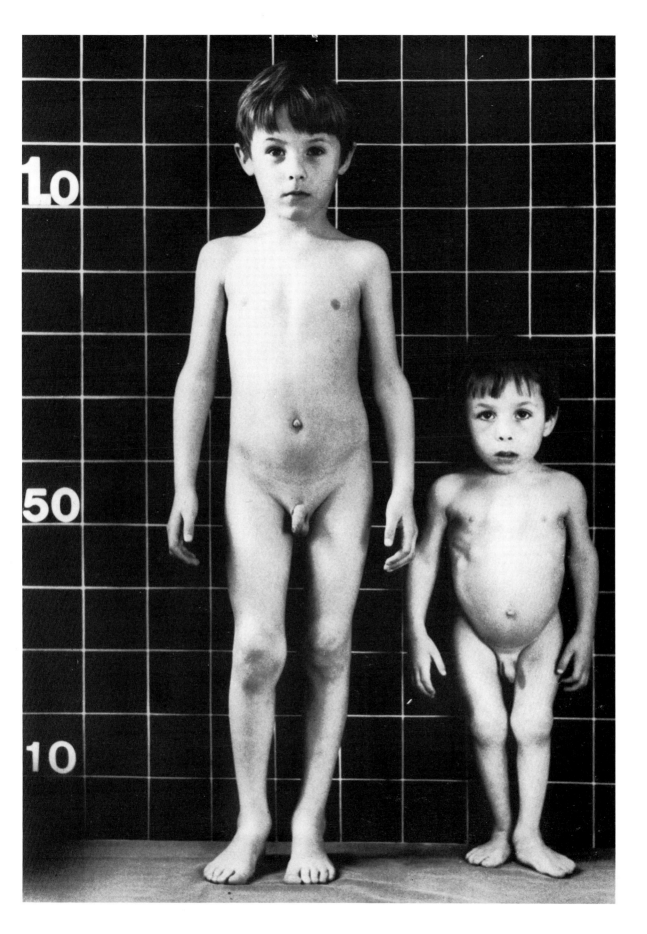

89. Syndrome of Hereditary Vitamin D Resistant Rickets

(Syndrome of Familial Hypophosphataemic Rickets; Phosphate Diabetes Syndrome)

A hereditary metabolic syndrome with growth deficiency and rachitic bone changes.

Main Signs:
1. Moderate growth deficiency with accentuated changes in lower extremities; pronounced bow-legs, less frequently knock-knees (1–3). Waddling gait, coxae varae. During childhood, the other rachitic bony changes (also rachitic rosary, swelling of the wrist and ankle joints, etc.).
2. Dental changes, such as enamel defects, delayed eruption, and premature loss.
3. Abnormal curvature of the spine in adulthood.
4. Possible craniosynostosis.

Supplementary Findings: Osteomalacia in adulthood, also bony protuberances at the site of tendon attachments.

Radiological changes as in vitamin D-deficiency rickets (4); however, not of the pelvis or vertebral column.

Hypophosphataemia, hyperphosphaturia – these together with slight growth deficiency being the only signs of the mild form of the disorder – and elevation of the serum alkaline phosphatase.

Manifestation: Biochemically, at birth or in the course of the first half year of life. Clinically, mostly in the 2nd and 3rd half-years of life and thereafter.

Aetiology: Sex-linked dominant hereditary disorder; correspondingly milder manifestations of the disorder in girls.

Frequency: Rather low.

Course, Prognosis: Improvement of the signs of florid rickets with the physiological slowing and the cessation of growth. Adult height between about 1.30 and 1.60 m. Frequent joint and back pain and complaints of stiffness during adulthood.

Differential Diagnosis: Vitamin D-deficiency rickets (here, prompt response to physiological doses of vitamin D; no family history) and other forms of rickets. Syndrome of metaphyseal chondrodysplasia of type Schmid (p.186) as well as cartilage-hair hypoplasia (p.188).

Treatment: Variously handled and assessed. With daily administration of vitamin D analogs (1α–OHD_3, $1,25$– $(OH)_2D_3$) and phosphate, carefully monitored with blood chemistries, some authors have seen good clinical and biochemical results; however, the hypophosphataemia could hardly be influenced. Some authors have reported a positive effect on growth in height. Orthopaedic–operative correction of the leg deformities preferably after cessation of growth.

Illustrations:
1–3 Two children (of different parents) at ages 5 years and 3 years. Both are 9 cm too short.
4 Radiological bone changes in a 1-year-old patient.

Reference:
Stanbury J. B., Wyngaarden J. B., Fredrickson D. S.: The Metabolic Basis of Inherited Disease. McGraw-Hill Book Company 1978, p.1537

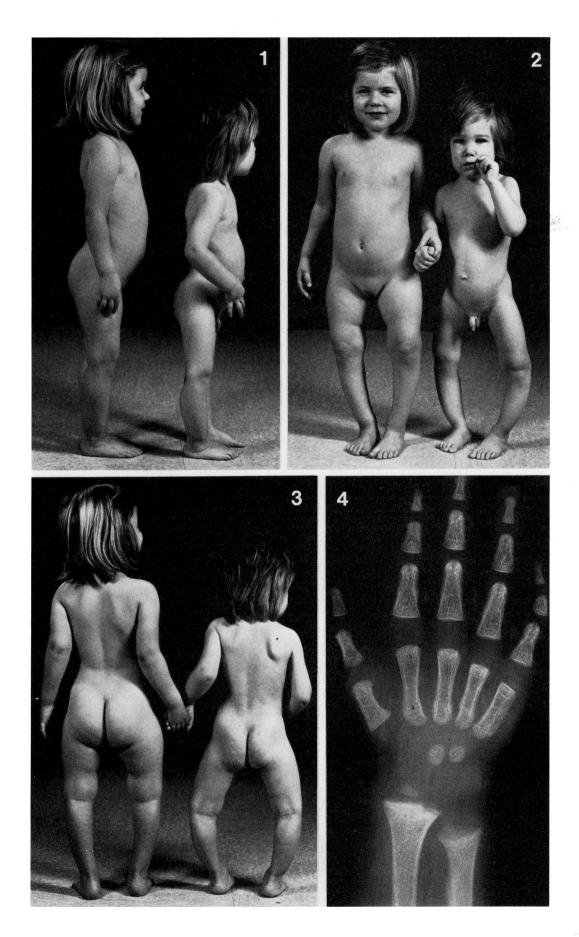

90. An Unfamiliar Growth Deficiency Syndrome with Striking Distal Inhibition of Ossification

A syndrome of growth deficiency, severe infantile scoliosis, and other skeletal anomalies, with severely delayed ossification in bones of the hands and feet.

Main Signs:
1. Marked growth deficiency.
2. Marked infantile scoliosis with corresponding abnormality of proportions and other secondary changes (**11–13**).
3. On X-ray, markedly delayed ossification in bones of the hands and feet ('empty wrist') (**6** and **7**).

Supplementary Findings: Normal mental development.

Radiologically, numerous wormian bones of the skull (**3** and **4**). Possible evidence of malformations of the vertebral column or other regions.

Manifestation: Birth or early childhood.

Aetiology: Uncertain; genetic basis probable.

Course, Prognosis: Undetermined; certainly very dependent on the osseous foundation and whether the scoliosis is accessible to therapy.

Treatment: Adequate orthopaedic care.

Illustrations:
1–13 A 4½-year-old boy, the 6th child of healthy consanguineous Turkish parents. A similarly affected sister: normal mental development; short stature; severe right convex scoliosis of the thoracic part of the spine, allegedly since the age of 3 years, with wedge-shaped vertebrae and synostoses; torsion defect of the lower leg. Other living siblings healthy. In the proband, the deformities of the spine and thorax (bulging rib cage, right side) are said to have been present at birth. Normal mental, delayed statomotor development. Now deficient growth, far below the third percentile, with short neck, abnormal course of the ribs, extremities relatively too long, and severe right convex scoliosis of the thoracic part of the spinal column (sloping of shoulders and pelvis). Round cranium with numerous wormian bones in the sagittal and especially the lambdoid sutures. Mild coxae varae; torsion defect of the upper and lower leg; patellae luxated laterally; pes adducti with diverse position anomalies of the toes. Radiologically practically 'empty wrists' and considerable delay of ossification in the metacarpals and phalanges but approximately normal epiphyses for age in the pelvis and knee regions. Also marked delay in development of the skeleton of the feet. Exhaustive chemical and endocrinological laboratory examinations negative.

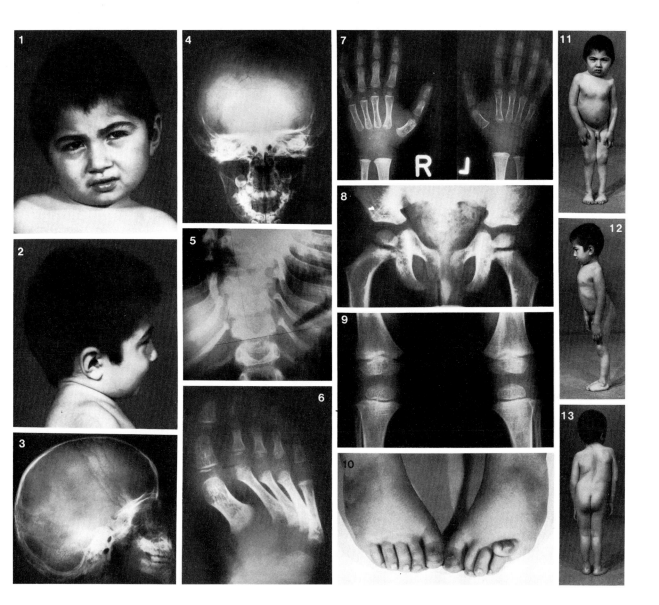

91. Joint Dysplasia – Small Stature – Erythema Telangiectasia

An unusual syndrome of multiple congenital joint dysplasias, small stature, and telangiectatic erythema of the face.

Main Signs:
1. Congenital, not completely symmetrical anomalies of the joints and skeleton: hip dysplasia, impaired extension of the knee joints, and – small – club feet, malformations of both distal humeri with luxation of the humeroulnar and radioulnar joints, relatively short forearms, limited mobility of the wrists, campto- and in part clinodactyly of fingers II–V (4 and 6–8). No fossettes cutanées.
2. Primary (+ secondary) growth deficiency under the third percentile (at 12 years, 2 months, about 1.30 m; twin brother 1.60 m).
3. Age 2-8 years, butterfly-like distribution of paranasal telangiectatic erythema of the face, suggested also on the forearms, that may have been aggravated by exposure to sunlight. (1 and 2; in 3 and 5 at 12 years, only slight residual spots on the left cheek.)

Supplementary Findings: Dolichocephaly; long, narrow face with prominent nose, slightly receding chin (3 and 5).

Kyphoscoliosis, lumbar hyperlordosis (4).

At well over 12 years, still no signs of onset of puberty.

X-ray of the hands and feet: Hypoplasia of the distal ends of the ulnae with absence of the styloid processes; considerable brachymesophalangia of the IInd–Vth fingers bilaterally, severe brachymesophalangia of the IInd–Vth toes.

Manifestation: Birth and later.

Aetiology: Uncertain.

Comment: Bloom syndrome (p.270) is apparently not present, and Larsen syndrome (p.304) could be ruled out. Classification as arthrogryposis multiplex congenita (p.302) did not seem to be justified here.

Treatment: Intensive orthopaedic–surgical as well as physiotherapeutic efforts required. Promotion of intellectual development, adequate vocational training, psychological guidance. Genetic counselling.

Illustrations:
1–8 A mentally normal girl, a twin child (brother quite unremarkable) of healthy, nonconsanguineous parents after two older healthy siblings. Father 47 years old at the proband's birth, mother 40 years. Unremarkable family history. Birth measurements 3000 g, 49 cm; no problems of any kind with rearing. 1 shows the girl as a pre-school child, 2 as a young school girl, 3–8 at almost 12¼ years. Flexion and adduction contractures of the hips with deviation of the thighs to the left; contracted talipes equinus. Chromosome analysis negative.

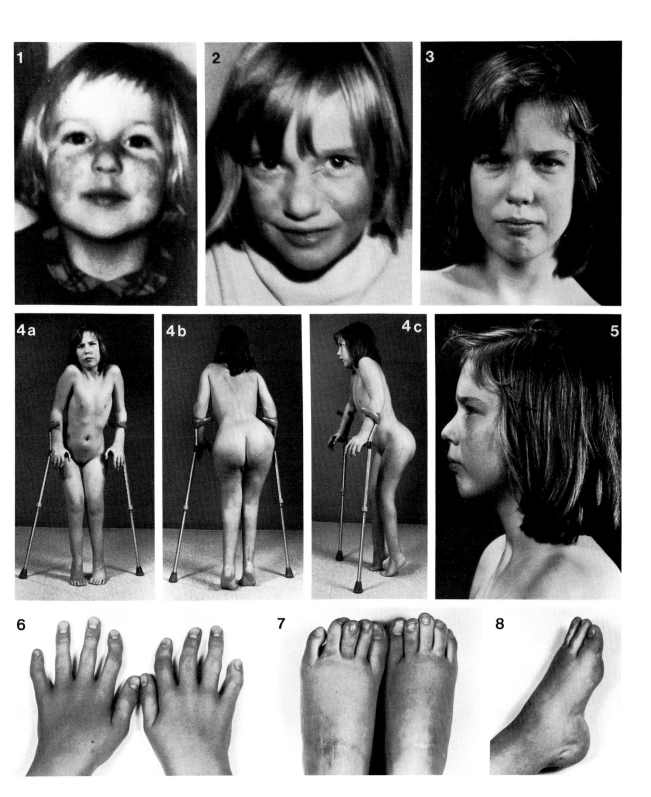

92. Hypochondroplasia

One of the achondroplasia-like hereditary short-limbed dwarfisms of mild expression.

Main Signs:
1. Dwarfism with disproportionately short extremities – more or less distinctly apparent – and broad, short hands (without 'trident' appearance) and feet (**1–6**). Adult height between about 1.15 and 1.50 m.
2. Cranium normal or oversized, often with protruding forehead. Root of the nose not low, and facial formation also essentially normal (**1–5**).
3. Limitation of motion of the elbow joints (with regard to full extension and supination). Frequent increase in lumbar lordosis (**4b**) as well as genua et crura vara (**2, 3,** and **4a**).

Supplementary Findings: Radiologically (**6** and **7**) the signs somewhat of an 'attenuated achondroplasia'. Square pelvis with narrow inlet (generally dystocia), short and broad femoral necks, disproportionately long fibulae, brachydactyly, etc.
   Occasional mental retardation.

Manifestation: Birth (length usually around 48 cm) and thereafter. Sporadic cases are first noted by family members in the course of the early pre-school years.

Aetiology: Hereditary disorder, autosomal dominant, of very variable expressivity – i.e., from very slight to very definite resemblance of achondroplasia. Many sporadic cases representing new mutations, frequently associated with increased paternal age.

Frequency: Not so rare.

Course, Prognosis: Normal life expectancy.

Differential Diagnosis: Achondroplasia (p.164; here typical facial dysmorphism, markedly shortened arms, trident hands, etc.), chondrodysplasia metaphysaria type Schmid (p.186; here quite different X-ray findings, etc.), and other forms of growth deficiency.

Treatment: Symptomatic. Genetic counselling.

Illustrations:
1–5 Children and adults with hypochondroplasia: 1-year-old and 11-year-old boys; mother and daughter; a 12-year-old and a 16-year-old girl.
6 X-rays of the left hand of a child at 6 and again at 13 years.
7 X-ray of the lower extremities of the girl in **3**.
(Pictures in part by kind permission of Professors J. Spranger, Mainz and D. Knorr, München.)

References:
Spranger J.W., Langer L.O., jr, Wiedemann H.-R.: Bone Dysplasias. An Atlas of Constitutional Disorders of Skeletal Development, Stuttgart and Philadelphia, G. Fischer and W.B. Saunders 1974
Oberklaid F., Danks M., Jensen F. et al: Achondroplasia and hypochondroplasia. J. Med. Genet. 16:140 (1979)
Hall Br.D., Spranger J.: Hypochondroplasia: Clinical and radiological aspects in 39 cases. Radiology 133:95 (1979)

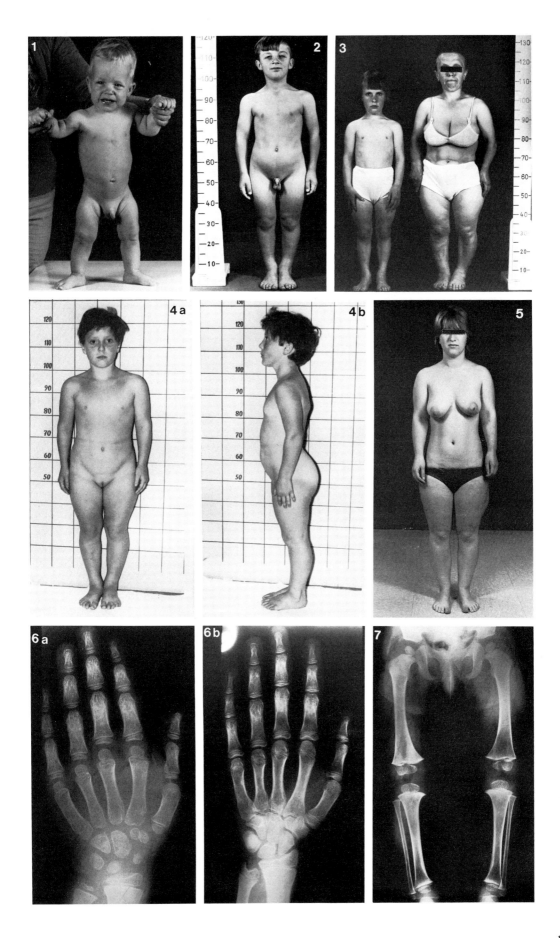

93. Syndrome of Metaphyseal Chondrodysplasia Type Schmid

(Metaphyseal Dysostosis Type Schmid)

An autosomal dominant hereditary syndrome of dwarfism with relatively short legs and crura vara, waddling gait, and a more or less pseudorachitic X-ray appearance of the metaphyses of the long bones.

Main Signs:
1. Short-legged dwarfism with unremarkable cranium, face, and trunk. More or less severely bowed legs (**1a** and **b**). Waddling gait. Large joints usually freely mobile. No muscular hypotonia.
2. Radiological shortening of the long bones with more or less rachitic-like changes of the metaphyses (but without mineral depletion) especially within the lower extremities, and here, most marked in the proximal femora. Coxae varae; short femoral necks (**1c**).

Supplementary Findings: Normal blood and urine analyses.

Manifestation: Second year of life.

Aetiology: Autosomal dominant hereditary disorder.

Frequency: Rare.

Course, Prognosis: Favourable. Even though the varus deformity of the lower extremities usually persists, joint function is generally normal. Adult height between about 1.30 and 1.60 m.

Differential Diagnosis: Syndrome of hereditary vitamin D-resistant rickets and other forms of rickets; here the corresponding biochemical abnormalities. Cartilage-hair hypoplasia: p.188.

Treatment: After closure of the epiphyses, osteotomy to correct the bowed legs. Vitamin D treatment contraindicated. Genetic counselling.

Illustrations:
1a–c   A child at 1 year (**a** and **c**) and 10 years. Micromelic dwarfism; crura vara; swelling of some joint regions. X-rays show broad, dense metaphyses with irregular borders; detached epiphyseal ossification centres of normal configuration.

Reference:
Spranger J.W., Langer L.O., jr, Wiedemann H.-R.: Bone Dysplasias. An Atlas of Constitutional Disorders of Skeletal Development. Stuttgart and Philadelphia, G. Fischer and W.B. Saunders 1974

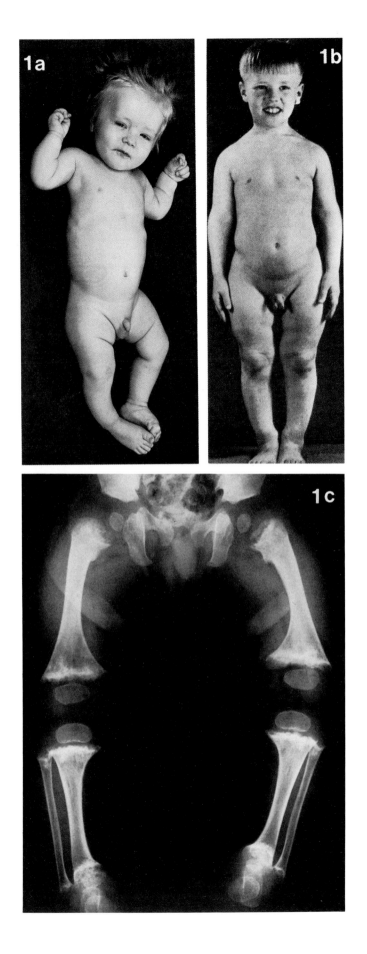

187

94. Syndrome of Cartilage-Hair Hypoplasia

(Syndrome of Metaphyseal Chondrodysplasia Type McKusick)

A hereditary syndrome, quite characteristic when fully expressed, comprising short-limbed dwarfism; fine, sparse hair; and short, stubby hands and feet.

Main Signs:
1. Dwarfism of the micromelic type with unremarkable cranium and facial configuration (**1a** and **b**).
2. Short, stubby hands and feet (**1a**) with hyperextensible wrist, ankle, and finger joints.
3. Sparse, fine, light, relatively brittle scalp hair; possibly also similar characteristics of the eyebrows, eyelashes, beard, and body hair.

Supplementary Findings: Possible moderately severe deformity of the thorax. Narrow pelvis. Slightly bowed legs (crura vara). Limited extension of the elbow joints. Short and possibly brittle finger- and toenails.

Radiologically, shortened tubular bones with metaphyseal dysplasia (**1c**), the metaphyseal irregularities generally seen more distinctly in the knee than in the proximal femora. Disproportionately long fibulae, especially distally.

Possible signs of malabsorption in early childhood (tending to improve spontaneously); also Hirschsprung's disease. Patients may show decreased resistance to viral infections.

Manifestation: Usually at birth.

Aetiology: Autosomal recessive hereditary disorder; very variable expressivity.

Frequency: Rare (apart from special isolates with inbreeding).

Course, Prognosis: Limited vitality and a decreased average lifespan have been noted. Adult height between about 1.10 and 1.45 m. Caesarian section because of narrow pelvis with pregnancy.

Differential Diagnosis: Metaphyseal chondrodysplasia type Schmid (p.186) does not show correspondingly short stubby hands and feet (and nail changes), but does show pronounced crura vara and on X-ray, more severe metaphyseal changes in the proximal femoral than in the knee joint areas; coxae varae; other mode of inheritance.

All forms of rickets can be clinically eliminated in the face of the fully expressed syndrome; in addition, they are easily ruled out biochemically.

Treatment: Avoidance of small pox vaccination and, as far as possible, of exposure to varicella. Genetic counselling.

Illustrations:
1a–d A now 23-year-old patient with the full picture of the cartilage-hair hypoplasia syndrome. Small size since birth; height now 130 cm. Short broad hands with short nails. Scalp hair short, brittle, thin, sparse, blond. Secondary hair growth scanty. Hyperextensible wrists; limited extension of the elbows.
1c Moderately severe metaphyseal irregularities of the knee at age 8 years.
1d The same joint at age 23 years. Each showing hypoplasia of the lateral portions of the femoral epiphysis.

References:
Wiedemann H.-R., Spranger J., Kosenow W.: Knorpel-Haar-Hypoplasie. Arch. Kinderheilkd. *176*:74 (1967)
Spranger J. W., Langer L. O., jr, Wiedemann H.-R.: Bone Dysplasias. An Atlas of Constitutional Disorders of Skeletal Development, Stuttgart and Philadelphia, G. Fischer and W. B. Saunders 1974

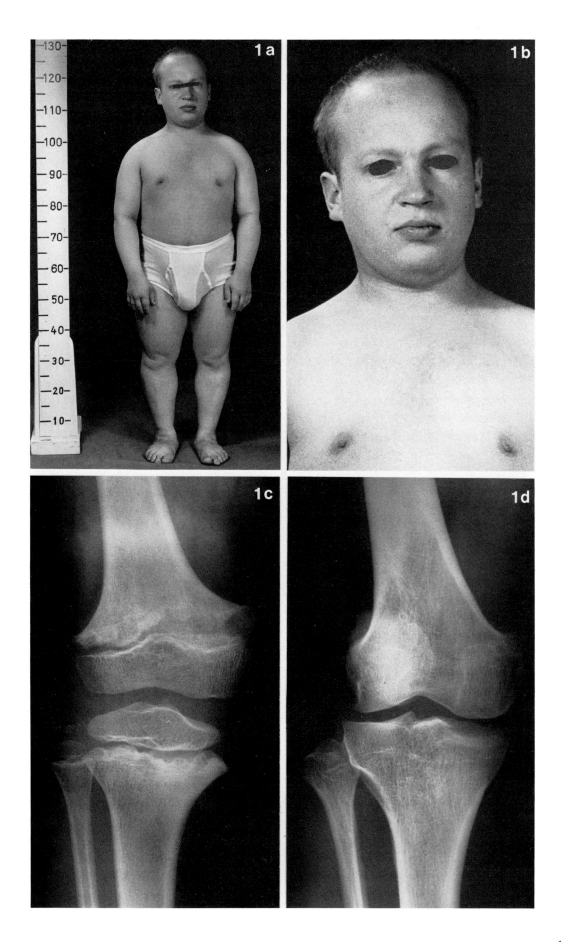

189

95. Metaphyseal Chondrodysplasia Type Wiedemann–Spranger

A congenital skeletal dysplasia with micromelic growth deficiency during the first decade of life, a more or less pseudorachitic X-ray appearance of the metaphyses of the long bones, a somewhat unusual appearance, and a good prognosis.

Main Signs:
1. Congenital disproportionate small size due to shortening especially of the proximal extremities and crura vara. Short neck (1). Limited motion of the hip joints; initially, swelling around the knee joints, wrists, and ankles.
2. Antimongoloid slant of the palpebral fissures (1 and 2).
3. Radiologically marked pseudorachitic structural anomalies of the metaphyses of the long bones (3 and 7) and on lateral view, deformities of the vertebral bodies in part suggesting a horizontal hourglass (5).
4. Gradual improvement of proportions (to yield an unremarkable neck, straightening of the legs, extensive compensation of the initial X-ray changes, 2, 4, 6, and 8) as well as catch-up growth.

Supplementary Findings: Hypermobility of the shoulders and wrists. Unremarkable slender hands and feet.

Frequent lumbar lordosis.

Slight delay in motor development, initially with a pronounced waddling gait.

No characteristic metabolic abnormalities.

Manifestation: Birth.

Aetiology: Little doubt of a genetic basis; mode of transmission uncertain.

Frequency: Probably low.

Course, Prognosis: Favourable. Height extensively compensated. No basis for decreased life expectancy.

Differential Diagnosis: Other metaphyseal chondrodysplasias (e.g., of type Schmid, p.186), which, however, are easily excluded because they are usually manifested later.

Treatment: Symptomatic.

Illustrations:
1–8 The 1st child of healthy, tall and well-proportioned, possibly consanguineous parents, birth about 6 weeks prematurely with *41* cm, 2000 g (3 and 7 at 5 months, 1 at 10 months, and 5 at 13 months; 4 and 8 at 13 years and 2 and 6 at almost 18 years). Gradual compensation of the growth deficiency during his early school years; attainment of 1.66 m adult height.

References:
Wiedemann H.-R., Spranger J.: Chondrodysplasia metaphysaria (Dysostosis metaphysaria) – ein neuer Typ? Z. Kinderheilkd. *108*:171 (1970)
Several similar observations have been made known to the first author in the meantime (Maroteaux and others)

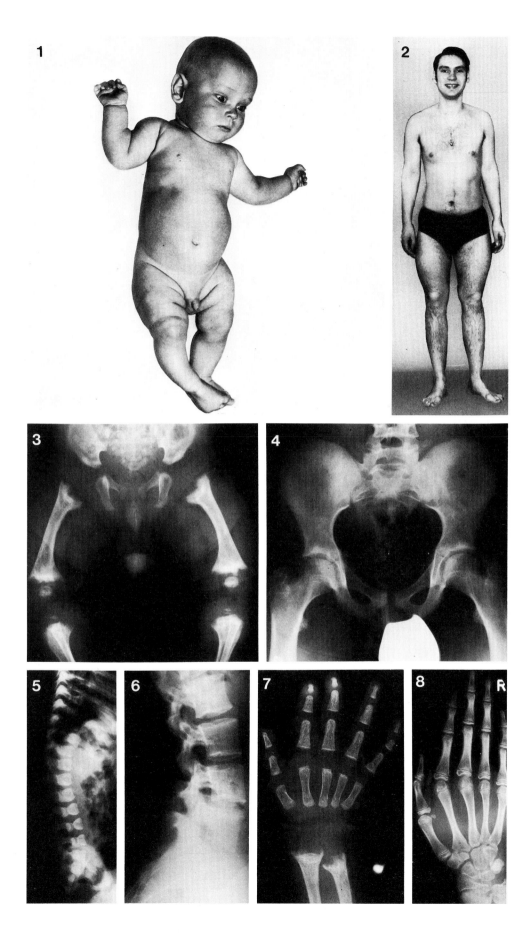

96. Pseudoachondroplasia Syndrome

In appearance, an achondroplasia-like growth deficiency or nanism, but of postnatal manifestation, with normal cranium and facial bones and with a marked disorder of epiphyseal ossification on X-rays.

Main Signs: Short-limbed dwarfism with disproportionately long trunk. Cranial and facial parts of the skull unremarkable. Lumbar hyperlordosis. Genua valga or bowed legs. Hypermobility of more or less all joints except for the elbow (and possibly the hip and knee) joints (1–3).

Supplementary Findings: Weakness of joint capsules and ligaments. Not infrequently development of scoliosis.

Normal mental development.

Radiological changes of the vertebral bodies, severe developmental defects of the femoral capital and other epimetaphyseal areas (4 and 5).

Manifestation: After the first year of life (second year of life or later) with the onset of a waddling gait and growth retardation (and the corresponding X-ray changes).

Aetiology: Monogenic hereditary disorder in a severe and also a mild form. Heterogeneity. The majority of the cases probably represent autosomal dominant new mutations.

Frequency: Not so rare.

Course, Prognosis: Normal life expectancy. Adult height between 0.90 and 1.40 m. Early development of arthroses, especially of the hip and knee joints.

Differential Diagnosis: Achondroplasia (p.164); congenital manifestation, abnormal cranial configuration, etc.); spondyloepiphyseal dysplasia congenita (p.174; congenital manifestation); hypochondroplasia (p.184).

Treatment: Symptomatic–orthopaedic. Corrective surgery of bowed legs toward the end of the growth period. Sooner or later, possible arthroplasties. Psychological guidance with the best possible vocational training. Genetic counselling.

Illustrations:
1   A 14-year-old boy.
2 and 3   Girls of about the same age. Height of the children well below the 3rd percentile (height difference from the average for age: for the girl in 3, about 40 cm; for the child in 1, about 70 cm). The boy in 1 was normally proportioned as an infant and walked without support at 9 months. Manifestation at about 2 years.
4 and 5   X-rays of the child in 3.

References:
Kopits S. E., Lindstrom J. A., McKusick V. A.: Pseudoachondroplastic dysplasia: pathodynamics and management. Birth Defects 10/12:341 (1974)
Spranger J. W., Langer L. O., jr, Wiedemann H.-R.: Bone Dysplasias. An Atlas of Constitutional Disorders of Skeletal Development. Stuttgart and Philadelphia, G. Fischer and W. B. Saunders, 1974
Hall J.: Pseudoachondroplasia. Birth Defects 11/6:187 (1975)
Heselson N. G., Cremin B. J., Beighton P.: Pseudoachondroplasia, a report of 13 cases. Br. J. Radiol 50:473 (1977)
Maroteaux. P.: Stanescu R., Stanescu V., et al: The mild form of pseudoachondroplasia. Eur. J. Pediatr. 133:227 (1980)
Horton W. A., Hall J. G., Scott Ch. I., et al: Growth curves for height for diastrophic dysplasia, spondyloepiphyseal dysplasia congenita, and pseudoachondroplasia. Am. J. Dis. Child. 136:316 (1982)

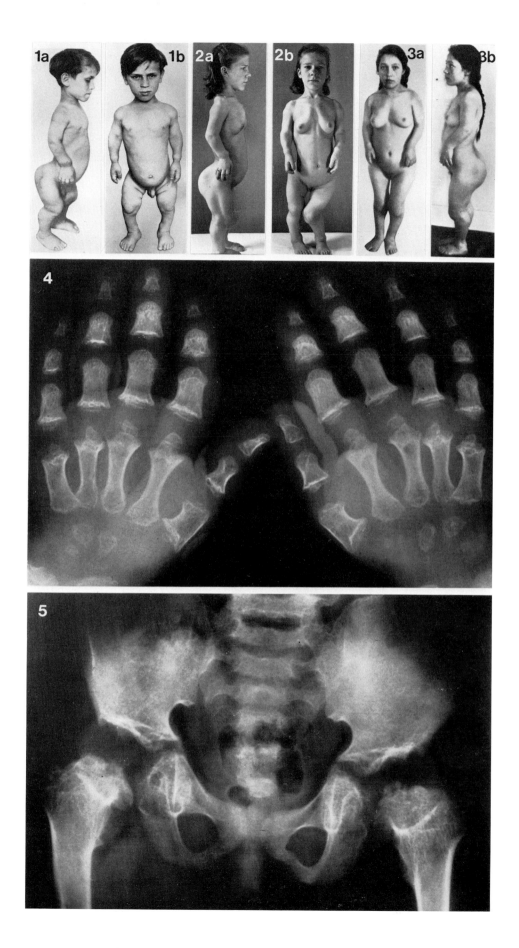

97. Syndrome of Progeria

(Hutchinson–Gilford Syndrome)

A highly characteristic syndrome of dwarfism and the appearance of premature (child-like) corporal 'senescence'.

Main Signs:
1. Growth deficiency manifest after the 1st year of life.
2. Concomitant, increasing 'senescence': loss of hair (3–5), of subcutaneous fat – including that of the auricles (7 and 8), of the normal thickness and elasticity of the skin; flexion contractures of the large joints (1 and 6) and of the finger joints; dystrophy of the nails (9); prominence of the scalp veins (4/5 and 7/8); development of a sharp, beaklike nose jutting out from the small face with receding chin, slightly protruding eyes, and (only relatively) large cranium, defining a 'bird face' (1 and 7); protruding abdomen.

Supplementary Findings: Possible skin changes of a diffuse scleroderma.

Radiologically, hypoplastic skeleton with persistence of the anterior fontanelle, wasting of the lateral portions of the clavicles and of the terminal phalanges (acromicria, 10); coxae valgae.

Teething anomalies.

Absence or delay of sexual development (1 and 6).

Possible hyperlipidaemia and -lipoproteinaemia.

Aetiology: Genetically determined syndrome, possibly autosomal recessive mode of inheritance.

Frequency: Very rare: roughly 1 case in about 250 000 live births. Up to 1980, about 75 observations had been reported (3 in Germany).

Course, Prognosis: Regularly premature development of atherosclerosis. Death usually in the 2nd decade of life as a result of arteriosclerotic complications (coronary occlusion).

Diagnosis, Differential Diagnosis: Easy to recognise in the fully developed clinical picture. Exclusion of the Cockayne (p.108), the Hallermann–Streiff–François (p.402), the connatal cutis laxa (p.198), and the Wiedemann–Rautenstrauch syndromes (p.196) should not cause any particular difficulties.

Treatment: Symptomatic the only possible (psychological guidance; possible wig, etc.).

Illustrations:
1 Progeria in a 17-year-old, from H. Gilford (1897/1904).
2–10 A German child at 10 months (2), 1½ years (3; growth deficiency, loss of hair), 3½ and 7½ years (4 and 5), and 14½ years (6–10). 6, Height of a 7-year-old, no signs of sexual maturation; tense, thin, yellow-brown, spotted, hyperpigmented skin; sclerosed A. radialis; calcification of one of the heart valves; cardiac death at 15¾ years.

References:
Wiedemann H.-R.: Syndrome mit besonderem 'Altersaspekt': Progeria (Hutchinson–Gilford–Syndrom). Handbuch der Kinderheilkunde, Bd 1, Teil 1, p.828ff, Heidelberg, Springer 1971
De Busk F.L.: The Hutchinson–Gilford progeria syndrome. J. Pediatr. 80:697 (1972)
Brown W.T., Darlington Gr.J., Arnold A., et al: Detection of HLA antigens on progeria syndrome fibroblasts. Clin. Genet. 17:213 (1980)

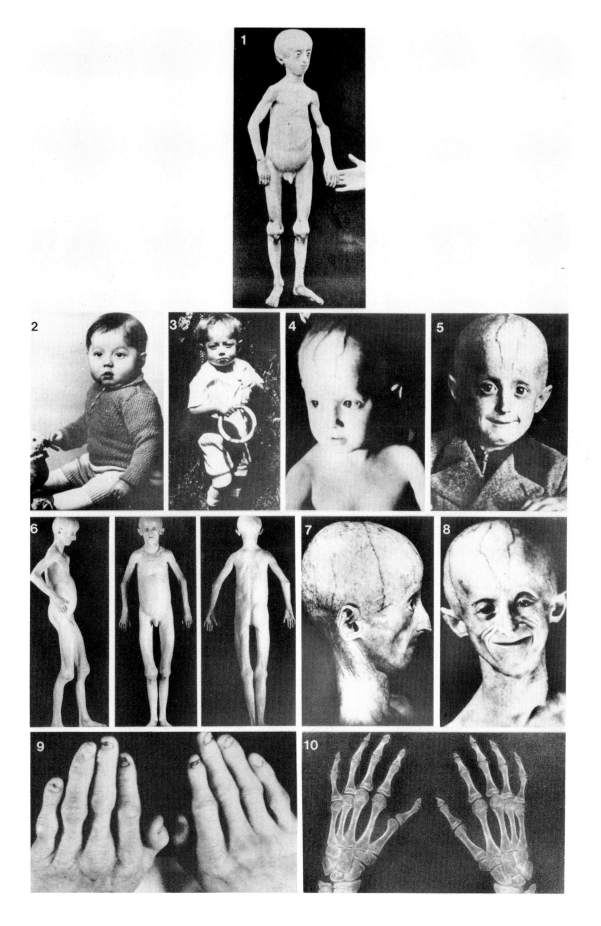

98. Congenital Pseudohydrocephalic Progeroid Syndrome

(Neonatal Progeroid Syndrome, Wiedemann–Rautenstrauch Syndrome)

A hereditary syndrome manifested at birth as pseudohydrocephalus, small senile-appearing face, 'congenital teeth', and extensive deficiency of adipose tissue.

Main Signs:
1. Along with a small, somewhat triangular-looking, senile-appearing face, a hydrocephaloid cranium with wide-open sutures, persistent anterior fontanelle, prominent venous markings, and more or less sparse hair (1–9). Relatively low-set ears, low-set eyes, scanty eyebrows and eyelashes (possible entropion). Small maxilla, protruding chin; 'congenital' incisors.
2. Striking general deficiency of subcutaneous fatty tissue, apart from the development of paradoxical accumulations of adipose tissue on the buttocks and flanks or in the anogenital area (10–13).

Supplementary Findings: Congenital small size in spite of term birth. Difficulties in rearing. Retarded growth and development.

Progressive development of a beak-like nose in infancy (4–6).

Delayed statomotor development. Mental development more or less severely impaired, but also possibly within normal limits.

Manifestation: Birth.

Aetiology: Hereditary defect, presumably autosomal recessive.

Frequency: Extremely rare; to date 5 cases have been published, a few further cases presumably of this syndrome are known to the authors.

Course, Prognosis: In part dependent on the presence and severity of mental retardation. Long-term observations are not yet available.

Differential Diagnosis: Primarily the Hallermann–Streiff–François syndrome (p.402) and congenital generalised lipodystrophy (p.202) must be ruled out, which is not difficult clinically. The Hutchinson–Gilford syndrome, the true progeria, is usually not manifest at birth, but develops during the early postnatal period (p.194).

Treatment: Symptomatic.

Illustrations:
1–3 Three different children, all a few weeks of age.
4–6 The development of a somewhat beak-like nose (4 and 5, the same child at 6 weeks and 8 months).
7–9 Three children at 8 months.
10–13 The absence of subcutaneous adipose tissue, with the exception of limited paradoxical caudal deposits of fat; the latter is especially apparent in 13.
(1, 7, 8, and 11 after Rautenstrauch et al – see below.)

References:
Rautenstrauch Th., Snigula Fr., Krieg Th., et al: Progeria: A cell culture study and clinical report of familial incidence. Eur. J. Pediatr. *124*:101 (1977)
Wiedemann H.-R.: An unidentified neonatal progeroid syndrome: Follow-up report. Eur. J. Pediatr. *130*:65 (1979)
Devos E. A., Leroy J. G., Fryns J. P., et al: The Wiedemann-Rautenstrauch or neonatal progeroid syndrome. Eur. J. Pediatr. *136*:245 (1981)
Snigula Fr., Rautenstrauch Th.: A new neonatal progeroid syndrome. Eur. J. Pediatr. *136*:325 (1981)

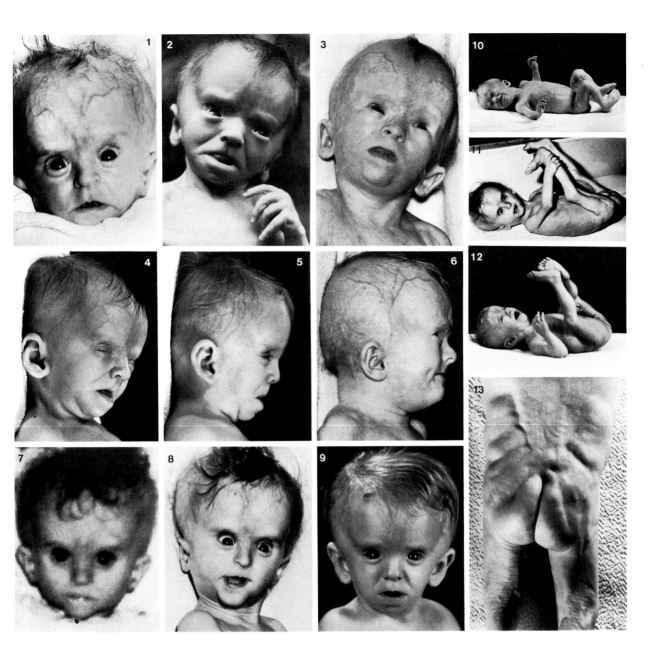

99. Connatal Cutis Laxa Syndrome

(Dermatochalasis Connata)

A hereditary syndrome of congenital cutis laxa with corresponding 'aged appearance' and optional further, more or less numerous defects.

Main Signs: Generalised cutis laxa; soft, loose, pendulous, wrinkled skin (1–3) which – especially on the face – may give the impression of premature ageing, even senescence (3a), and may appear grotesque.

Supplementary Findings: Depending on the biological type (see below), congenital small size, postnatal delay in growth and general development, deficient subcutaneous adipose tissue, and muscular weakness, Hypertelorism (3a), microgenia (1c) as well as other skeletal dysmorphisms and deformities, delayed closure of the fontanelles, luxatio coxarum, general hyperextensibility of the joints and tendency to luxation. Internal changes may include laxity of the vocal cords, emphysema of the lungs, vascular wall aneurysms and vascular stenoses, multiple gastrointestinal diverticula, hernias, and prolapses. Thus, laxity of the skin may be only one, external sign of a systemic mesenchymal disorder.

Manifestation: Birth.

Aetiology: The syndrome (a still poorly understood 'potpourri') comprises a number of monogenic hereditary disorders; thus, heterogeneity. Probably several autosomal recessive hereditary types of different expression and course, a – more favourable – autosomal dominant type, and probably also X-chromosomal biological types.

Formal Pathogenesis: Histologically, deficiencies of elastic fibres have been demonstrated repeatedly, in part as more or less generalised elastolysis (degeneration and decomposition). In many cases demonstration of defects of (different) enzymes or enzyme inhibitors or copper metabolism, with the basic defects still unknown.

Frequency: Low. About a hundred reports in the literature.

Course, Prognosis: Dependent on the type. Potentially early lethal course especially with the recessive types (e.g., as a result of cor pulmonale).

Differential Diagnosis: The Ehlers–Danlos syndrome (p.272) with cutis hyperelastica can be readily excluded.

Treatment: Whether to use cosmetic plastic surgery in mild forms of the disorder should be considered very carefully. Genetic counselling.

Illustrations:
1–3   A congenitally undersized 6-year-old boy (his first-born brother died post partum with the identical clinical picture). Growth deficiency of about 15%; markedly delayed closure of the fontanelles; luxatio coxarum bilaterally, general ligament, capsule, and muscle weakness with further luxations. Hypoplasia of the iris, tortuous fundic vessels. Sudden death at age 7 years.

References:
Wiedemann H.-R.: Über einige progeroide Krankheitsbilder und deren diagnostische Einordnung. Z. Kinderheilkd. *107*:91 (1969)
Beighton P.: Cutis laxa. A heterogeneous disorder. Birth Defects. *10*:126 (1974)
Wilsch L., Schmid G., Haneke E.: Spätmanifeste Dermatochalasis. Dtsch. med. Wochenschr. *102*:1451 (1977)
Agha A., Sakati N. O., et al: Two forms of cutis laxa presenting in the newborn period. Acta Paed. Scand. *67*:775 (1978)

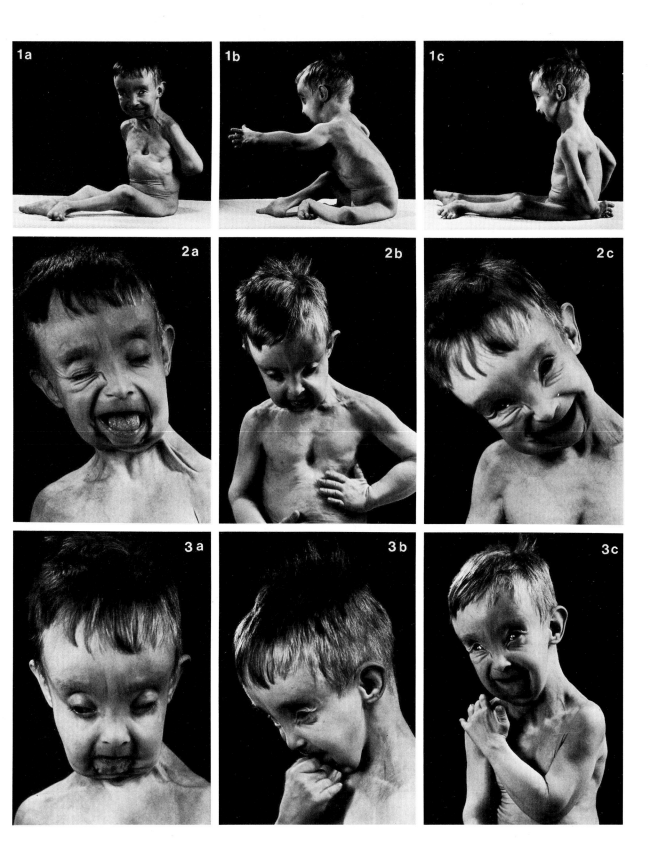

100. An Obscure Progeroid Syndrome with Cardiac Anomaly

A syndrome of 'too old' appearance, generalised leanness, scanty hair growth, peculiarities of the joints, cardiovascular anomalies, and retarded maturation.

Main Signs:

1. Narrow face, appearing generally 'too old', with hypotelorism; short palpebral fissures; deep-set eyes; protruding, narrow, and slightly aquiline nose; prominent ears; high palate; and (initial, pronounced) microretrognathia inf. (**1–3, 5,** and **6**). Dimple on the chin (**2** and **5**).

2. Premature closure of the fontanelles and continuing small size of the cranium (at 14 years 52.5 cm). Mental development normal for age.

3. Extremely scanty development of scalp hair, eyebrows, and eyelashes during infancy (**1–3**). Subsequently also, relatively thin and delicate hair growth, and at 14 years barely incipient growth of secondary hair and deficiency of other signs of maturity (**4–6**).

4. Generally extremely little development of subcutaneous fatty tissue and musculature (weight of this 1.60 m tall, and therefore of normal height, 14-year-boy only 35 kg).

5. Since birth, knee and elbow joints not fully extensible; other large joints hyperextensible. Unusually long fingers and toes, especially in infancy (**7** and **8**), with 'acrogeria' (**7–9**); at 14 years, slight flexion contractures of the distally tapered distal phalanges. Asymmetrically elevated shoulders with prominent shoulder blades; increased thoracic kyphosis. Dimples over most of the large joints.

6. Cardiac anomaly (ventricular septal defect, subvalvular pulmonary stenosis – both corrected surgically at 14 years – pulmonary vascular anomalies); there was no decrease of maximum physical performance.

Supplementary Findings: Ophthalmological examination negative.

Radiologically no skeletal malformations; slight delay of ossification.

Laboratory analyses negative. Karyotype 44 + XY. Unilateral cryptorchidism.

Manifestation: Birth.

Aetiology: Unknown.

Course, Prognosis: Apparently favourable.

Differential Diagnosis: Many similarities with the observation of Ruvalcaba et al (see below) are noted; however, here the progeroid manifestations occurred considerably later.

Treatment: Symptomatic.

Illustrations:

1–9 The 2nd child of young, healthy, apparently nonconsanguineous parents (1st child unremarkable). Pregnancy normal, birth at term with normal measurements. **1, 3, 7,** and **8** show the proband at age 6 months, the remaining at 14 years. In **2** the remainder of an ossified cephalohaematoma on the left.

Reference:
Ruvalcaba R. H. A., Churesigaew S., Myhre S. A., et al: Children who age rapidly – Progeroid syndromes. Clin. Pediatr. *16*:248 (1977)

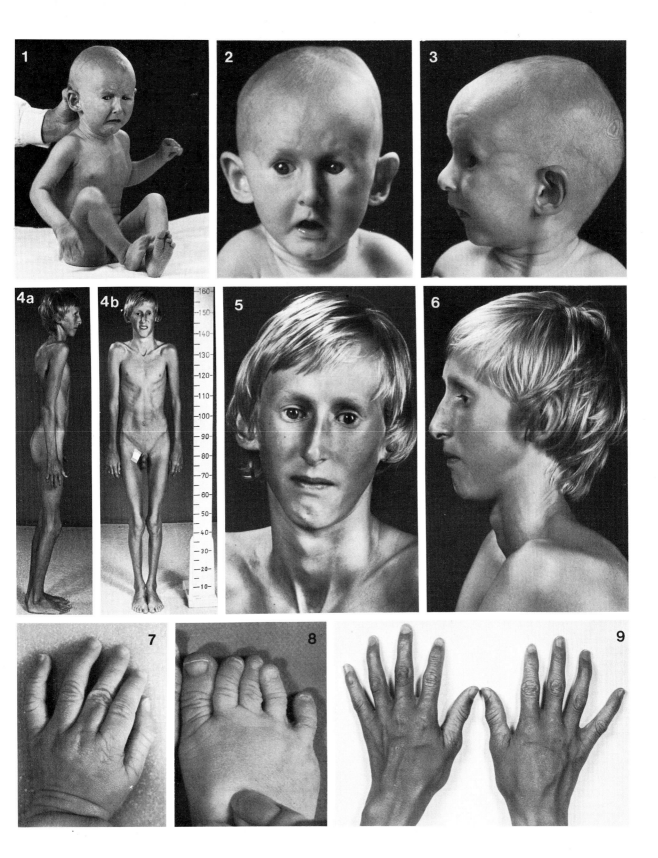

101. Syndrome of Congenital Generalised Lipodystrophy

(Berardinelli–Seip Syndrome)

A hereditary disorder with generalised deficiency of adipose tissue beginning at an early age, muscular hypertrophy, 'gigantism', acromegaly, encephalopathy, and other anomalies.

Main Signs:
1. Generalised lipoatrophy (**1** and **2**).
2. Muscular hypertrophy, which may lend a more or less athletic appearance in childhood.
3. Hyperpigmentation, acanthosis nigricans; overabundant, curly scalp hair (**2**) or general hypertrichosis; dilated cutaneous veins (**1b** and **2b**).
4. Congenital excessive length or macrosomia or several years of postnatal gigantism. Acromegalic facial dysmorphism, relatively large auricles, abnormally large hands and feet (**1b** and **2b**) as well as possible hypertrophy of the penis or clitoris.
5. 'Encephalopathy' of a non-progressive nature with about half of the cases showing mental retardation (mild to severe) associated with regularly demonstrable partial dilation of the cerebral ventricles or cisterns.

Supplementary Findings: Usually hepatomegaly (fatty liver), frequently also cardiomegaly, nephromegaly.

The postnatal gigantism is accompanied by corresponding acceleration of ossification and dentition.

Elevated basal metabolic rate. Disorders of carbohydrate and fat metabolism; extreme insulin resistance, hyperlipaemia.

Development of a nonketotic diabetes mellitus lipoatrophy (approximately after the beginning of the 2nd decade of life).

Manifestation: Birth and thereafter.

Aetiology: Autosomal recessive inherited disorder (the effect assumed to be mediated by hypothalamic dysfunction).

Frequency: Rare; from 1954 to 1968, somewhat over 40 observations were described in the literature.

Course, Prognosis: Premature closure of the epiphyses; normal adult height. Onset of puberty at approximately the expected age. Prognosis clouded, especially with regard to the diabetogenous vascular complications.

Differential Diagnosis: Acquired generalised lipodystrophy, partial lipodystrophies.

Treatment: Symptomatic, including psychological guidance and possible cosmetic measures. Genetic counselling.

Illustrations:
1 and 2 Typically affected siblings (1¼ and 6 years old). Considerably too large – the 6-year-old showing the bone age of a 12-year-old; hepatomegaly in both children; enlargement of the 3rd ventricle and of the basal cisterns, respectively, on pneumoencephalograms.
(By kind permission of Prof. M. Seip, Oslo.)

References:
Seip M.: Generalised lipodystrophy. Ergeb. Inn. Med. Kinderheilkd. N. F. *31*:59 (1971)
Wiedemann H.-R.: Dienzephale Syndrome des Kindesalters. Pädiat. Prax. *11*:95 (1972)

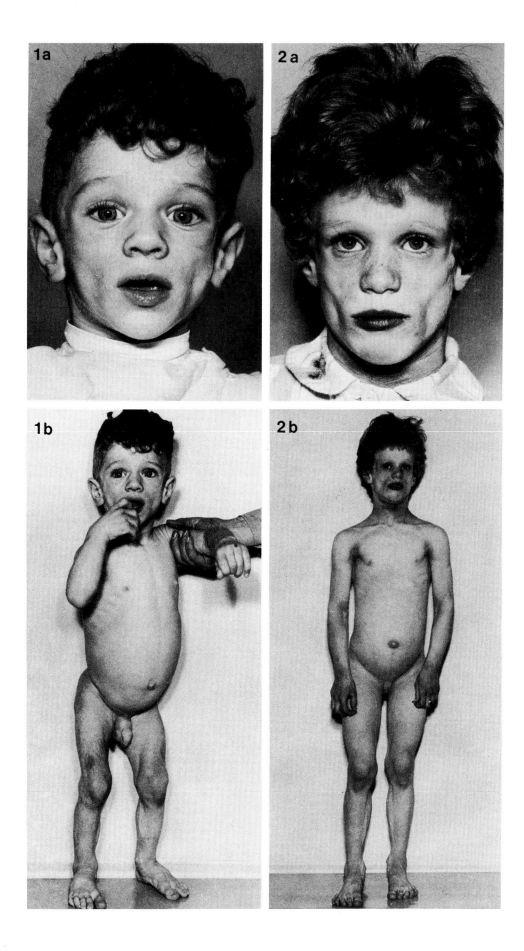

102. Syndrome of a Partial Lipodystrophy Combined with Juvenile Diabetes Mellitus in Monozygotic Twin Brothers

A lipodystrophy beginning in the lower extremities and following in the upper extremities or face, associated with juvenile diabetes mellitus.

Main Signs:
1. Lipoatrophy of insidious onset in the 2nd or 3rd year of life (child in **1** = proband I) and in the 4th year of life (child in **2** = proband II), affecting the right foot and lower leg beginning distally in proband I, and both feet, lower legs, and lower areas of the thighs, beginning distally in proband II. In the meantime, advanced lipoatrophy of the thighs of proband II and new areas of lipoatrophy on both hands, the distal half of both forearms, and in the buccal areas bilaterally (right side more than the left; disfiguring severity). Perhaps corresponding onset in the buccal area in proband I.
2. Insulin-dependent, well-controlled diabetes mellitus in both children (manifest in proband I at 3½ years, in proband II at 13 months with pre-coma).

Supplementary Findings: In the regions devoid of fat, thin skin with very prominent veins (**1** and **2**).

Normal musculature.

In part, the lipoatrophy is directly preceded by 'transient itchy flushing of the skin' as well as painless nodular indurations of the tissue.

Differentiating laboratory findings in the children. In proband II, in conformity with the greater acuteness of the process, considerable increase of the gamma globulins and of the IgG; C_3 complement elevated.

Manifestation: Early childhood.

Aetiology: Not settled. Genetic basis assumed since the affected are monozygotic twins. More exact nature of the process still open.

Comment: Highly unusual course for a lipodystrophy; the combination with juvenile diabetes mellitus is just as unusual.

Course, Prognosis: Further progression of the lipoatrophy must be expected.

Differential Diagnosis: Other forms of lipodystrophy.

Treatment: Only symptomatic possible (including immunosuppression).

Illustrations:
1 and 2 Four-year-old monozygotic twin brothers, normally developed for their age, in whom subjective well being is unaffected; no further internal or neurological findings. No acceleration of growth in height, ossification, or dentition. These are the 2nd and 3rd children of young, healthy, nonconsanguineous parents; a 16-year-old brother of the father has been affected with insulin-dependent diabetes mellitus since his 12th year of life.
(By kind permission of Prof. J. Schaub, Kiel.)

Reference:
Peters M. S., Winkelmann R. K.: Localised lipoatrophy (atrophic connective tissue disease panniculitis). Arch. Dermatol. *116*:1363 (1980)

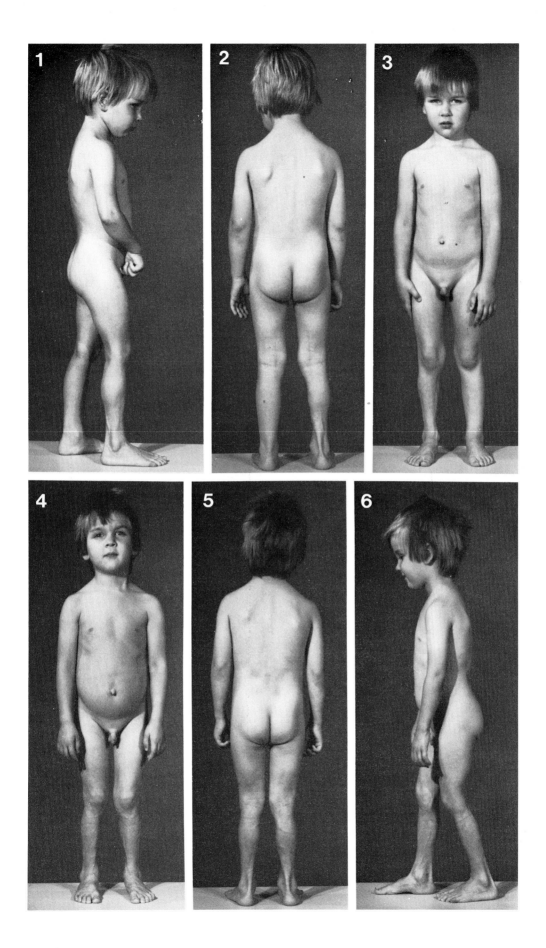

103. Diencephalic Syndrome of Infancy

(Russell)

A syndrome of severe wasting of fatty tissue, pseudoanaemic pallor, good food intake with vomiting, feeling of well-being to euphoria, and active, lively to hyperactive behaviour.

Main Signs:
1. Progressive emaciation (**1**) in spite of good food intake.
2. Unaffected cheerfulness to euphoria.
3. Increased liveliness to hyperactivity.
4. Emesis (occasionally or frequently). Marked pallor without anaemia.
5. Nystagmus (in 50%).

Supplementary Findings: Excitability, tremor, sweats.
Possible accelerated growth with acromegalic features (hands, feet, genitalia) (**1a**).
Characteristically, definite neurological signs tend to be absent for a long time.

Manifestation: From early infancy up to the end of the 2nd year of life (rarely later).

Aetiology: Often a slowly growing glioma in the anterior hypothalamus.

Frequency: Rare. About 80 cases described in the literature.

Course, Prognosis: To a great extent dependent on the time recognised and on the treatment (see below).
Average survival of untreated cases from the time of manifestation, about 12 months.

Diagnosis: In suspected cases CCT, and in some cases further neuroradiological studies as well as CSF protein determination and cytology.

Treatment: In some cases surgery and/or cobalt irradiation (on the average effecting considerable prolongation of life).

Illustrations:
1a–c A 2-year-old boy with 'diencephalic lipodystrophy' of several months duration (3.4 kg underweight in relation to height; dystrophy, 'tobacco-pouch buttocks'). Cranium normal for age (but appearing relatively too large). Large ears, thick protruding lips, large penis, and large feet. Pseudoanaemic pallor. Lively, mobile, friendly behaviour (**1a**). Superficially, neurologically unremarkable. Suspected tumour on brain scintiscan and angiography. Operatively confirmed hypothalamic spongioblastoma.

References:
Wiedemann H.-R.: Diencephale Syndrome des Kindesalters. Pädiatr.Prax. *11*:95 (1972)
Burr I.M., Slonim A.E., Danish R.K., Gadoth N., Butler I.J.: Diencephalic syndrome revisited. J.Pediatr. *88*:439 (1976)
Andler W., Stolecke H., Sirang H.: Endocrine dysfunction in the diencephalic syndrome of emaciation in infancy. Helv.Paediatr.Acta *33*:393 (1978)
Drop SLS., Guyda H.J., Colle E.: Inappropriate growth hormone release in the diencephalic syndrome of childhood: Case report and a 4 year endocrinological follow-up. Clin.Endocrinol. *13*:181 (1980)

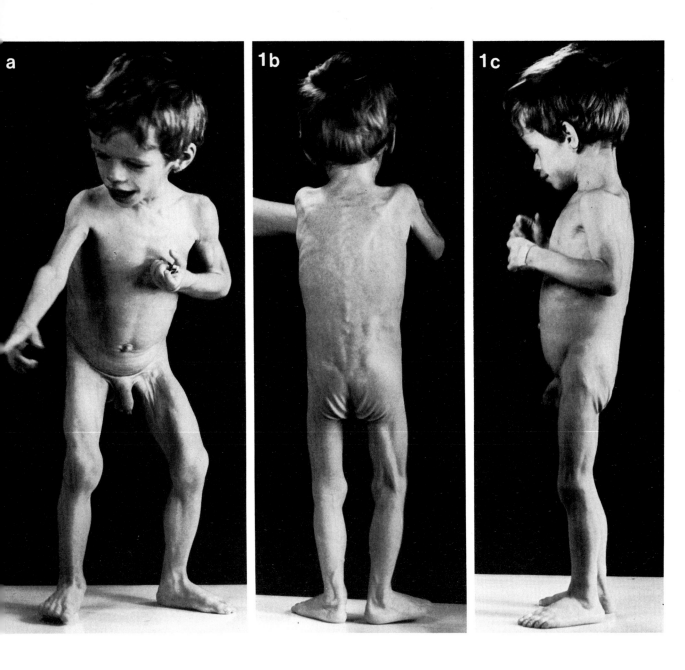

104. Prader–Willi Syndrome

A syndrome of mental retardation, growth deficiency, obesity, and hypogonadism – after initial marked muscular hypotonia in infancy.

Main Signs: Small stature (3–6), increasing obesity, psychomotor retardation (usually imbecility); in boys, hypogenitalism with scrotal hypoplasia and frequent cryptorchidism (3, 5, 6, and 7), in girls labia minora often absent and labia majora underdeveloped; hypogonadism in both sexes.

Supplementary Findings: A relatively narrow forehead, frequent strabismus, possibly almond-shaped eyes and a triangular, open mouth may yield a quite typical facies in the young child. Possible enamel hypoplasia; early severe caries (8 and 9).

Small hands and feet. Very frequently development of kyphoscoliosis.

Development of a diabetic metabolic condition; later (the second decade of life) diabetes mellitus, without tendency to ketosis.

Manifestation: Congenital muscular hypotonia frequently with severe hypokinesia (1 and 2) and respiratory and feeding problems. Gradual improvement of tone after about the second half of the first year of life. Adiposity and growth deficiency manifested after infancy or early childhood.

Aetiology: Probably genetically determined or partly determined syndrome with development via hypothalamic dysfunction. As a rule, sporadic occurrence. A whole series of cases have shown abnormalities of chromosome 15; this finding requires further careful observation.

Frequency: Not at all rare, at least 1:10 000.

Course, Prognosis: Frequent increase in obesity, which can barely be controlled and may reach grotesque proportions. Shortened life expectancy. Often *pubertas tarda et incompleta*; in males, no change of voice. Frequent psychosocial problems in adolescence and adulthood. Infertility.

Diagnosis, Differential Diagnosis: Initially, other forms of muscular atonia (see, e.g., pp.376, 386) must be ruled out. Later, differentiation facilitated by the two-phase course, e.g., a history of congenital muscular atony and initial difficulties with rearing. Thus, e.g., Laurence–Moon–Bardet–Biedl syndrome (here additionally polydactyly, retinitis pigmentosa, p.210) or Frölich adiposogenital dystrophy (here no mental retardation, but progressive cerebral signs) as well as the Cohen syndrome (p.212) are readily eliminated.

Treatment: Limitation of the polyphagia as far as possible, also keeping the disposition to diabetes in mind. In some cases special nursery schools, special schooling, etc.

Illustrations:

1 and 2 A 4-month-old infant with severe muscular hypotonia, adynamia, hypokinesia, and hyporeflexia; weak cry, suck, and swallowing; hypomimia with triangular, open ('fish') mouth; microgenia; psychomotor retardation. (**3** and **7**, same child as **1** at age 5 years.)

3–6 Children of ages 5, 5, 6, and 7 years, all mentally retarded, with short stature, their heights differing from medians for their ages by respectively 6.5, 9, 11, and 24 cm. All three boys have cryptorchidism. Hyperglycaemia of the boy in **6** since age 4 years, manifest diabetes mellitus since his 6th year of life.

8 Same child as in **6**.

References:

Prader A., Labhart A., Willi H.: Ein Syndrome von Adipositas, Kleinwuchs, Kryptorchismus und Oligophrenie nach myatonieartigem Zustand im Neugeborenenalter. Schweiz. Med. Wochenschr. 86:1260 (1956)

Stephenson J. B. P.: Prader–Willi syndrome: Neonatal presentation and later development. Develop. Med. Child Neurol. 22:792 (1980)

Holm V. A., Sulzbacher S., Pipes P.-L. (eds): The Prader–Willi syndrome. Baltimore, University Park Press (1981)

Laurance B. M., Brits B., Wilkinson J.: Prader–Willi syndrome after age 15 years. Arch. Dis. Childh. 56:18 (1981)

Ledbetter D. H., Riccardi V. M., Airhart S. D., et al: Deletions of chromosome 15 as a cause of the Prader–Willi syndrome. N. Engl. J. Med. 304:325 (1981)

Ledbetter D. H., Mascarello J. T., Riccardi V. M., et al: Chromosome 15 abnormalities and the Prader–Willi syndrome: A follow-up report of 40 cases. Am. J. Hum. Genet. 34:278 (1982)

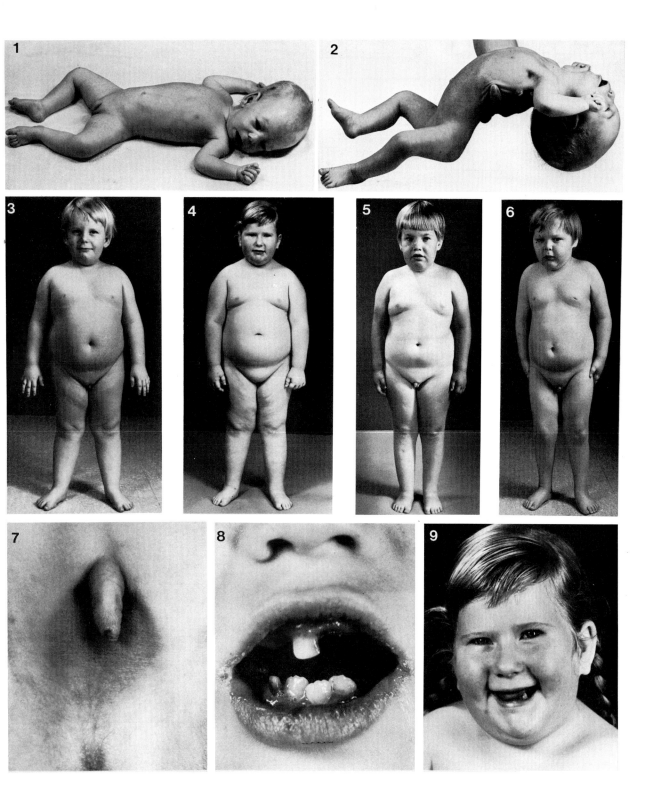

105. Laurence–Moon–Bardet–Biedl Syndrome

(Laurence–Moon Syndrome)

A hereditary syndrome of polydactyly, hypogenitalism, obesity, impaired vision, and mental retardation.

Main Signs:
1. Obesity, usually from the 3rd/4th year of life on, frequently increasing (1).
2. Hypogenitalism (with normal and low gonadotropin levels). Small genitalia (4), testes undescended, bifid scrotum, hypospadias. Little or no development of the secondary sex characteristics, amenorrhoea.
3. Distinct mental retardation. Occasionally impaired hearing and neurological abnormalities.
4. Ulnar or fibular polydactyly, varying between rudimentary appendages and functioning 6th fingers or toes (2 and 3), preferentially on the feet. (All in all not a very constant anomaly.)

Supplementary Findings: Growth deficiency, usually moderate.

Retinitis pigmentosa (or also sine pigmento) as the most constant sign; optic atrophy, occasionally cataract, microphthalmos, coloboma of the iris; myopia.

Possible urinary tract abnormalities, nephropathy and uraemia; also congenital cardiac abnormality.

Manifestation: Hexadactyly from birth, retinitis pigmentosa and obesity in early childhood, hypogenitalism from birth on.

Aetiology: Autosomal recessive hereditary disorder with markedly varied expressivity, even within a family.

Frequency: Less than 1:160 000.

Course, Prognosis: Determined by the severity of mental retardation and the progression of the retinitis. In one study, threequarters of the patients were blind by age 20.

Differential Diagnosis: Prader–Willi syndrome (p.208; no retinitis, no polydactyly).

Treatment: Symptomatic. Genetic counselling.

Illustrations:
1–4   A 7-year-old boy. Overweight since infancy. Debility. Retinitis pigmentosa.

References:
Bauman M.L., Hogan G.R.: Laurence–Moon–Biedl syndrome. Am.J.Dis.Child. *126*:119 (1973)
Hurley R.M., Dery P., Nogrady M.B., et al: The renal lesion of the Laurence–Moon–Biedl syndrome. J.Pediatr. *87*:206 (1975)
Otherwise any comprehensive internal medicine, neurology, or paediatric textbook.

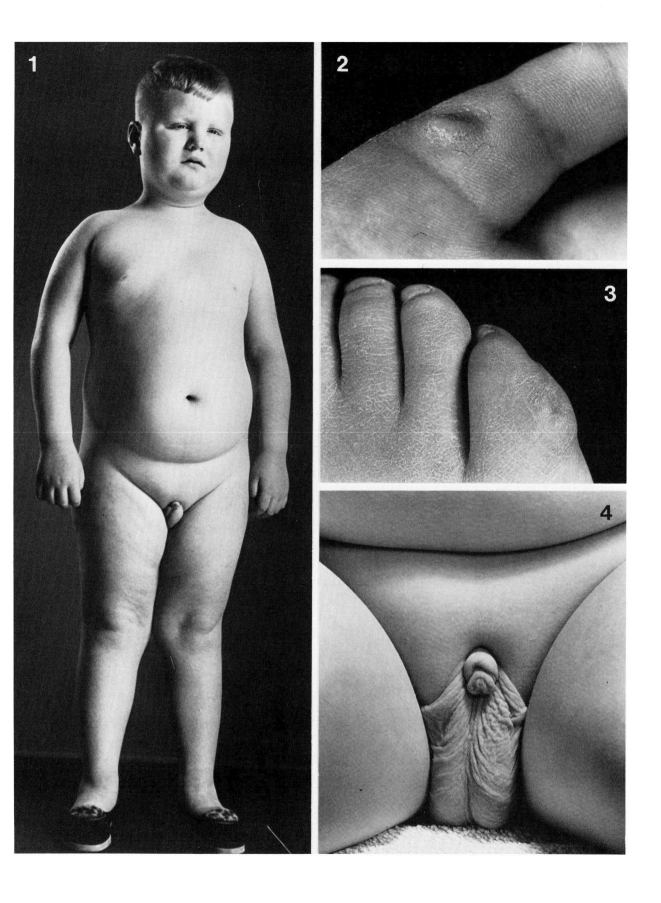

106. Cohen Syndrome

A syndrome of characteristic facies, microcephaly with mental retardation, muscular hypotonia, small stature, obesity, and hand and foot anomalies.

Main Signs:
1. Facies: Broad and prominent nasal root with possible slight antimongoloid slant of the palpebral fissures; more or less prominent large ears; protrusion of the premaxilla, middle incisors, and upper lip with high narrow palate, short philtrum, and open mouth; micrognathia inferior (1–3).
2. Slight microcephaly. Mental retardation (IQ between about 30 and 70).
3. Muscular hypotonia and flabbiness.
4. Short stature.
5. Mild to moderate obesity of the trunk (1).

Supplementary Findings: Hands and feet may be unusually narrow with long slender fingers and toes; possibly also syndactyly, simian crease, and other anomalies.

Possible strabismus, refractive error, among other ocular anomalies.

Possible development of scoliosis, hyperextensibility of joints.

Manifestation: Birth and later. Obesity usually from mid-childhood.

Aetiology: Hereditary defect of variable expression, presumably autosomal recessive.

Frequency: Rare.

Differential Diagnosis: Primarily the Prader–Willi (p.208) and Bardet–Biedl syndromes (p.210).

Treatment: Symptomatic.

Illustrations:
1–3   The 1st and 2nd children of healthy, young, nonconsanguineous parents. The 11-year-old girl and her 10-year-old brother are mildly microcephalic, mentally retarded, short, and obese and show the characteristic facies. Hypotonia in the boy; in the girl, a focal seizure disorder since early childhood.
(By kind permission of Prof. F. Majewski, Düsseldorf.)

References:
Cohen M. M., jr, Hall B. D., Smith D. W., et al: A new syndrome with hypotonia, obesity, mental deficiency, and facial, oral, ocular, and limb anomalies. J. Pediatr. *83*:280 (1973)
Ferré P., Fournet J. P., Courpotin C.: Le syndrome de Cohen... Arch. Fr. Pédiatr. *39*:159 (1982)
Goecke T., Majewski F., Kauther K. D., et al: Mental retardation... (Cohen Syndrome). Eur. J. Pediatr. *138*:338 (1982)

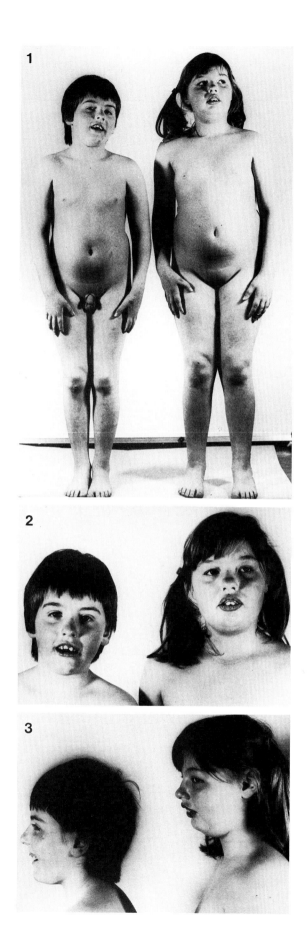

107. Klippel–Feil 'Syndrome'

A malformation complex involving either exclusively or especially the cervical vertebrae, with short neck and possibly disorders of mobility, posture and neurological function.

Main Signs:
1. Short neck (**1a, b**) to 'necklessness', with low posterior hairline. Usually limited motion of the head, painless, especially sidewards (**1a**). Thorax in some cases barrel-shaped, with high, rounded hump. Possible elevation of the shoulders.
2. Radiologically: Block vertebrae for a variable extent of the cervical spine (possibly also wedge-shaped or hemivertebrae or anomalies of the neural arches), in some cases in combination with malformations in lower sections of the vertebral column and with diverse anomalies of the ribs (**2** and **3**).

Supplementary Findings: Possibly more extensive disorders of posture and motion, and irritation or functional disorder of nerves.

Cleft palate.

Occurrence of congenital anomalies of the urogenital tract and of cardiac defects.

Hearing impairment or even deafness not extremely rare.

Manifestation: Birth and later, depending on the severity of the malformations.

Aetiology: Not uniform. Mostly isolated cases. Autosomal dominant occurrence has been observed.

Frequency: Rare (estimation about 1:50 000).

Prognosis: Dependent on the severity of the anatomical defect.

Treatment: For the most part symptomatic–orthopaedic. Early audiometric examination and adequate treatment as required.

Illustrations:
1a and b A 6-month-old infant with short neck, limited mobility of the head sidewards, somewhat barrel-shaped chest; otherwise, normal psychomotor development.
2 AP X-ray of the child showing hemi- and partial block vertebrae formation at the junction of the cervical and thoracic columns and hypoplasia of the upper ribs bilaterally.
3 Lateral X-ray of the cervical vertebrae of a 12-year-old girl with Klippel–Feil syndrome. Extensive block vertebrae with partial inclusion of vertebral arches and spinal processes.

References:
Gunderson C.H., Greenspan R.H., Glaser G.H., Lubs H.A.: The Klippel–Feil syndrome. Genetic and clinical reevaluation of cervical fusion. Medicine 46:491 (1967)
Palant D.I., Carter B.L.: Klippel–Feil syndrome and deafness. Am. J. Dis. Child. *123*:218 (1972)
Helmi C., Pruzansky S.: Craniofacial and extracranial malformations in the Klippel–Feil syndrome. Cleft Palate J. *17*:65 (1980)

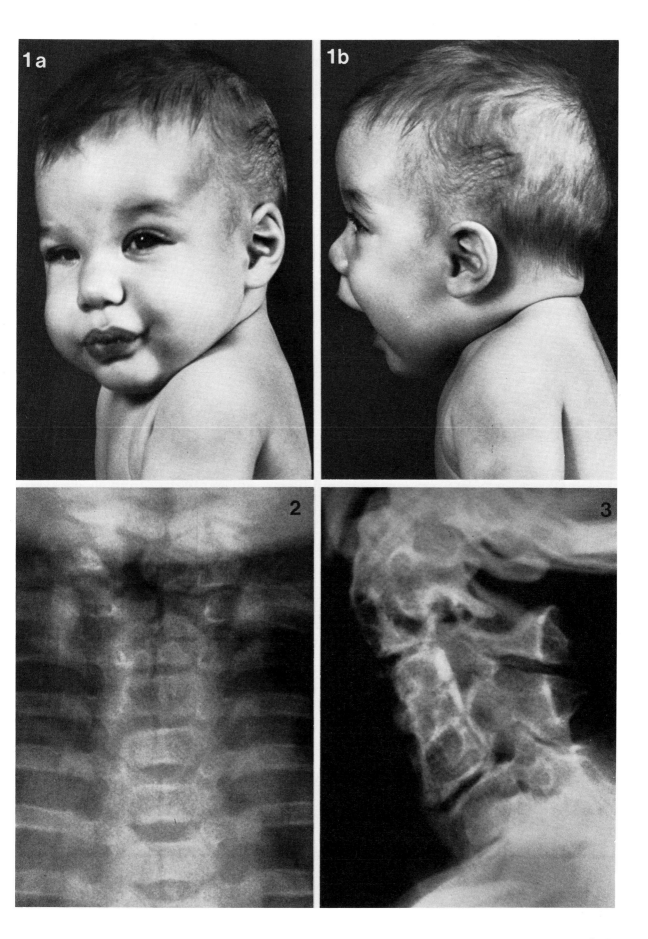

108. Wildervanck Syndrome

(Cervico-oculo-acoustic Syndrome)

A complex of anomalies including short neck, similar to that of 'Klippel–Feil' syndrome (p.214), facial anomalies, and hearing impairment.

Main Signs:
1. Those of the Klippel–Feil syndrome (p.214).
2. In most cases facial asymmetry, possibly with torticollis, uni- or bilateral abducens paralysis and bulbar retraction, hypoplasia of the upper jaw and micrognathia inferior, narrow and possibly cleft palate.
3. Uni- or bilateral moderate to severe sensorineural or conductive hearing impairment. Occurrence of inner and external ear malformations.

Supplementary Findings: Mental retardation may be present. Unilateral epibulbar dermoids may occur.

Manifestation: Birth; hearing impairment possibly later.

Aetiology: Genetic situation not clear. Since the vast majority of those affected are females, sex-linked dominant has been considered, although a multifactorial occurrence has also been discussed.

Frequency: Not so rare.

Course, Prognosis: Life expectancy favourable, after a possibly difficult neonatal course.

Diagnosis, Differential Diagnosis: Exclusion of the Goldenhar syndrome (p.40) may be very difficult, if not impossible, as in the case shown. Similar problems may be encountered in ruling out Klippel–Feil syndrome (p.214). Exclusion of dysostosis mandibulofacialis is not difficult (p.36).

Treatment: If necessary, initial care as with the Robin anomaly (p.52). Early audiometric testing, prompt application of speech and hearing aids as required. In given cases orthopaedic, cosmetic–surgical orthodontic corrections.

Illustrations:
1–6 A 6-year-old girl with a faciovertebral anomaly complex. Bony malformation at the atlantooccipital junction, block formation of cervical vertebrae 2–4 and synostoses of the spinous processes to C6. Low posterior hairline, marked limitation of motion at the neck. Mild facial asymmetry. Left palpebral fissure relatively narrow and somewhat oblique (no epibulbar dermoid). Hypoplasia of the upper jaw (which has a double row of teeth), narrow palate, immobile palatum molle, well-corrected horizontal clefts of the cheeks. Unremarkable external ears. Conductive hearing impairment.

References:
Sherk H. H., Nicholson J. T.: Cervico-oculo-acusticus syndrome. J. Bone Jt. Surg. 54A:1776 (1972)
Konigsmark Br. W., Gorlin R. J.: Genetic and Metabolic Deafness, W. B. Saunders Co., Philadelphia 1976

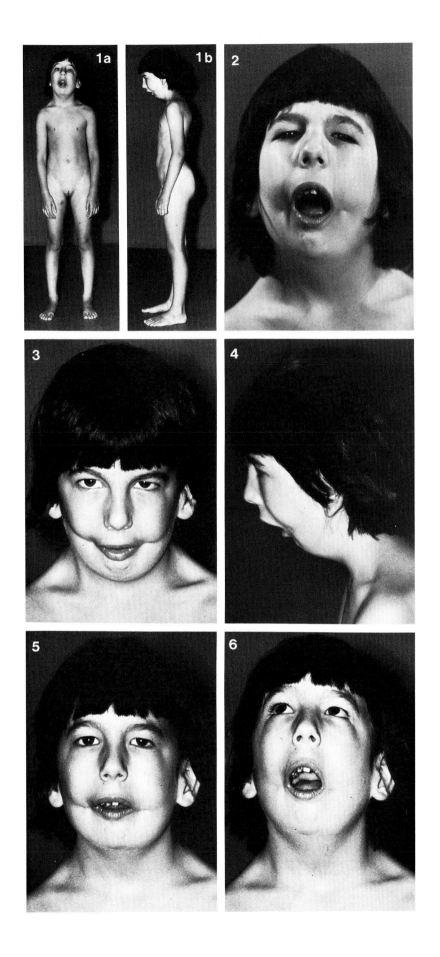

109. Aplastic Abdominal Musculature 'Syndrome'

(Furchennabel* 'Syndrome'; Prune Belly 'Syndrome')

A congenital condition in males showing a slack, wrinkled abdominal wall; undescended testicles; and urinary tract abnormalities. (Occurrence of analogous abdominal muscle dysplasia in females exceptionally.)

Main Signs:
1. A thin, loose, and (especially in early life) wrinkled and shrivelled ('prune-like') abdominal wall with persistent furrow-like umbilicus (2), protruding (1) in part over 'flabby' abdominal organs. (Basis: hypo- and aplasia of the abdominal wall musculature, which is not necessarily symmetrical.)
2. Bilateral cryptorchidism.
3. More or less extensive and severe anomalies of the urinary tract: megalocystis, megaloureter, hydronephrosis (3).

Supplementary Findings: Quite frequently malrotation, as well as other, additional dysplasias (e.g., of hips, feet, or heart).

Manifestation: Birth.

Aetiology: Not settled. Probably heterogeneous (according to an old and renewed interpretation, proceeding from intrauterine urethral obstruction – to which male fetuses are much more disposed) pathological complex. A few familial observations. The increased risk for further offspring is a few percent.

Frequency: About 1:40 000 live births. In the literature up to 1972, well over 250 cases described.

Course, Prognosis: Dependent on the severity of the anomalies. A high percentage of those affected die within the first years of life.

Treatment: Exact definition of the urodynamics. If the case requires, prompt primary decompression, e.g., by means of cystostomy. Treatment of urinary tract infection. Further care by a paediatric urologist. Genetic counselling (see below); prenatal diagnosis via ultrasonography (megalocystis? fetal ascites?) with subsequent pregnancies.

Illustrations:
1–3 A male infant; 3, the urogram of the child as a newborn, showing extreme bilateral megaureter. The 2nd child of healthy parents (the first pregnancy ended with a stillbirth in the 7th month, for unexplained reasons). At birth of the proband, after an unremarkable pregnancy, extensive aplasia of the abdominal wall musculature, megalocystis, megaloureter and bilateral cryptorchidism. Resection of a urethral polyp at 4 months. Apart from numerous urinary tract infections, normal development of the child so far, who in the meantime is several years old.

*Umbilical slit

References:
Pagon R. A., Smith D. W., Shepard Th.: Urethral obstruction malformation complex: A cause of abdominal muscle deficiency and the 'prune belly'. J. Pediatr. *94*:900 (1979) + ibid *96*:776, 777 (Letters to the Editor).
Aaronson I. A., Cremin B. J.: Prune belly syndrome in young females. Urol. Radiol. *1*:151 (1979/80)
Kösters S., Horwitz H., Ritter R.: Typische röntgenologische Veränderungen an Nieren und Harntrakt beim Bauchmuskelaplasie-Syndrom. Pädiatr. Prax. *22*:125 (1979/80)

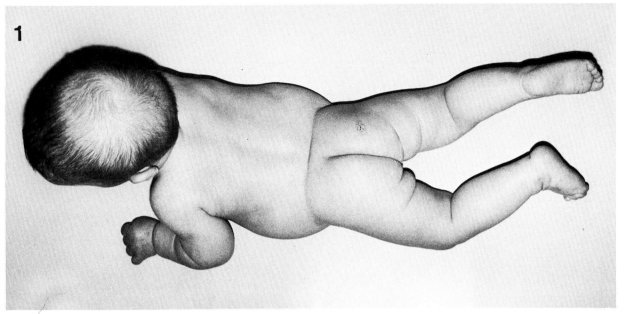

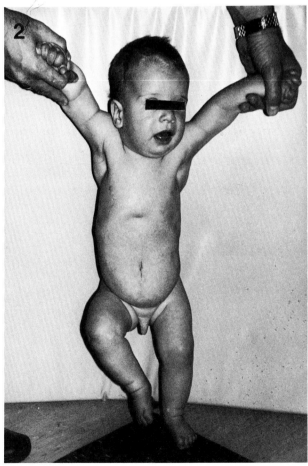

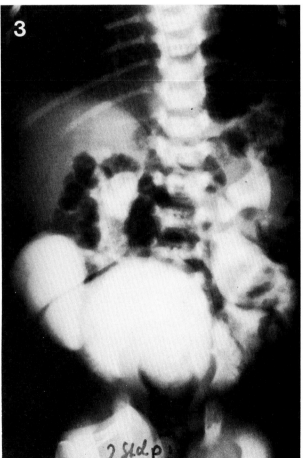

110. Syndrome of Early Manifested Polycystic Kidney Degeneration

A clinical picture of early abdominal distension, palpable 'giant kidneys', and more or less protracted course with development of hypertension.

Main Signs:
1. Protuberant and more or less widely bulging abdomen with markedly enlarged kidneys (**1,2**).
2. Possible analogous involvement of other large inner organs, especially the liver.
3. As a rule, more or less rapid development and progression of renal insufficiency.

Supplementary Findings: Confirmation by ultrasonography or IV pyelogram (**2**).

Presence or development of corresponding urinary, serum, or circulatory findings.

Manifestation: Birth or later.

Aetiology: Genetic basis, heterogeneity. Clinical differentiation from the less favourable so-called infantile (with autosomal recessive inheritance) and more favourable adult (autosomal dominant) cases may be difficult – if not impossible, since the latter may also be manifest in early childhood – in case the mode of inheritance is not clear.

Frequency: Not so rare.

Course, Prognosis: Shortened life expectancy; the more so, the earlier the manifestations.

Comment: The patient presented *could* have the so-called 'adult form' of polycystic kidney degeneration as the result of a new mutation.

Treatment: Symptomatic. In the late phase, dialysis, transplantation as required. Genetic counselling. In case of further pregnancy in the mother, prenatal diagnosis by means of ultrasonography.

Illustrations:
1 and 2 The 1st child of young, healthy, nonconsanguineous parents. Birth after an unremarkable pregnancy, approximately at term, with 3170 g, from breech presentation.

Markedly protuberant abdomen and symmetrical firm kidney 'tumours' extending from the costal arch into the true pelvis. IV pyelogram on the 7th/8th day of life: after 2 hours, widely separated, markedly dilated renal pelvic systems recognisable and 19 hours post infusion, strong presentation of renal parenchymal shadows of 10:6 cm diameter, with caudally converging axes (**2**). Cystographically no peculiarities of the efferent urinary tract. During a 10-week hospital stay, oedema, increased urea nitrogen, and haematuria or erythrocyturia, lymphocyturia, and slight proteinuria. With symptomatic treatment, clearing of these signs and subsequently good progress. **1** shows the proband at 3 years, 4 months. At 5 years, 7 months 112.5 cm and 20.5 kg (average for age); palpable kidney enlargement, liver 3 cm below the costal arch; urine negative; blood pressure (antihypertensive therapy) normal, occasionally to 135/80 mm Hg. In the meantime, the boy is about to start school and has three healthy brothers.

References:
Shokeir M. G. K.: Expression of the 'adult' polycystic renal disease in the fetus and newborn. Clin. Genet. *14*:61 (1978)
Chilton S. J., Cremin B. J.: The spectrum of polycystic disease in children. Pediatr. Radiol. *11*:9 (1981)
Koletzko S., Koletzko B., Orlowski M., et al: Fehldiagnose 'Polyzystische Nieren'... Monatschr. Kinderheilkd. *130*:299 (1982)

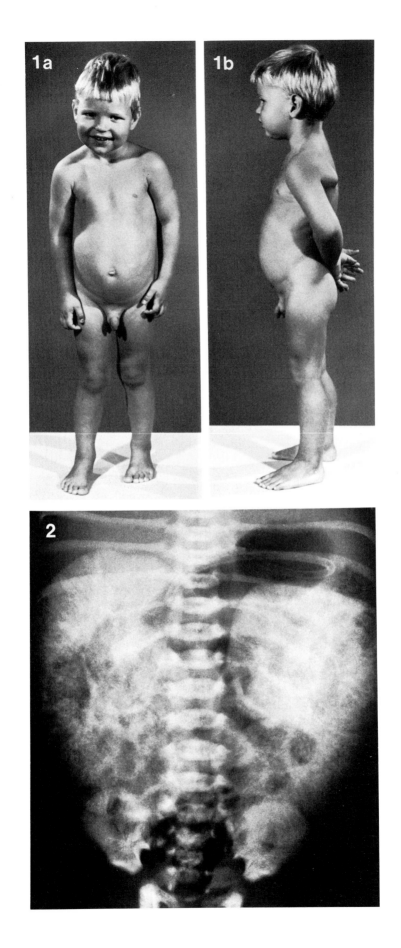

111. Gaucher Disease Type I

('Classic', Chronic Visceral Form of Gaucher Disease)

A chronic 'storage' disease, sparing the nervous system, with hepatosplenomegaly, dyshaematopoiesis, and characteristic 'orthopaedic complications'.

Main Signs:
1. Hepatosplenomegaly, which may be extreme (**1b**).
2. Dyshaematopoiesis ('splenogenic marrow depression': thrombocytopenia, leucopenia, anaemia); pallor, possibly haemorrhages.
3. Periodic bone and joint pain, especially involving the long bones, pseudoosteomyelitic or pseudoarthritic, in some cases pathological fractures, some with aseptic osteonecrosis; epiphysiolysis. Preferred sites: femur; especially characteristic: necrosis of the head of the femur (**1c** and **2**); also, destruction of vertebral bodies and other areas.
4. Children often show growth deficiency, delayed maturation (**1a**).

Supplementary Findings: Mental development and nervous system normal.

Possible gold-brownish skin coloration, especially of the face, neck, hands, and extensor surfaces of the lower legs and – in adults – yellowish spots ('pinguecula') on the sclerae.

Elevation of the (tartrate-resistant) acid serum phosphate; Gaucher cells demonstrable in bone marrow punctures or other organ preparations or – simpler and conclusive – demonstration of cerebroside-beta-glucosidase defect in leucocytes.

Manifestation: Any age (from early childhood) possible.

Aetiology: Autosomal recessive hereditary disorder occurring especially in Ashkenazic Jews. Probable heterogeneity.

Course, Prognosis: Patients may live to an old age. The sequelae of fractures of the neck of the femur with necrosis of the femoral head, when there is irreversible damage, are often regarded as the greatest problem in adulthood.

Treatment: Careful orthopaedic supervision. Exemption from school sports. Furtherance of intellectual development and adequate vocational training. For acute attacks of pain, immobilisation suffices. For previous hip damage, possible surgical correction of position, with more extensive revision at a later date. Splenectomy for marked signs of abdominal displacement and marked dyshaematopoiesis. Psychological guidance. Genetic counselling. Prenatal diagnosis.

Illustrations:
1 and 2 A 14-year-old girl (one parent Ashkenazi). Left-sided 'coxitis' at 5 years, further attacks of hip pain on the left at 11 and, bilaterally, at 13 years. Protuberant abdomen due to hyperlordosis (**1b**) and organomegaly. Splenectomy carried out (typical Gaucher histology); hepatomegaly to the level of the umbilicus. 'Dystrophic growth deficiency' (here below the 3rd percentile) with excessive length of the extremities; delayed puberty (no menarche to date); bone age retarded about 3 years. 'Limping' for months: dislocated left hip with necrosis of the left femoral head and severe destruction of the neck of the femur (in the meantime correction of position has been accomplished); in addition, storage focus in the right femur below the lesser trochanter (**2**); no further skeletal foci determined (nor changes in the lungs). Enzyme defect demonstrated by leucocyte test.

References:
Any comprehensive paediatric or internal medicine text book. In addition:
Tjhen K. Y., Zillhardt H. W.: M. Gaucher Typ 1. Pädiatr. Prax. *18*:247 (1977)
Goldblatt J., Sacks S., Beighton P.: The orthopaedic aspects of Gaucher disease. Clin. Orthopaed. *137*:208 (1978)

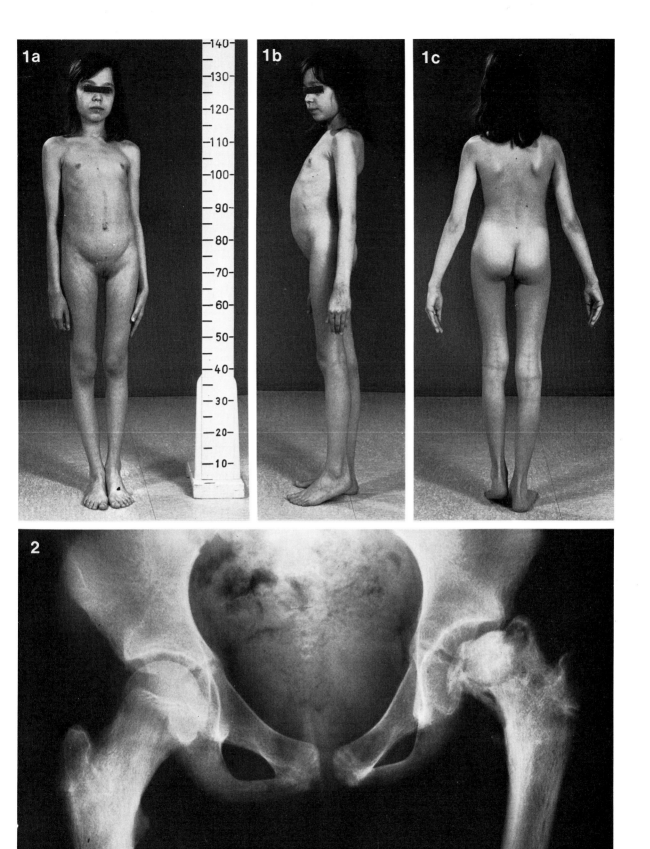

223

112. Caudal Dysplasia Syndrome

(Syndrome of Sacrococcygeal Agenesis; Caudal Regression Syndrome)

A malformation syndrome of hypo- or aplasia of the caudal vertebrae of various degrees of severity – with developmental defect of the corresponding segment of spinal cord – and hypo- or dysplasia of the pelvis and the lower extremities.

Main Signs:
1. Shortening, narrowing, or atypical configuration of the lower portion of the trunk, especially apparent dorsally, the buttocks often presenting a flat surface with dimples and a shortened gluteal fold (**1b**). Distinctly disproportionate short stature possible due to short trunk and relatively excessive length of the extremities, especially the upper (**1a** and **b**).
2. Weakness and atrophy, possibly also malformation or hypoplasia of the legs. Hips often dislocated (**2** and **3**). Flexion contractures of the hips and knees. Club feet. Frequent paralysis of the muscles of the pelvic floor and sphincters, with urinary and faecal incontinence; areflexia of the lower extremities (motor and sensory defects need not be parallel). Neurological impairment may vary between total paralysis below the defect and a slight disorder of bladder control.

Supplementary Findings: Radiologically, lumbosacrococcygeal vertebral defects of various grades of severity and possibly malformation and narrowing of the pelvis with narrowly spaced hypoplastic ilia, which are closely approximated dorsally (**2** and **3**). In some cases dislocated hips, femoral hypoplasia.

Possible malformation of the gastrointestinal tract, of the large parenchymatous abdominal organs, or the heart, among others.

Possible maternal diabetes.

Manifestation: Birth.

Aetiology: Not uniform. Mostly isolated cases. A good 15% of the affected have mothers with diabetes mellitus; in these cases the syndrome falls within the framework of 'diabetic embryopathy'.

Frequency: Not so rare. The majority of cases are not associated with maternal diabetes; ca. 1% of children of diabetic mothers are affected.

Course, Prognosis: Dependent on the severity of the dysplasia and on the quality and consistency of care and on necessarily multidisciplinary rehabilitation.

Illustrations:
1–3 A now 14-year-old mentally normal girl, whose mother had been diabetic for 13 years at the time of the patient's birth. Growth deficiency of about 20 cm from the average for age due to caudal shortening of the trunk. Narrowly spaced ilial wings; abnormal configuration of the lower back and gluteal region (**1b**) with shortened gluteal folds and dimples at birth. Waddling gait with complete luxation of the hip bilaterally; contracted knee joints; muscular atrophy and abundant fat in the lower extremities, the former especially of the calves; absent patellar reflex; intact sensation of the legs. Incontinent of urine (no longer of faeces). Relatively good physical rehabilitation after surgery for club feet and other orthopaedic care, after surgery for congenital valvular and subvalvular pulmonary stenosis and an atrial septal defect, and under paediatric urological care. Very good psychosocial adjustment. X-rays (**2** and **3** at respectively 5½ and 8 years): absence of the 4th and 5th lumbar vertebrae, all of the sacrum, and the coccyx. Dorsal parts of the ilia small and directly approximated dorsally with small heart-shaped pelvis and extremely narrow pelvis minor. Severe dysplasia of the hip joint bilaterally; lateralised ossification centres of the femoral heads, coxae varae.

References:
Price D. L., Dooling E. C, Richardson jr E. P.: Caudal dysplasia (caudal regression syndrome). Arch. Neurol. *23*:212 (1970)
Amendt P., Goedel E., Amendt U., Becker G.: Mißbildungen bei mütterlichem Diabetes mellitus unter besonderer Berücksichtigung des kaudalen Fehlbildungs syndroms. Zbl. Gynäkol. *96*/30:950 (1974)
Andrish J., Kalamchi A., MacEwen G. D.: Sacral agenesis: A clinical evaluation of its management, heredity, and associated anomalies. Clin. Orthopaed. *139*:52 (1979)
Stewart J. M., Stoll St.: Familial caudal regression anomalad and maternal diabetes. J. Med. Genet. *16*:17 (1979); and ibid. *17*:57 (1980)

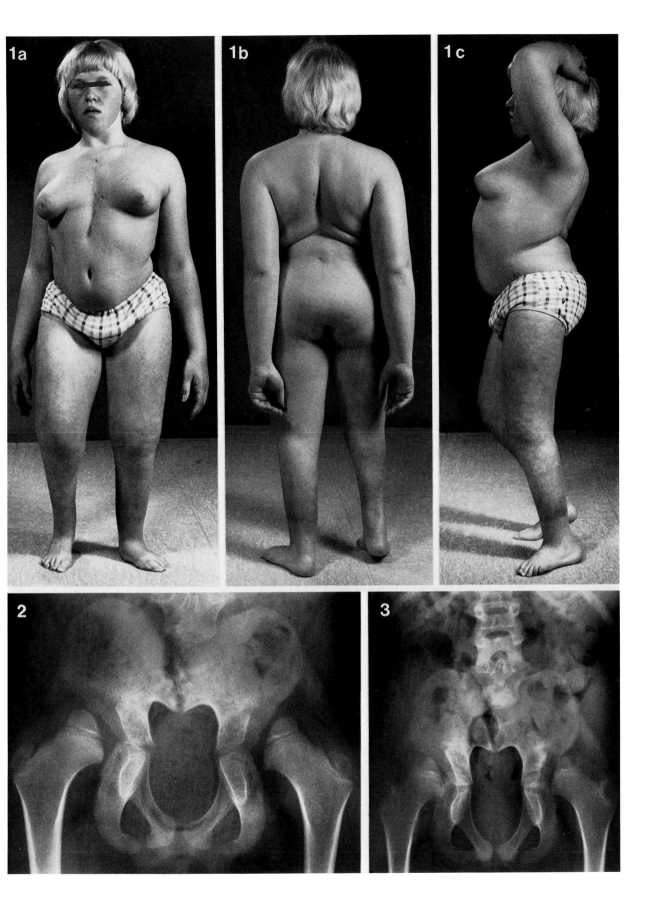

225

113. Gingival Fibromatosis–Hypertrichosis Syndrome

A hereditary syndrome of early manifested generalised hypertrichosis and gingival fibromatosis.

Main Signs:
1. Generalised hypertrichosis, the hair usually being dark (also in otherwise light-complexioned families) (**1** and **3**).
2. Gingival fibromatosis, which more or less covers and constrains the teeth, delays eruption, overgrows the crowns, and may bring about loss of teeth (**4–6**). In some cases protrusion of the lips and jaws and other secondary mechanical effects.

Supplementary Findings: Epilepsy and/or mental retardation are often present in the – less frequent – sporadic cases (see below; recessive hereditary form?).

Manifestation: Development of generalised hypertrichosis in the first two years of life; the gingival changes also in infancy or early childhood.

Aetiology: Hereditary disorder, usually autosomal dominant. Possibly also an autosomal recessive form; thus heterogeneity.

Frequency: Low.

Prognosis: Favourable with respect to the gingival fibromatosis, assuming adequate treatment. Crucial in the prognosis is the patient's mental development.

Comment: In a special form, in which the mode of inheritance is not absolutely clear and which cannot be identified with certainty prior to sexual maturity, female carriers develop mammary fibroadenomatosis with a tendency to malignant degeneration.

Treatment: Very meticulous oral hygiene; gingivectomy; in some cases extraction of teeth and prosthetic measures. Depilation. Genetic counselling.

Illustrations:
1–4 A boy with typical development of the syndrome; very heavily-developed eyebrows, hyperplasia of the eyelashes (three rows), simulated small size of the teeth.
5 and 6 Gingival hyperplasia in another case.
(All photographs by kind permission of Prof. B. Leiber, Frankfurt a.M.)

Reference:
Witkop C.J., jr: Heterogeneity in gingival fibromatosis. Birth Defects VII, 7:210 (1971)

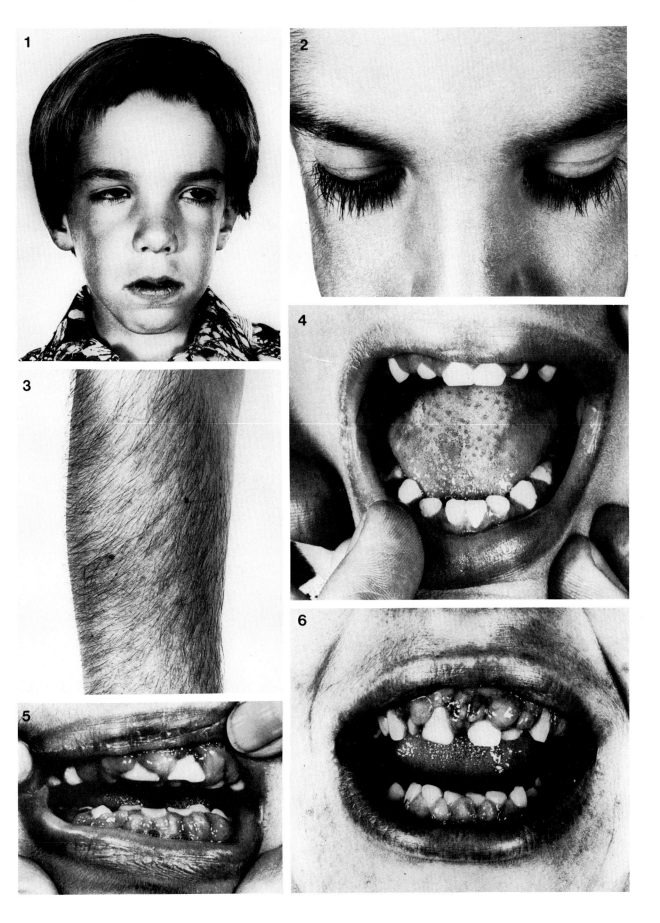

227

114. 'Syndrome' of Giant Hairy Naevus with Satellite Naevi

Congenital extensive naevocytic naevus possibly associated with leptomeningeal melanocytosis (then: 'neurocutaneous melanoblastosis').

Main Signs: More or less intensive black-brown, bilaterally symmetrical or asymmetrically distributed changes ('bathing suit'-, 'bathing trunk'-, 'cap-', 'neck poultice'-, 'stocking'-naevus, etc.), flush with the skin or partially elevated, nodose, wartlike, and more or less coarsely haired, with multiple corresponding smaller naevi (**1** and **2**).

Supplementary Findings: Development of hydrocephalus and/or cerebral seizures or other neurological or psychological signs of irritation or damage should suggest progressive meningocerebral involvement.

Manifestation: Hairy naevus present at birth. Although cerebral signs may appear as early as infancy, they generally begin at a pre-school age, and occasionally not until much later.

Aetiology: Unclear. Usually sporadic occurrence, familial as an exception (in which case family members repeatedly show only multiple small corresponding naevi); possible multifactorial inheritance. Basic defect unknown.

Frequency: Up to 1978 (at least) 70 cases of neurocutaneous melanosis, 28 of these with malignant meningeal meningioma (see below), were reported in the literature.

Course, Prognosis, Treatment: CNS involvement or its progression may lead to death in infancy or early childhood. (Extensive hairy naevi of the head or neck region are said to be regularly combined with meningeal melanocytosis, thus less favourable.) The risk of developing a malignant melanoma is increased in the region of the skin naevus as well as in the correspondingly affected intracranial area – this not infrequently is manifest within the first five years of life. *The treatment* of choice is extirpation of the entire giant skin naevus (as well as the satellites) with grafting; when not feasible, as often the case, the most extensive possible excision. Such a surgical procedure is perhaps more successful if not carried out until after infancy. Definite cosmetic improvement may be accomplished by planing. A more recent recommendation is immediate postpartum abrasion! Considering the associated risk, a hairy naevus requires regular careful follow-up; the patient and in some cases family members require appropriate psychological guidance and help.

Illustrations:

1a–d A neonate with 'bathing trunk' naevus pigmentosus et pilosus and numerous satellite naevi. Relatively large cranium. Up to that time, no pathological growth of the skull or other neurological signs.
2a–c A 6½-year-old boy. Hairy naevi with satellites. Recent onset of focal seizures.

References:
Voigtländer V., Jung E. G.: Giant pigmented hairy nevus in two siblings. Humangenetik. *24*:79 (1974)
Lamas E., Diez Lobato R., et al: Neurocutaneous melanosis. Acta Neurochirurgica *36*:93 (1977)
Solomon L. M.: The management of congenital melanocytic nevi. Arch., Derm. *116*:1017 (1980)
Hecht F., LaCanne K. M., Carroll D. B.: Inheritance of giant pigmented hairy nevus...Am. J. Med. Genet. *9*:177 (1981)
Fleissner J., Kleine M., Bonsmann G., et al: Dermabrasion eines großflächigen kongenitalen Pigmentnävus...Pädiat. Prax. *26*:505 (1982)
Konz B.: Problem der angeborenen pigmentierten Nävi. Pädiatr. Prax. *26*:106 (1982)

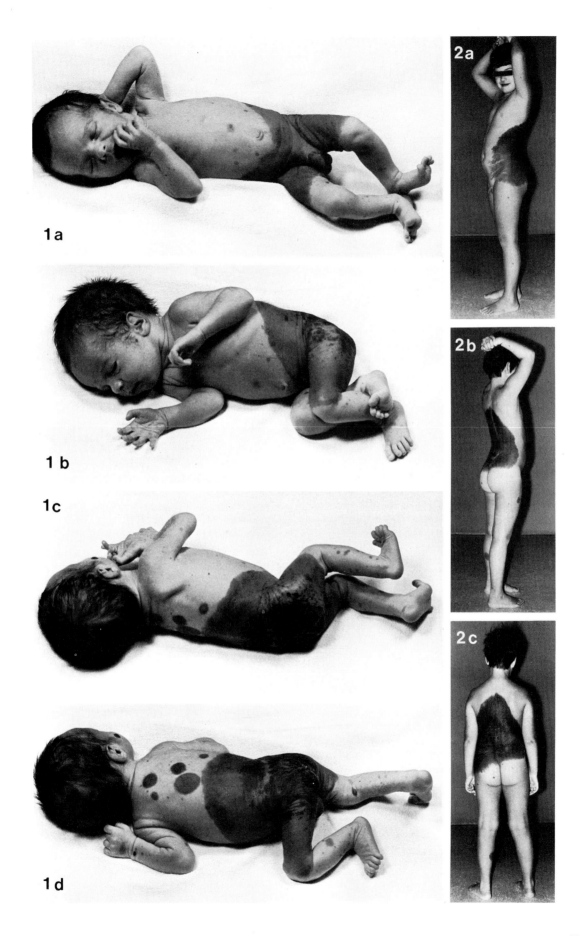

115. Schimmelpenning–Feuerstein–Mims Syndrome

(Syndrome of Linear Naevus Sebaceus)

A syndrome of linear sebaceous naevus of Jadassohn usually involving the middle of the face, cerebral seizures, and mental retardation.

Main Signs:

1. Sebaceous naevus of Jadassohn; uni-, but also bilateral; localised mainly on the cranium (with focal alopecia), around the ears, on the forehead and temples, and often extending to the tip of the nose or on to the rest of the face, possibly also elsewhere on the body; changes varying from narrow, barely apparent to broad, conspicuous stripes. Yellow-brown appearance; greasy, warty consistency (1–3). Frequently additional, more or less diffuse, pigmented naevi (1 and 2).

2. Cerebral seizures, usually in the form of focal epilepsy, of variable severity and with various effects.

3. Mental or psychomotor retardation of any grade of severity (possibly even absent). Frequently more or less severe behavioural abnormalities.

Supplementary Findings: Congenital involvement of one or both eyes in about 50% of cases: coloboma of the iris (sometimes also of the chorioretina or lid), lipodermoid of the conjunctiva and possibly the cornea.

Frequent markedly asymmetrical development of the two sides of the cranium and face. Hemimacrocephaly, eye anomalies, dilation of the ventricles and focal EEG findings with cerebral involvement of a probably hamartomatous nature (and atrophy): then, as a rule ipsilateral to the main naevus involvement.

Frequent proliferation of the oral mucous membrane and more or less severe dysodontiasis (5).

Possible osteodystrophy with numerous 'spontaneous' fractures (Milkman phenomenon).

Possible growth deficiency.

Manifestation: The naevus is usually present at birth (further pigmentary changes and verrucous deformity of the naevus usually occur later). Cerebral seizures, mostly of a focal nature, often starting in early infancy (but sometimes much later). Mental retardation may be manifest sooner or later, depending on the grade of severity.

Aetiology: Considered open. Genetic basis highly likely, possibly autosomal dominant mode of inheritance of a pleiotropic gene with relatively low penetrance. Most cases have been sporadic.

Frequency: Low; up to 1980, about 50 case reports in the literature.

Course, Prognosis: Seizures and developmental defects are especially likely when linear sebaceous naevus occurs in the middle of the face. The course of the disorder varies greatly and depends on the severity of mental retardation and epilepsy. The former need not be severe; the latter may improve spontaneously or may be controlled medically. The Jadassohn naevus is subject to verrucous hyperplasia in childhood and adolescence and may pose a serious cosmetic problem (1). The dentition may also be problematic starting at an early age (5).

In adulthood malignant tumours, e.g., basal cell epithelioma, may be expected to develop in the naevus (approximately 15% of cases). In addition, the syndrome as such may be accompanied by the development of tumours (hamartoma of the kidney, nephroblastoma, cystic adenoma of the liver, fibroangioma, and osteoclastic tumours of the jaw have been found in isolated cases).

Differential Diagnosis: Syndrome of encephalocraniocutaneous lipomatosis, p.234.

Treatment: Symptomatic. If, or as far as, possible, early extirpation of the naevus. Anticonvulsive medication if required. Dental treatment. Cosmetic care in some cases.

Illustrations:

1–5 A 12-year-old, the 2nd child of young, nonconsanguineous parents, after a healthy girl. Congenital sebaceous naevus of Jadassohn distributed in broad stripes bilaterally and asymmetrically on the face, the scalp – with alopecia –, and neck (1; post planing; 3), and also in narrow streaks on the abdomen and right leg and foot, with spotty hyperpigmentation of parts of the trunk and arms (2). Left-sided focal seizure disorder manifested in the 2nd year of life; dilatation of the left cerebral ventricle; mental retardation (Hawik—IQ 78). Additional findings: crossed neurogenic hemihypotrophy (left sided on the cranial and facial part of the skull and including the tongue, 1b, 4 and 5; thereafter on the right, 2a) with dysphagia as well as abnormal motor function and dysreflexia on the hypotrophic side. Extensive proliferation of the oral mucous membranes, bipartite uvula, extremely numerous 'spontaneous' fractures and Looser's transformation zones quite preponderant on the hypotrophic, right side of the body. Short stature, below the 3rd percentile (parents relatively small). Ophthalmological examination negative. Father of the proband has a neuromotor disability, one arm full of diverse naevi, and a family history of focal seizure disorders.

References:
Schimmelpenning G. W.: Klinischer Beitrag zur Symptomatologie der Phakomatosen. Fortschr. Röntgenstr. 87:716 (1957)
Feuerstein R. C., Mims L. C.: Linear nevus sebaceus with convulsions and mental retardation. Am. J. Dis. Child. 104:675 (1962)
Wauschkuhn J., Rhode B.: Systemisierte Talgdrüsen-, Pigment- and epitheliale Naevi mit neurologischer Symptomatik: Feuerstein-Mimssches Neuroektodermales Syndrom. Hautartzt 22:10 (1971)
Barth P. G., Valk J., Kalsbeek G. L., et al: Organoid nevus syndrome (linear nevus sebaceus of Jadassohn). Neuropädiatrie 8:418 (1977)

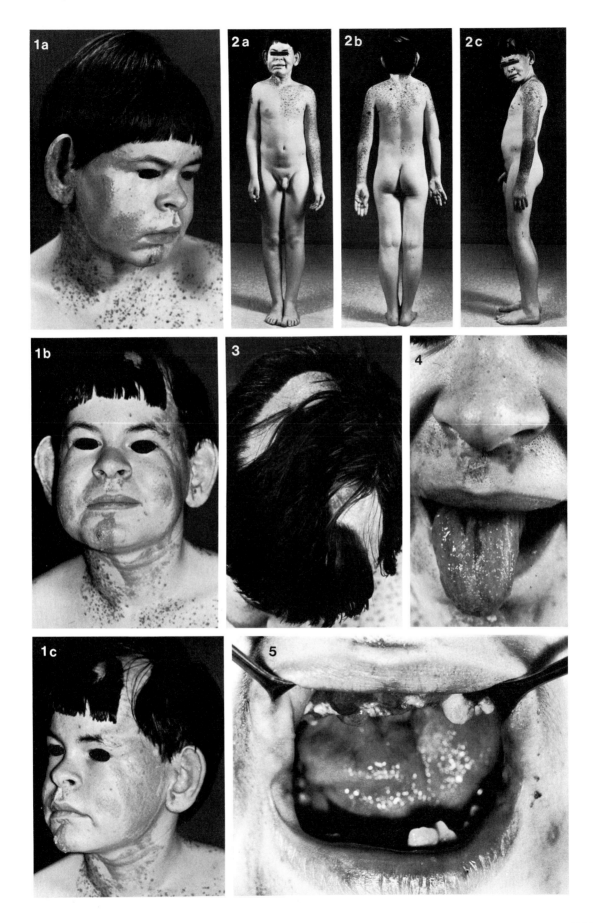

116. Syndrome of Partial Macrosomia, Linear Naevus, Macrocranium with Signs of Cardiac Overload Due to Intracranial A-V Shunt, Parietal Soft Tissue Swelling with Alopecia, Psychomotor Retardation, and Growth Deficiency

A syndrome of congenital macrosomia of a lower extremity, linear verrucous naevus on the trunk, macrodolichocephaly with signs of cardiac overload (without evidence of cardiac malformation) associated with intracranial A-V fistula, biparietal soft tissue swelling with alopecia, psychomotor retardation, and short stature.

Main Signs:

1. Congenital macrosomia of the left leg (1), a cavernous haemangioma of the thigh having been removed when the patient was 2 years old. At age 3 years, the left leg 2 cm longer than the right; at 4 years, 4 cm. Left leg lividly discoloured; pad-like swelling, especially on the back of the foot. Secondary flexion contractures of the hip and knee joints. Systolic murmur over the femoral artery, but absence of a significant A-V fistula on angiogram.

2. Linear hyperpigmented verrucous naevus of the thorax, extending to the midline and then continuing downwards (1 and 3) (biopsy scar above): epitheliomatous naevus.

3. Macrodolichocephaly (at 2¾ years, 53 cm; at 4¾ years, 55 cm) with signs of cardiac overload and cardiomegaly with barrel-shaped chest, without evidence of cardiac malformation. Continuous systolic–diastolic murmur over the cranium. Demonstration of an intracranial A-V fistula with a large aneurysm of the great vein of Galen and dilatation of the neighbouring venous sinuses (4).

4. Biparietal soft tissue swelling with alopecia, present since the first weeks of life (2). (Biopsy: 'anetoderma').

5. Stato- and psychomotor retardation with muscular dystonia. (No cerebral seizure disorder.)

6. Short stature (below the 3rd percentile).

Supplementary Findings: High forehead with bossing. Antimongoloid slant of the palpebral fissures, especially on the right.

High and narrow palate; uvula fissa.

Bony protuberance on the lateral rim of the left orbit: on X-ray of the skull, irregular translucent areas and densities of the parietal cortex. Oval cystic translucency distally on the left femur.

Slight pareses of the left facial and abducens nerves with strabismus. Ocular fundi hyperpigmented, otherwise negative.

Manifestation: Birth and later.

Aetiology: Uncertain; presumably a genetic basis.

Course: Death of the child at 5 years as a result of intracranial bleeding.

Comment: The clinical picture of this child suggests the Schimmelpenning–Feuerstein–Mims syndrome (p.230) or the encephalocraniocutaneous lipomatosis syndrome (p.234) and also bears a resemblance to a condition observed by Goldschmidt et al (see below); however, it does not completely fit any of these. Cf. also p.24 and p.300.

Illustrations:

1–4 A 3-year-old boy, the first child of young, healthy, nonconsanguineous parents. Semeiotic data as above.

(By kind permission of Prof. P. Heintzen and Dr E. Stephan, Kiel.)

References:
Goldschmidt H., Thiede G., Pfeiffer R. A., et al: Hemihypertrophie, Naevus sebaceus, multiple Knochenzysten und zerebroretinale Angiomatose: eine komplexe Phakomatose. Helv. Paediatr. Acta 31:487 (1976)

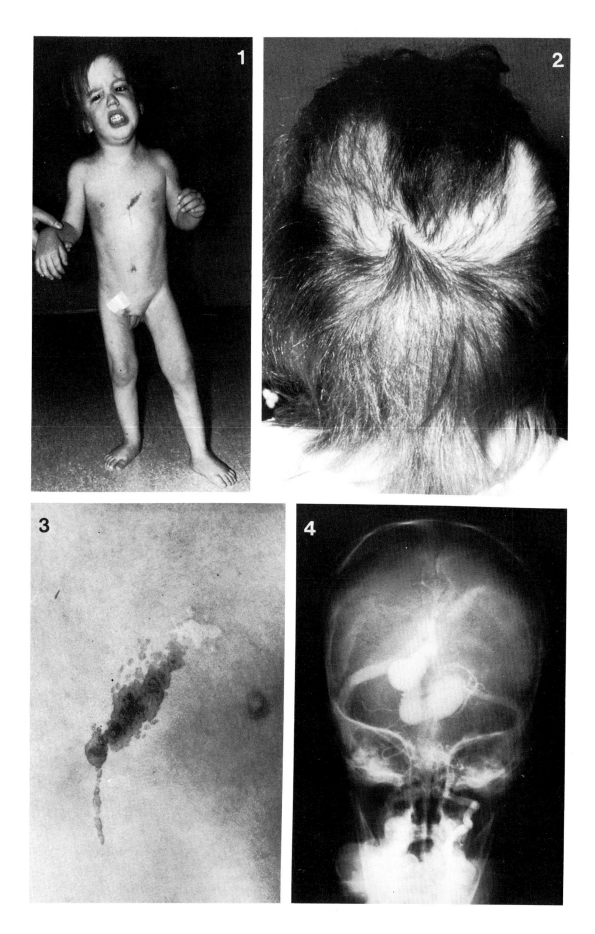

117. Syndrome of Encephalocraniocutaneous Lipomatosis

A syndrome of macrocephaly, soft tissue tumours of the cranium and eyes, focal cerebral seizures, and psychomotor retardation with unilateral porencephalic cyst, and cerebral hemiatrophy with lipomatosis.

Main Signs:
1. Congenital or postnatally manifest macrocrania, sometimes quite asymmetrical and possibly showing definite progression and signs of hydrocephaly (1–5).
2. Soft tissue swellings, slight or marked, single or multiple, uni- or bilateral, of the parietooccipital, frontotemporal, or other parts of the cranium or facial part of the skull; alopecia of the affected area; lipomatous on biopsy (1–5). Bony swelling possible.
3. Possible soft tissue tumours involving conjunctiva, sclera, cornea, and/or eyelids; lipodermoid on biopsy.
4. Early manifested focal cerebral seizures.
5. Psychomotor retardation of various grades of severity, in some cases with hemispasticity, etc.
6. A unilateral porencephalic cyst of variable size communicating with the ventricular system with unilateral atrophy of the brain can be demonstrated. At autopsy, sometimes more or less widespread intracranial (and possibly also intraspinal) lipomatosis, possibly involving the cranial bones.

Supplementary Findings: Possibly small 'connective tissue naevi' or angiofibroma, fibrolipoma present additionally in the facial–cranial area.

Possible xanthochromia and increased protein in the cerebrospinal fluid.

Manifestation: Birth and postnatally.

Aetiology: Uncertain; genetic basis may be assumed.

Frequency: Rare, to date only a few cases described in the literature.

Course, Prognosis: Unfavourable.

Differential Diagnosis: Schimmelpenning–Feuerstein–Mims syndrome p.230. Definite overlap with this syndrome, but the highly characteristic pathological findings would seem to justify separate classification.

Treatment: Symptomatic.

Illustrations:
1–5 The first child of young, healthy, nonconsanguineous parents; (1 and 2) at 4 weeks, 3–5 at 2½ years. Congenital macrodolichocephaly (41.5 cm) with signs of increased intracranial pressure, xanthochromia and increased protein in the cerebrospinal fluid. Congenital severe soft tissue swelling of the left cheek; (haematoma on the right upper lid). Early focal cerebral seizures. Psychomotor retardation with signs of cerebral palsy. Ophthalmological examination showing localised chorioretinal accumulations of pigment in the left eye, otherwise negative. Computed tomography study showing severe porencephalic dilatation of the left ventricular system. Ventricular-cardiac shunt. Head circumference at 2½ years, 62.5 cm; very high forehead. Extirpation of the lipoma from the left cheek. Death of the child at 3¼ years.
(By kind permission of Prof. H. Doose, Kiel.)

References:
Haberland C., Perou M.: Encephalocraniocutaneous lipomatosis. Arch. Neurol. *22*:144 (1970)
Fishman M. A., Chang Ch.S.C., Miller J. E.: Encephalocraniocutaneous lipomatosis. Pediatrics *61*:580 (1978)
Sanchez N. P., Rhodes A. R., Mandell F., et al: Encephalocraniocutaneous lipomatosis: a new neurocutaneous syndrome. Br. J. Dermatol. *104*:89 (1981)

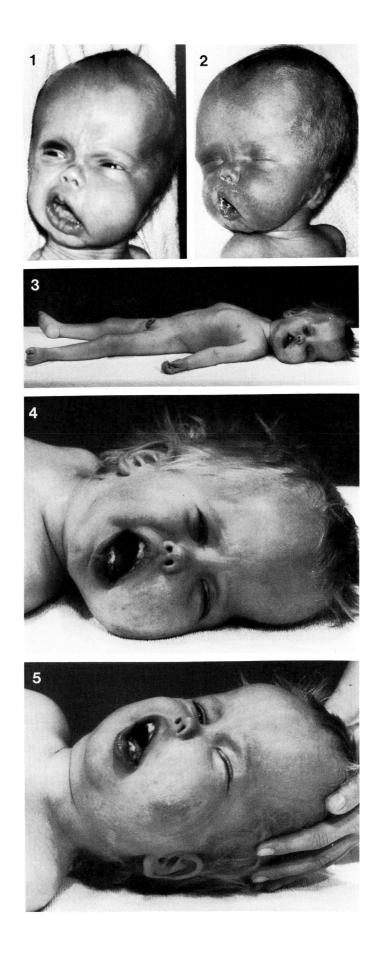

118. McCune–Albright Syndrome

(Albright Syndrome, Weil–Albright Syndrome)

A characteristic syndrome of fibrous bone dysplasia, irregular brown hyperpigmentation of the skin, and precocious puberty (almost exclusively in girls).

Main Signs:
1. Café au lait- or dark-coloured hyperpigmented areas with irregular, sharp maplike borders (**1**), often unilateral along the midline, preferentially on the buttocks, thighs, back, and neck.
2. Precocious menarche, followed by premature development of the secondary characteristics. (In boys precocious puberty only exceptionally.)
3. Spontaneous fractures and/or more or less marked skeletal deformity, both more frequent on the lower extremities, especially the proximal femur, with polyostotic fibrous dysplasia-type lesions and corresponding X-ray findings (**2**).

Supplementary Findings: In some cases accelerated growth in height and skeletal maturity; premature closure of the epiphyses may eventually result in short stature.

Serum calcium and phosphate levels normal; alkaline phosphate normal or elevated.

Manifestation: Pigment spots present at birth or shortly thereafter; subsequent proportional growth. Menarche possibly occurring in infancy (regular menses usually not until a few years later); further sexual characteristics subsequently appear more or less rapidly. The bony defects become manifest mainly during the 1st decade of life.

Aetiology: Unknown; sporadic occurrence.

Frequency: Rare (up to 1966 about 130 case reports in the literature).

Course, Prognosis: Usually slow progression of the number and size of the bony changes during the growing years; as a rule the changes become stationary in the 2nd–3rd decade of life. Life expectancy normal (in a few cases development of sarcoma during adolescence). Fractures tend to heal well.

Treatment: Generally limited to prevention of stress damage, care of pathological fractures, and orthopaedic care of skeletal deformities. Attempts at therapeutic application of ionising radiation contraindicated. Perhaps administration of gestagen.

Illustrations:
1 and 2 A 13¼-year-old girl: Pigment anomalies since birth, vaginal bleedings since infancy, secondary characteristics since early childhood. X-ray: polyostotic fibrous dysplasia with foci in the pelvis and upper leg, left tibia, left scapula, the proximal humeral metaphyses, and both temporal bones.
2 Pelvis oblique and tilted; coxa vara; pathological fracture of the left femoral neck medially; cystic and honeycomb-like changes in the ileosacral area bilaterally, in the region of the left anterior iliac spine, and in both proximal femora with the epiphyses largely spared, and with monocystoid expansion affecting the left diaphysis, which is dilated and shows thinning of the cortex.

References:
Boenheim F., McGavack Th. H.: Polyostotische fibröse Dysplasie. Erg. Inn. Med. Kinderheilkd. *3*:159 (1952)
Hauke H.: Osteofibrose. Handbuch der Kinderheilkunde, Bd 6, p.389 ff. Heidelberg, Springer 1967
Spranger J. W., Langer L. O., jr, Wiedemann H.-R.: Bone Dysplasias. An Atlas of Constitutional Disorders of Skeletal Development, Stuttgart and Philadelphia, G. Fischer and W. B. Saunders 1974
Giovannelli G., Bernasconi S., Banchini G.: McCune–Albright syndrome in a male child: A clinical and endocrinologic enigma. J. Pediatr. 92:220 (1978)

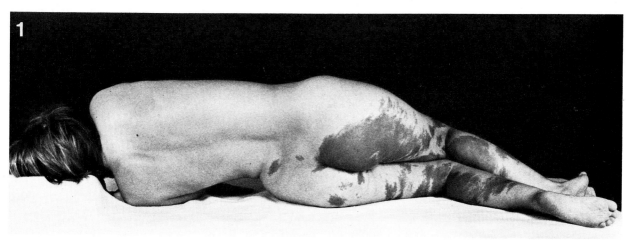

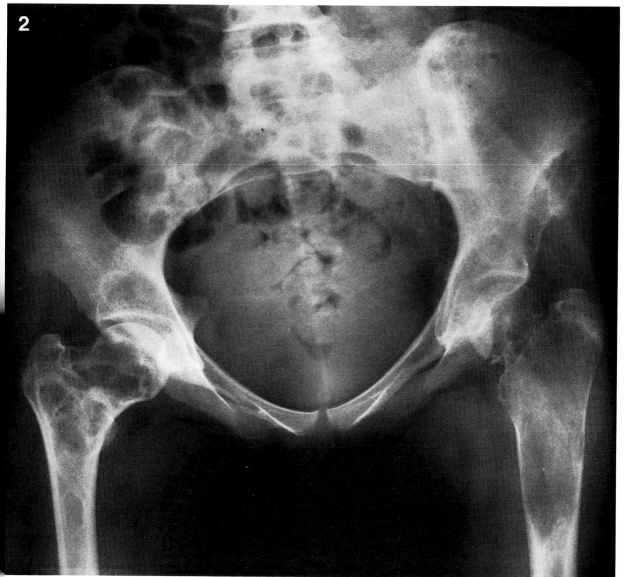

119. Miescher Syndrome

(Bloch–Miescher Syndrome, Mendenhall Syndrome)

A syndrome closely resembling a congenital generalised lipodystrophy and comprising congenital acanthosis nigricans, hypertrichosis, failure to thrive and growth deficiency, dysmorphisms especially in and around the jaw and oral cavity, insulin-resistant diabetes mellitus, and a characteristic general appearance.

Main Signs:
1. Acanthosis nigricans especially of the neck, axillary, inguinal, and genital regions (**2–4** and **6–8**).
2. Lanugo-type hypertrichosis of the trunk (**5**), possibly also on the extremities; in some cases overabundant scalp hair (**3** and **7**).
3. Deficient physical – possibly also mental – development, with decreased adipose tissue (**2**), aged appearance (**4, 7,** and **8**), and short stature.
4. Relatively coarse facial features due to protruding chin (**3, 4, 7,** and **8**), poorly formed, malpositioned teeth (**9** and **11**), and large relatively low-set ears (**7** and **8**).

Supplementary Findings: High palate; fissured tongue (**10**); milky opacity of the oral mucous membranes, which are coarse and velvety.

Stubby fingers and toes.

Goitre (**3** and **4**), often nodular.

Insulin-resistant diabetes mellitus with little tendency to ketosis.

Manifestation: Birth and subsequent years; manifestation of diabetes during childhood or adolescence.

Aetiology: Genetically determined syndrome; probably autosomal recessive transmission.

Frequency: Very low.

Course, Prognosis: Decrease in intensity and extent of the acanthosis nigricans possible after many years. Diabetes relatively mild.

Illustrations:
1–11 Siblings with the Miescher syndrome. Latent diabetes mellitus in the father. Both children of short stature. The distinctly more severely affected 13½-year-old boy shows manifest diabetes and nodular goitre; the 11½-year-old girl, latent diabetes. (**6, 10,** and **11** are of the boy; **9,** of the girl).

References:
Miescher G.: Zwei Fälle von congenitaler familiärer Akanthosis nigricans, kombiniert mit Diabetes mellitus. Derm. Z. *32*:276 (1921)
Mason H. H., Sly G. E.: Diabetes mellitus: Report of a case resistant to insulin…JAMA *108*:2016 (1937)
Mendenhall E. N.: Tumor of pineal body with high insulin resistance. J. Indiana. M. A. *43*:32 (1950)
Rabson S M., Mendenhall E. N.: Familial hypertrophy of pineal body…Am. J. Clin. Pathol. *26*:283 (1956)
Wiedemann H.-R., Spranger J., Mogharei M., et al: Über das Syndrom…und Miescher-Syndrom im Sinne dienzephaler Syndrome. Z. Kinderheilkd. *102*;1 (1968)
Seip M.: Generalised lipodystrophy. Ergeb. Inn. Med. Kinderheilkd. *31*:59 (1971)
Dumas R., Rolin B., de Paulet P. Cr., et al: Trois observations de diabéte lipoatrophique familial. Ann. Pédiatr. *21*:625 (1974)
Barnes N. D., Palumbo P. J., Hayles A. B., et al: Insulin resistance, skin changes and virilization…Diabetologia *10*:285 (1974)
West R. J., Lloyd J. K., Turner W. M. L.: Familial insulin-resistant diabetes, multiple somatic anomalies…Arch. Dis. Child. *50*:703 (1975) relative to the latter: Holmes J., Tanner M. S.: Premature eruption and macrodontia associated with insulin resistant diabetes…Br. Dent. J. *141*:280 (1976) + West R. J., Leonard J. V.: Familial insulin resistance…Arch. Dis. Child. *55*:619 (1980)
Colle M., Doyard P., Chaussain J.-L., et al: Acanthosis nigricans, hirsutisme et diabète insulino-resistant, Arch. Franc. Pédiatr. *36*:518 (1979)

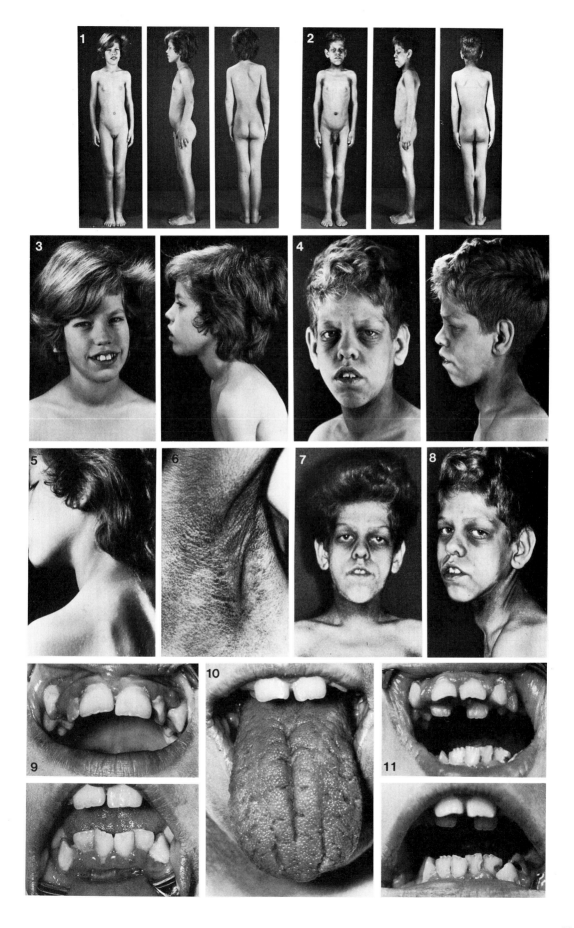

120. Syndrome of Multiple Lentigines

(LEOPARD Syndrome)

A complex hereditary syndrome involving skin, heart, and other areas and with relatively typical facial dysmorphism.

Main Signs:
1. Multiple lentigines of the skin (dark brown, up to 5 mm in diameter), most common on the back of the neck and upper trunk (3–6). Face, scalp, palms, soles, and genitalia may also be affected. Mucous membranes not involved.
2. Cardiac anomaly (7) – usually mild pulmonary stenosis or (and) subaortic stenosis or hypertrophic obstructive cardiomyopathy – with diverse ECG changes (e.g., conduction disturbances).
3. Ocular hypertelorism and 'coarse facies' (2): large pinnae, pouting lips, protruding lower jaw.

Supplementary Findings: Growth and skeletal abnormalities: growth deficiency; possible anomaly of the thorax (funnel or pigeon breast), scapulae alatae, kyphosis, and general weakness of the the connective tissues.

Genital dysplasia (cryptorchidism, hypospadias) as well as delayed puberty may be features. Sometimes inner ear hearing impairment or deafness.

Mild mental retardation noted in a few cases.

Manifestation: Lentigines present at birth or appearing during the first years of life, increasing continuously (3 and 4). Hearing impairment may be congenital or of early onset. Cardiac disorder according to severity.

Aetiology: Monogenic hereditary disorder, autosomal dominant, with high penetrance. Variable degree of expressivity.

Frequency: Rare (about 100 cases reported up to 1978).

Course, Prognosis: Increasing development of lentigines. Degree of impairment otherwise dependent essentially on the type, development, and possible operative correction of the cardiac defect as well as on a possible hearing or mental impairment; furthermore, on the extent of a possible growth deficiency and of a delay in sexual maturation.

Differential Diagnosis: von Recklinghausen's neurofibromatosis (p.248). Occasionally additional single (and rather dark!) 'café au lait spots' are found with the LEOPARD syndrome. Noonan syndrome (p.132).

Comment: The designation LEOPARD syndrome has its origin in the initials of the most important signs of the syndrome: **L**entigines; **E**lectrocardiographic conduction defects; **O**cular hypertelorism; **P**ulmonary stenosis; **A**bnormalities of genitalia; **R**etardation of growth; **D**eafness.

Illustrations:
1–7 An affected child at ages 7½ (1 and 3), 10 (4), 11 (2, 5, and 6), and 12 years (7). Note increased coarsening of the facial features (1 and 2) and increase in number of lentigines (3 and 4). Cardiac defect recognised since birth; shown in later studies to comprise marked stenosis of the pulmonary valve along with a left heart anomaly (probably severe subaortic stenosis); X-ray: marked enlargement and deformity of the heart shadow (7); ECG: pathological right heart pattern with deep Q_3 and extremely high ventricular peaks on the limb leads; extreme right and left hypertrophy with ventricular conduction defect and severe impairment of repolarisation. Lentigines increasing continuously since birth. No hearing impairment. Increasing growth deficiency (at 7½ about 17 cm, at 12 years about 20 cm from the average for age). Slight mental retardation (special school). High narrow cranium (2), epicanthi, ogival palate, short neck (5 and 6), scapulae alatae, coxae valgae. Death due to heart failure in the middle of the 2nd decade of life.

Reference:
Voron D., Hatfield H., Kalkhoff R.: Multiple lentigines syndrome. Am. J. Med. 60:447 (1976)

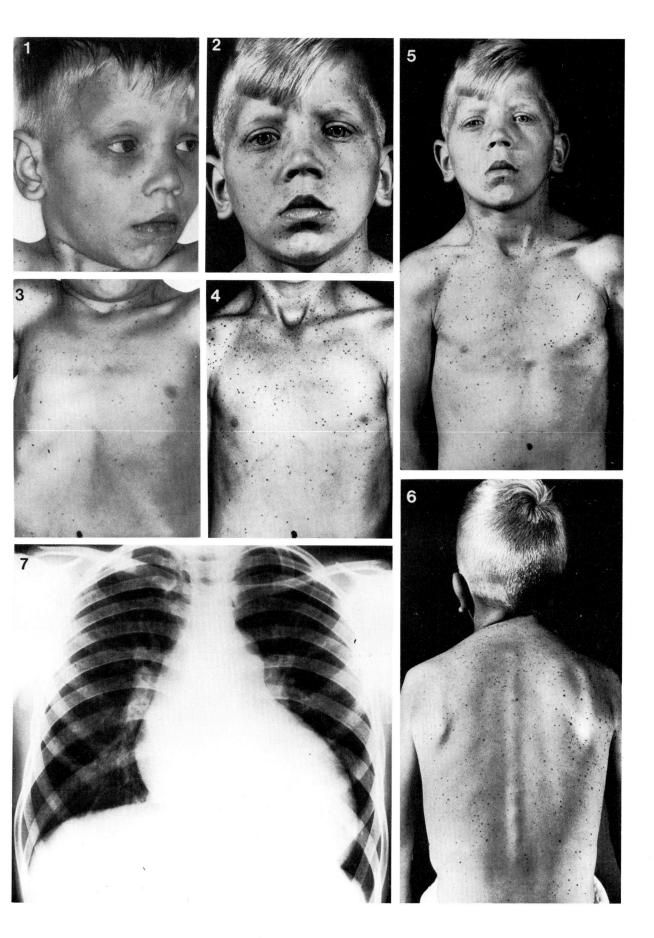

121. Peutz–Jeghers Syndrome

(Syndrome of Mucocutaneous Pigmentation and Intestinal Polyposis; Pigment Spots –Polyposis Syndrome)

An autosomal dominant hereditary disorder of conspicuous pigmentations predominantly on the face and oral mucosa associated with intestinal polyposis.

Main Signs:
1. Dark, brown or grey blue-black pigmented spots on the skin of the face – especially around the orifices, on the oral mucosa, extremities (including the nail beds), and occasionally other areas (**1–5**).

Supplementary Findings: With the appropriate studies, more or less extensive polyposis of the gastrointestinal tract – especially the jejunum – and less often of the mucosa of the respiratory and/or urogenital tracts.

Manifestation: The melanin spots may be present congenitally; otherwise they appear in early childhood. Manifestations of intestinal polyposis – colicky pain, intestinal bleeding with possible eventual anaemia, in some cases recurrent signs of intussusception – also frequently in early childhood.

Aetiology: Autosomal dominant hereditary disorder with high penetrance of the pathological gene.

Frequency: Not so rare; a few hundred cases have been reported.

Course, Prognosis: The extent of the pigmentation on the oral mucosa does not predict the extent of the visceral polyposis. The pigmented spots of the skin tend to fade after early adulthood. Possible malignant transformation of the intestinal polyps, although the risk is relatively low. Occasional development of ovarian tumours.

Differential Diagnosis: Freckles: Other distribution and no mucous membrane involvement. The latter is also true for the LEOPARD syndrome (p.240). Addison disease: Diffuse pigmentation of the skin and more pronounced in skinfolds (oral mucosa may show similar spots, however).

Treatment: Intussusception, etc., may require surgery, resection of polypous segments of the intestine may be necessary. Genetic counselling.

Illustrations:
1–5 A 9-year-old boy. Pigmented spots recognised since the 2nd year of life. Since school age, recurrent signs suggesting ileus. Polyposis also demonstrated in the stomach and large intestine. Father of the boy died of ileus secondary to intestinal polyposis; allegedly he had shown no pigmental skin anomalies.

References:
Jeghers H., McKusick V. A., Katz K. H.: Generalised intestinal polyposis and melanin spots of the oral mucosa, lips and digits. A syndrome of diagnostic significance. N. Engl. J. Med. *241*:993 (1949)
Klostermann G.: Pigmentfleckenpolypose. Thieme, Stuttgart 1960
Long J. A., jr, Dreyfuss J. R.: The Peutz–Jeghers syndrome: A 39-year clinical and radiologic follow-up report. N. Engl. J. Med. *297*:1070 (1977)

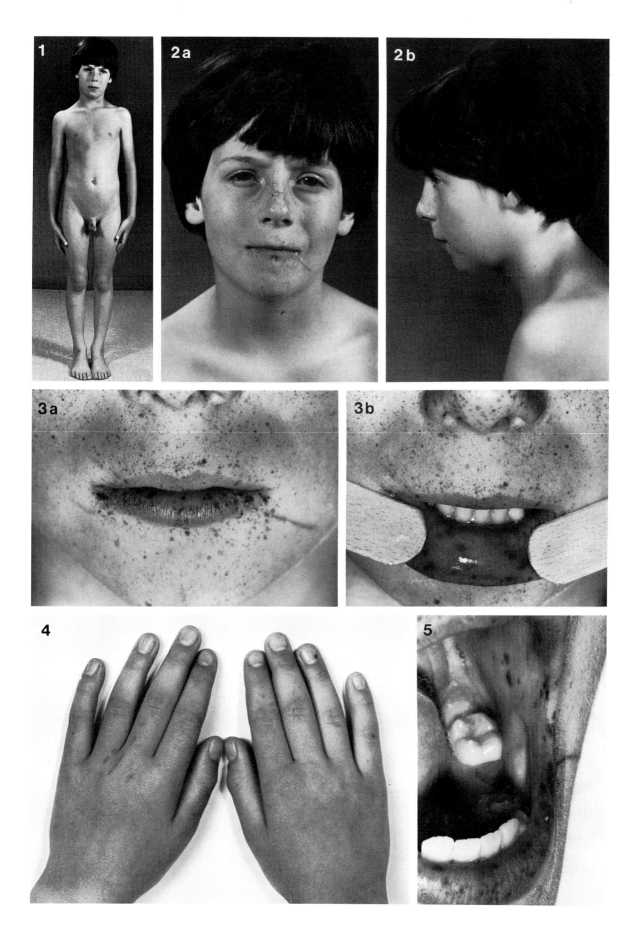

122. Rothmund–Thomson Syndrome

(Syndrome of Congenital Poikiloderma)

A hereditary syndrome of early manifested 'mottling' of the skin frequently combined with development of cataracts, growth deficiency, and further anomalies.

Main Signs:

1. 'Poikiloderma' (mottled skin) as a result of erythema with subsequent spotty atrophy and hyper- and depigmentation and reticular telangiectasia, in the facial area, ears, back of the hands, underarms, and extensor surfaces of the legs as well as other areas exposed to light. Photosensitivity. Possible extensive absence of the eyebrows (as a sign of atrophy), involvement of the prolabium, eventual development of spotty hyperkeratoses of the backs of the hands and feet (**1–2**).

2. Bilateral cataract in some cases.

3. Possible growth deficiency (very variably expressed); 'triangular face' with protruding forehead and depressed nasal root; small hands and feet with brachydactyly.

Supplementary Findings: Frequent generalised or partial hypotrichosis, anomalies of the nails and teeth.

Cryptorchidism and other signs of hypogonadism.

Possible skeletal anomalies, especially of the extremities (e.g., hypo- or aplasia of the 1st rays of the upper extremities).

Manifestation: Development of the skin disorder in early childhood (from early infancy), of cataracts between about the 2nd and 8th years of life.

Aetiology: Hereditary disorder with autosomal recessive transmission; (uniform syndrome? heterogeneity?). Substantially more females affected.

Frequency: Rare (about 80 cases have been described).

Course, Prognosis: Life expectancy not affected – unless skin cancer is induced as a result of (rather unusual) marked photosensitivity together with atrophy of the skin and hyperkeratoses.

Differential Diagnosis: Bloom syndrome (p.270).

Treatment: Symptomatic. Protection from the sun. In some cases oncological follow-up. Genetic counselling.

Illustrations:

1 and 1a A 5-year-old girl affected with typical congenital poikiloderma.

2 A 4½-year-old.

(By kind permission of Prof. H. Reich, Münster i. W.)

Reference:
Rodermund O.-E., Hausmann D.: Das Rothmund-Syndrom. Z. Hautkr. *52*:129 (1977)

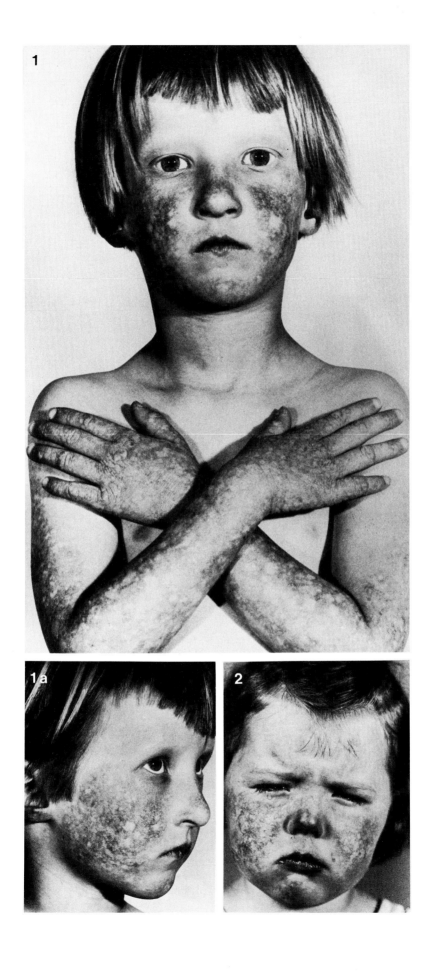

123. Xeroderma Pigmentosum

A hereditary syndrome of hypersensitivity to sunlight and photophobia beginning at an early age, development of pigment anomalies, and early development of skin cancer or precancerous lesions.

Main Signs:
1. Hypersensitivity to sunlight and photophobia (to the ultraviolet region of light) from birth on.
2. Development of hyper- and depigmentation (1 and 2).
3. Development of precancerous lesions and of skin cancer in the light-damaged areas.
4. Especially endangered areas are the lips and the eyes (with possible development of keratitis and corneal scars, and of malignant growths on the conjunctiva and eyelids).

Manifestation: Photophobia from birth; skin changes from early to late infancy.

Aetiology: Hereditary defect, autosomal recessive.

Frequency: Relatively rare in Europeans.

Course, Prognosis: Unfavourable.

Treatment: As far as possible, avoidance of exposure to sunlight; regular application of a sunscreen salve (Contralum®*) to protect the skin from light rays; early excision of precancerous lesions. Genetic counselling for the parents.

Illustrations:
1 and 2   A 5-year-old boy. Hypersensitivity to sunlight from a young age; starting in the 2nd year of life, appearance of pigmental moles and telangiectases on the face and hands. Now all sunlight-exposed areas of the skin covered with small hyper- or depigmented spots and telangiectases. Up to this age, 10 precancerous lesions. Additional development of numerous haemangiomas and multiple keratoacanthomas.
(By kind permission of Prof. R. Happle, Münster i. W.).

References:
Any textbook of dermatology.

*A special salve for treating Xeroderma Pigmentosum, manufactured in Germany but available in other countries.

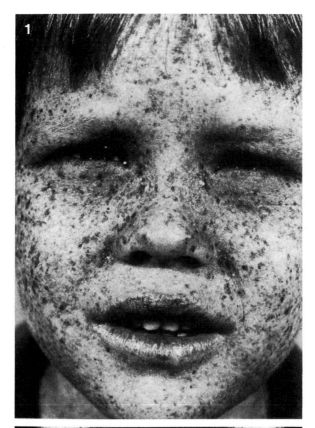

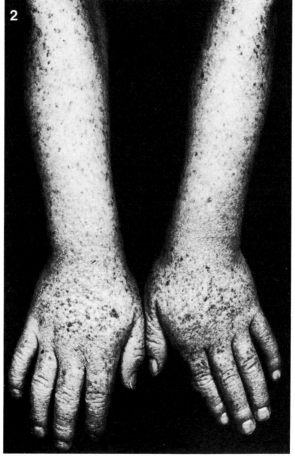

124. Syndrome of von Recklinghausen Neurofibromatosis

A characteristic hereditary syndrome of multiple café-au-lait spots, skin tumours, and skeletal, neurological, and other signs.

Main Signs:
1. More or less abundant café-au-lait spots, especially on the trunk; also various other pigmentation anomalies (**1–9** and **12**).
2. Multiple fibromas or neurofibromas and other dysplastic intra- and subcutaneous growths along the nerve trunks and in other regions (**11** and **12**).
3. Frequent development of neurological and/or ophthalmological defects (e.g., as a result of nerve compression) (**1** and **2**).
4. Frequent skeletal anomalies such as congenital pseudarthrosis, club foot, lux. coxae, spina bifida or development of kyphoscoliosis or (on X-rays) cystic-sclerotic lesions (**9**, **3**, and **4**). Possibly partial macrosomia (**1** and **10**).
5. Mental retardation not uncommon; possible seizure disorder.

Supplementary Findings: Not infrequently macrocranium. Frequent changes of and about the eyes (neurofibroma of the eyelid, corneal clouding, Lisch nodules of the iris, or others).

Possible development of endocrinological disorder (e.g., precocious puberty).

Manifestation: At and after birth. However, during childhood, at first often only café-au-lait spots or freckle-like pigmentations are detectable. Increase in the size and number of these signs during the first two decades of life.

Aetiology: Autosomal dominant hereditary disorder with high penetrance but very variable expressivity. About half of the cases are due to new mutations.

Frequency: Relatively high. Estimation: 1 case in every 2500–3300 births.

Course, Prognosis: In principle, progression is to be expected. Dysplastic blastomas may develop, also on deep-lying peripheral nerves, on sympathetic nerves, on the spinal roots, cranial nerves, or retina, in the brain or intraspinally, on the adrenals, kidneys, or other locations. And danger of later development of malignancy in these sites in over 5% of cases.

Diagnosis: Five or more café-au-lait spots of more than 1.5 cm diameter are considered diagnostic of neurofibromatosis. Pigmented spots in the axilla are also of diagnostic value.

Differential Diagnosis: Syndrome of multiple lentigines (p.240), possibly also McCune–Albright syndrome (p.236).

Treatment: Symptomatic. Genetic counselling.

Illustrations:
1 A pre-school child from a neurofibromatosis kindred. Clusters of café-au-lait spots; small tumours on the head and left leg; tumorous macrosomia of the right leg (histologically: neurofibromatosis); also intraspinal space-occupying lesion; hypertrophy of the clitoris; lux. coxarum.
2 and 12 A patient aged 5 years; fibroma of the left upper thigh, multiple smaller tumours and xanthoma tuberosum. Macrocephaly, ataxia; debility. Coxa vara; cryptorchidism. Neurofibromatosis kindred.
3 A patient aged 10 years; multiple café-au-lait spots, kyphoscoliosis, erethistic mental retardation.
4 A patient aged 13 years; hyperpigmented areas to the size of the palm of a hand, fibroma, tumid deformity of the nose, a hump on the thoracic vertebrae, debility.
5–8 A patient aged 12 years; short stature, kyphosis, typical bilateral nodules of the iris; pigment anomaly of the fundus.
9 A patient aged 5 years, from a neurofibromatosis kindred and with a sacrococcygeal deformity, café-au-lait spots, growth deficiency, congenital heart defect, hypertelorism, strabismus, prominent optic disc on the left, mentally retarded.
10 Macrodactyly of the left hand in a 12-year-old patient studded with café-au-lait spots; hypertelorism, facial scoliosis, ogival palate; fibromatosis.
11 The lower back of a woman from a neurofibromatosis kindred.

References:
Any paediatric, neurology, or dermatology textbook.
Riccardi V. M.: von Recklinghausen neurofibromatosis. N. Engl. J. Med. (1981): 1617; complementary letter texts: ibid. (1982): 1177/1188

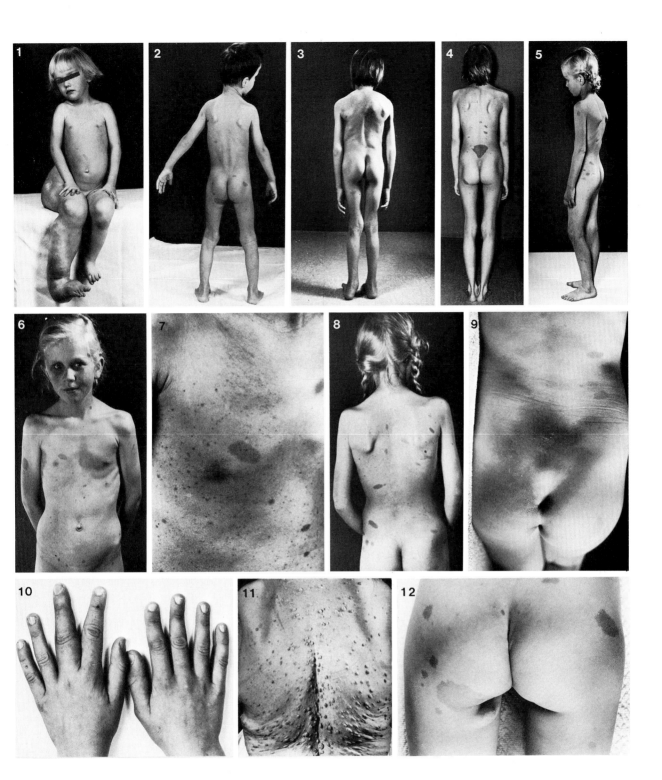

125. Goltz–Gorlin Syndrome

(Focal Dermal Hypoplasia)

A complex mesoectodermal hereditary syndrome characterised by focal dermal atrophy with hernias of adipose tissue, associated with a multitude of possible skeletal, dental, ophthalmological, and other anomalies.

Main Signs:

1. Approximately lentil-sized areas of dermal atrophy in an irregular – in part netlike, wormlike, or striped – or a systematic distribution in addition to corresponding larger foci with hernias of adipose tissue (**1**). Additionally, displacement of pigment, telangiectases, scars (from congenital skin defects) and possible papillomas of the lips, gums, or genital and/or anal areas.
2. Skeletal anomalies: syndactyly (**2** and **3**); hypo- or aplasia of rays of fingers and/or toes (**5**) and more extensive dysmelias. Hypo- and aplasia of the trunk skeleton, in some cases with subsequent kyphoscoliosis, etc.
3. Malpositioning and hypo- and aplasia of the teeth. Hypo- and dysplasia of the nails (**2b** and **5**). Disorder of hair growth (hypotrichosis or localised alopecia).
4. Possible anomalies of the eyes such as coloboma, aniridia, microphthalmos, or others.

Supplementary Findings: Microcephaly, mental retardation; short stature, asymmetry or hemihypoplasia; anomalies of the ears, and many other developmental defects.

Radiologically, characteristic longitudinal striation of the metaphyses of the long bones.

Manifestation: Skin changes usually present at birth; some possibly developing soon thereafter from affected erythematous regions. Papillomas often not manifest until later on.

Aetiology: Genetically determined syndrome; predominantly sporadic cases, girls almost exclusively affected. The prevalent assumption is of X-linked dominance with almost certain lethal effect of the mutant gene in males in utero.

Frequency: Rare; up to 1978 somewhat more than 65 cases had been reported (of these, 9 were boys).

Course, Prognosis: Dependent on the type and severity of extracutaneous involvement.

Differential Diagnosis: Mainly the Bloch–Sulzberger syndrome (p.254).

Treatment: Symptomatic (multidisciplinary care as required by the case at hand). Genetic counselling.

Illustrations:

1–5 The 2nd child of healthy, young, nonconsanguineous parents. Typical skin changes quite pronounced on the right as are the associated anomalies (**2, 4** – diaphragmatic hernia –, **5**). Partial syndactyly II/III and clinodactyly of the right hand (**2b**), aplasia of the 12th rib on the right, aplasia of two rays of the right foot (**5**). X-ray: typical 'osteopathia striata'.

References:
Braun-Falco O., Hofmann C.: Das Goltz-Gorlin syndrome. Hautarzt 26:393 (1975)
Happle R., Lenz W.: Striation of bones in focal dermal hypoplasia Br. J. Dermatol. 96:113 (1977)
Fryns J. P., Dhondt F., Lindemaus L., et al: Focal dermal hypoplasia (Goltz's syndrome) in a male. Acta Paed. Belg. 31:37 (1978)

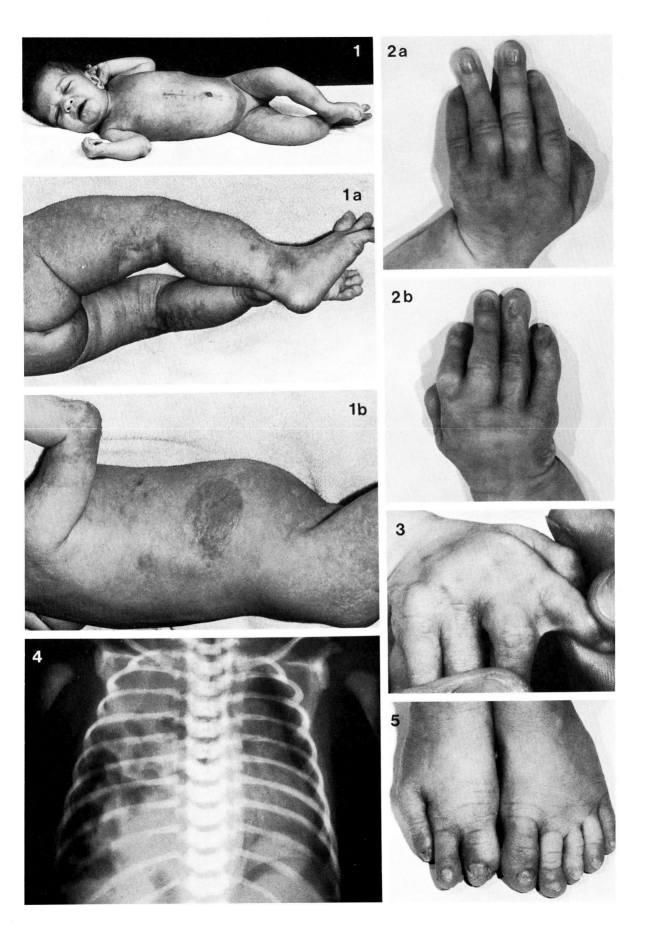

126. Syndrome of Hemihypoplasia and Symmetrical Localised Dermal Atrophy of the Hands and Feet

A congenital picture of general hemihypoplasia, symmetrical foci of atrophied skin and subcutaneous fat on the hands and feet, and other anomalies.

Main Signs:
1. Right-sided hemihypotrophy affecting the entire body half clinically and radiologically, with marked shortening of the tibia (humerus, radius, and ulna of about 4–5 mm, femur about 6 mm, fibula about 7 mm, and tibia about 11 mm compared with the other side) (**1–4**).
2. Atrophy of subcutaneous tissue and of the (wrinkled, thin) overlying skin, symmetrically over the extensor surfaces of the wrist and ankle joints, more pronounced on the right than the left (**3** and **4**). No hernias of adipose tissue; no telangiectases. Skin on the right side of the abdomen somewhat less pigmented than on the left; fine, diffuse haemangioma-like changes on the back, more pronounced on the right than the left; one café-au-lait spot each on the left shoulder, the left elbow, and the right upper arm.

Supplementary Findings: Flat face with widely spaced eyes, epicanthus.

Supernumerary nipple on the left.

Short thumbs bilaterally, deep insertion of the halluces; toes malpositioned and in part crooked, more severe on the right than the left.

X-ray: Distinct aortic configuration of the heart. Kidneys normal on pyelogram. Skeletal survey negative for calcium flecks ('stippling') and longitudinal striation of the metaphyses.

Manifestation: Birth.

Aetiology: Unknown.

Comment: A Goltz–Gorlin syndrome (p.250) had to be considered in the case presented here; however, in addition to other signs, the characteristic adipose tissue hernias and striations of the metaphyses on X-ray are not present. The skin lesions show at most superficial resemblance to the dermal scars resulting from varicella infection of the embryo, as has been described on numerous occasions, and there was no evidence at all of such an infection.

Illustrations:
1–4 A 7-month-old child, the 2nd of healthy parents. Birth at term after an unremarkable pregnancy. Birth measurements 48 cm, 2800 g, and 34 cm head circumference. Statomotor development slightly retarded, apparently normal mental development. Measurements (including head circumference) in the low normal range. Optic fundi negative; neurological examination negative. Chromosome analysis negative. Laboratory chemistries and serological examinations negative.

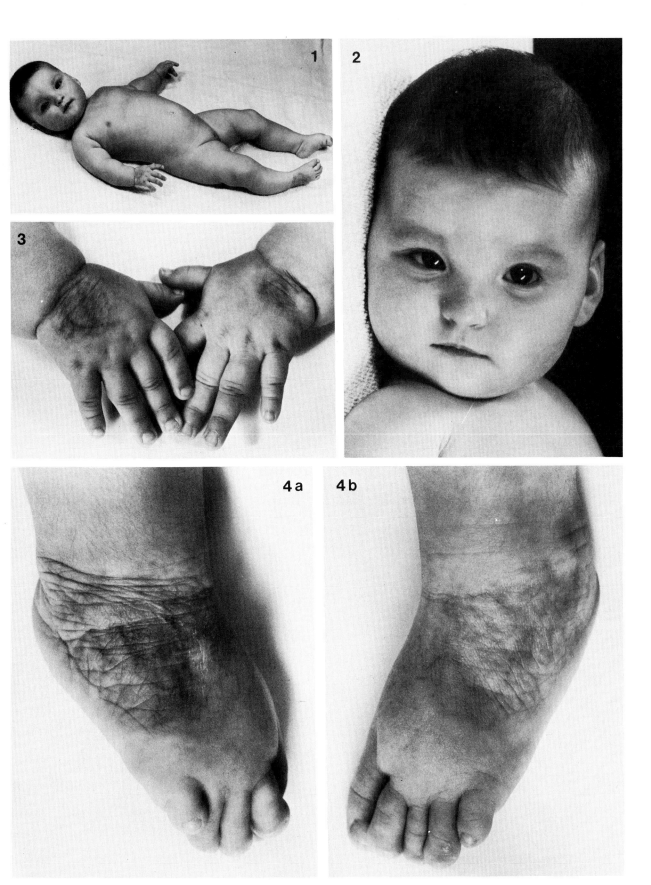

253

127. Syndrome of Incontinentia Pigmenti

(Bloch–Sulzberger Syndrome)

A hereditary dermatosis – herpetiform dermatitis, patchy or verrucous hyperkeratosis and/or streaky hyperpigmentation – associated with anomalies of the teeth, central nervous system, and eyes.

Main Signs:

1. The skin manifestations may be divided into three stages:

I. Nodules, vesicles, and pustules on an erythematous base, frequently linearly distributed, usually sparing the face, present at birth or appearing during the first months of life, persisting or taking an intermittent course over several months (**1**).

II. Patchy or verrucous pigmented hyperkeratoses following the lesions of stage I, likewise usually lasting several months (**2 and 3**).

III. Dirty brown, streaky garland-like distribution of hyperpigmentation, frequently symmetrical, preferentially affecting the sides of the trunk, axillas, groins, and thighs (**3–6**).

The stages occur consecutively, overlapping each other. Stage III may occur on previously normal skin, usually healing completely by the 3rd decade of life, occasionally with residual depigmentation.

2. Dental anomalies almost always present (delayed eruption of teeth, malformed teeth, hypodontia). Frequent focal alopecia, less frequently deformities of the nails.

Supplementary Findings: Anomalies of the eyes in about one-third of cases (strabismus, cataract, pseudoglioma, and others) and involvement of the central nervous system (spastic tetraplegia, seizures, mental retardation, and other), microcephaly.

In stage I, up to 50% blood eosinophils; eosinophilic granulocytes in the vesicles.

Manifestation: Stage I, at birth and early infancy. Stage II, principally in the 2nd–6th weeks; and stage III, in the 12th–26th weeks of life.

Aetiology: X-linked dominant hereditary disorder. The mutated gene is usually lethal in utero for males; thus almost exclusively females affected.

Frequency: About 1:40 000 girls. Over 650 cases, 16 of them in males, became known within 50 years.

Course, Prognosis: When severe neurological manifestations are not present, life expectancy unaffected.

Differential Diagnosis: Goltz–Gorlin syndrome (p.250).

Treatment: Not known, nor can the skin lesions be modified. Genetic counselling.

Illustrations:

1 Patient 1 at age 2 weeks; male (!) infant, but with Klinefelter syndrome (XXY sex chromosomes). Dental germs present. Neurologically unremarkable.

2 and 3 Patient 2 at age 2 months and 16 months. Hypodontia. Cerebral seizure disorder since 7 weeks of age. Normal intelligence.

4 Patient 3 at age 19 months, normal psychomotor development. Delayed eruption of teeth, hypodontia.

5 and 6 Patient 4 at age 12 years. Dental anomalies, microdontia, cerebral seizure disorder since age 4 weeks, right-sided spastic hemiparesis.

References:

Carney R. G., jr: Incontinentia pigmenti. Arch. Derm. *112*:535 (1976)

Hohenauer L., Wilk F.: Incontinentia pigmenti. Pädiatr. Prax. *19*:417 (1977/78)

Korting G. W., Bechtold M.: Alternierende Manifestationsäquivalente der Incontinentia pigmenti in 2 Generationen. Med. Welt. *31*:759 (1980)

Lenz W., Ullrich E., Witkowski R., et al: Halbseitige Incontinentia pigmenti…Pädiatr. Pädol. *17*:187 (1982)

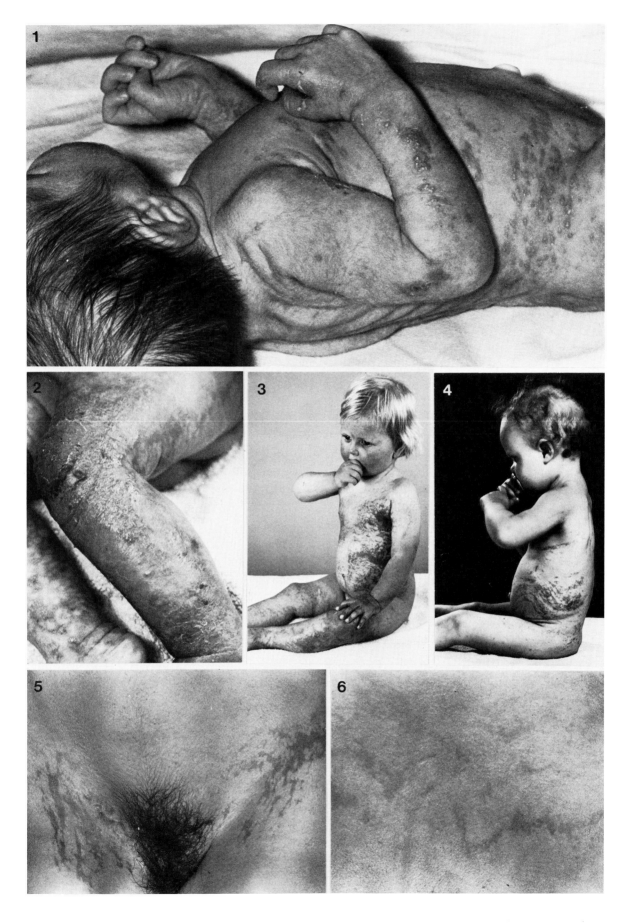

128. Hypomelanosis Ito

(Ito Syndrome; Incontinentia Pigmenti Achromians)

A hereditary neurocutaneous syndrome of streaky, patchy, or spray-like depigmentation of the integument, frequently associated with further, diverse anomalies.

Main Signs:
1. Systemic leucodermia in the form of bizarre, more or less symmetrically distributed (but occasionally unilateral) depigmented streaks, patches, whorls, or sprays (**1–3**). Occurring most commonly on the trunk (not crossing the midline), less frequently the face; distributed predominantly axially and on the flexion surfaces of the extremities. Apart from the hypopigmentation and occasional hyperkeratosis follicularis, the skin is unremarkable. Not preceded or accompanied by vesico-bullous or verrucous alterations.
2. Associated anomalies of a noncutaneous nature in about half of the cases. Especially: cerebral seizures or seizure disorders; stato- and/or psychomotor retardation; ophthalmological findings (strabismus, myopia, fundal changes, and others); dyscranias (macrocrania and others).

Supplementary Findings: Possible hypertelorism, anomalies of the auricles, 'unusual' or 'coarse' facies, in some cases with hypertrichosis; high palate or cleft palate. Hamartomatous excrescences on the upper and lower incisors.

Legs possibly of unequal lengths, or other marked asymmetries; scoliosis, hip dysplasia, and other skeletal anomalies.

Manifestation: Birth or infancy or early pre-school age. The skin changes appear lighter and more marked in persons of a dark than in those with a light complexion (in case of doubt: Wood's lamp). In early childhood the depigmentations may at least appear to spread.

Aetiology: Genetically determined syndrome; for the most part autosomal dominant inheritance assumed (with irregular penetrance and variable expressivity); however, not all questions settled here.

Frequency: Considered rare; to date about 40 cases have been reported in the literature.

Course, Prognosis: Dependent on the presence and severity of associated anomalies. The depigmented skin areas may darken with time.

Differential Diagnosis: Bloch–Sulzberger syndrome (p.254), which has been described as the 'negative' of the Ito syndrome. However, as a rule incontinentia pigmenti entails hyperpigmentation as the residual of an inflammatory process (with a different histological picture and mode of inheritance).

Treatment: Symptomatic. Genetic counselling.

Illustrations:
1–3 A 5½-year-old boy with typical Ito syndrome. Depigmentation noted in the 1st year of life, subsequently increasing and spreading. In early infancy, abnormal growth of the cranium (hydrocephalus), insertion of a shunt.

A focal cerebral seizure disorder from early infancy, eventually well controlled. Tapetoretinal degeneration with visual acuity below 0.1; strabismus, nystagmus. Hearing normal. Delayed statomotor, good intellectual development. Sturdy, stocky body build and dark complexion. No hyperpigmented lesions. Follicular hyperkeratoses on the arms and back. Foci of alopecia on the top of the head; mild hypertrichosis on the face and back. Macrocranium; CCT now negative. Impaired motor coordination, more marked on the right than the left; EEG still showing focal changes. IQ (verbal part) 112. Slight antimongoloid slant of the palpebral fissures, epicanthi, high palate, malocclusion, long narrow, peglike anterior teeth. Short broad neck with low posterior hairline. Increased dorsal kyphosis and compensatory lumbar lordosis. Elevation of the right gluteal fold, hypoplasia of the right gluteal region. Loose excessive tissue in the left flank. Scrotum palmatum (surgically corrected); small penis with true phimosis. Small hands with abnormal abduction of the thumbs; small feet with zygodactyly. (In part, by kind permission of Prof. H. Doose, Kiel.)

References:
Pfeiffer R.-A., Happle R., Stupperich G.: Das Syndrom von Ito…Klin. Pädiatr. *188*:181 (1976)
Schwartz M. F., jr, Esterly N. B., Fretzin D. F., et al: Hypomelanosis of Ito…J. Pediatr. *90*:236 (1977)
Ortonne J.-P., Coiffet J., Floret D.: Hypomélanose de Ito. Ann. Dermatol. Venereol. *106*:47 (1979)
Happle R., Vakilzadeh F.: Hamartomatous dental cups in hypomelanosis of Ito. Clin. Genet. *21*:65 (1982)

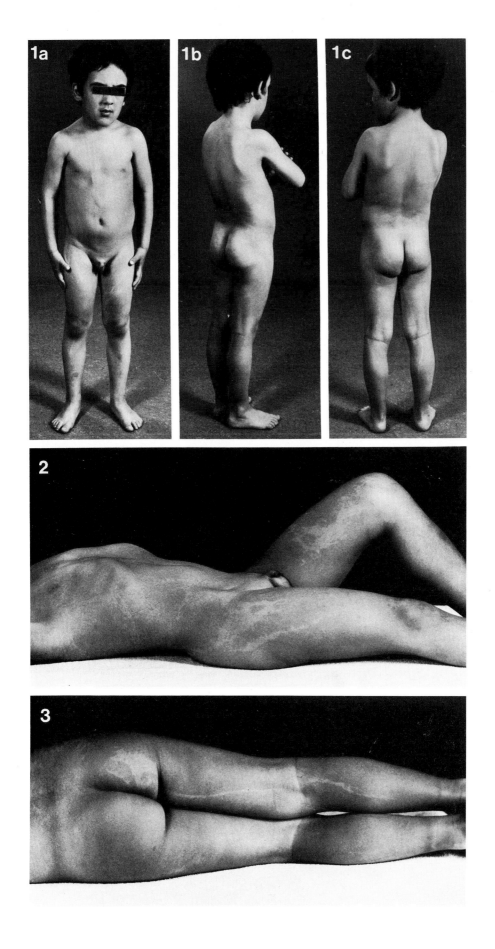

257

129. Syndrome of Tuberous Sclerosis

(Bourneville Syndrome)

A characteristic hereditary syndrome comprising skin changes, mental retardation, and epileptic manifestations.

Main Signs:
1. Skin changes: (a) varying numbers of 'white spots': irregular, but sharply outlined, often leaf- or lance-shaped areas of depigmentation of 0.5–3 cm diameter on the trunk and/or extremities (1). (b) Butterfly-like (localised paranasally and on the cheeks and chin) yellow-reddish nodular rash (so-called adenoma sebaceum, type Pringle; 2–6). (c) Possibly fibroepithelioma, shagreen skin (lumbosacral, also facial), sub- or periungual angiofibromas (8a and b).
2. Mental retardation – frequent and often severe.
3. Seizure disorder (at first very often as jacknife or salaam seizures; then possibly grand mal or any of the other forms). Possible spastic paresis.

Supplementary Findings: Occasionally conjunctival nodules or tumours of the eyelid. Frequent mushroom or mulberry-like papules on the optic disc or elsewhere on the fundus.

Not infrequently pit-like enamel defects of the teeth, depigmented tufts of hair. Frequent kidney tumours (usually bilaterally (9); frequently angiomyolipoma) and/or rhabdomyoma of the heart.

Tumour-like cerebral cortical nodules, ventricular or subependymal hamartoma (7) – possibly resulting in obstructive hydrocephalus, malignant degeneration, or other problems – with marked tendency to calcify.

Manifestation: White spots usually the first cutaneous abnormality, frequently from birth (detectable in up to 90% in the first years of life, later less frequently). Usually early onset of seizures (first 2 years of life). 'Adenoma sebaceum' rarely occurs in early infancy, but usually later (2–6).

Aetiology: Autosomal dominant hereditary disorder, variable expressivity. Frequent new mutations.

Frequency: Not rare; estimated at 1:20000–40000.

Course, Prognosis: Essentially progressive. The mental status – in many cases normal – may deteriorate at any time (whereas seizures are more readily controlled or decrease with increasing age). Death (in status epilepticus, from a cardiac rhabdomyoma, or as a result of renal tumours) not infrequently before adulthood.

Diagnosis: Jacknife or salaam seizures and white spots in the very young child should suggest tuberous sclerosis. In light-skinned individuals, a Wood's lamp may be needed to identify the white spots with certainty. Computer tomography greatly facilitates the early detection of focal intracranial densities. Also in potential gene carriers.

Treatment: Symptomatic (possibly including cosmetic skin surgery). Genetic counselling.

Illustrations:
1, 5, 6, and **8a** A child at ages 10 and 12 years. Multiple white spots on the trunk, increasing adenoma sebaceum, periungual fibroma of the big toe. Fine spotty skin depigmentation and fibromatous plaques. Increased intracranial pressure, unilateral protrusio bulbi, diplopia and facial paresis; intracranial calcification; space-occupying lesion in one kidney.
2 and 8b A 4-year-old boy with initial Pringle naevus, subungual fibroma, white spots, macrocephaly, choreoathetosis.
3 A 3-year-old patient with distinct Pringle naevus, white spots, hamartoma in the nasal meatus; macrocephaly, markedly decreased visual acuity, nystagmus, strabismus; tumours of the eye-grounds.
4 and 9 A 7½-year-old patient, microcephaly, secondary increase in intracranial pressure; palpable kidney tumours; possible cardiac involvement.
7 PEG of a 7-year-old patient with white spots, Pringle naevus, shagreen skin, and fundal involvement; indentation of the right lateral ventricle from the side by a prominence of soft-tissue density.

Mental retardation and a history of epilepsy in all 5 children (in 3, onset with infantile spasms).

References:
Any paediatric, internal medicine, neurology, or dermatology textbook

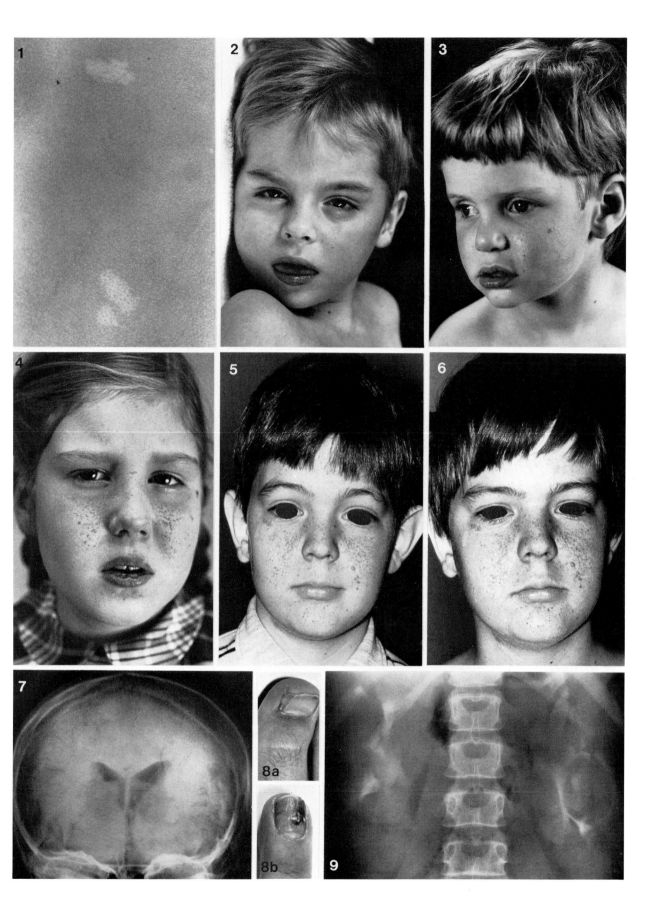

130. Waardenburg Syndrome Types I and II

A hereditary syndrome of facial anomalies, partial albinism, and in some cases deafness.

Main Signs: Lateral displacement of the inner canthi of the eyes ('dystopia canthorum' resulting in short palpebral fissures) and of the lacrimal points, both in type I only; high, broad nasal root and bridge of the nose (**1**); eyebrows quite pronounced medially, with possible synophyrs; strands of white hair over the mid-forehead (**1 and 2**) and/or other signs of partial albinism; in some cases congenital inner ear hearing impairment (apparently much more frequent in type II, without dystopia canthorum; often bilateral and severe; in about 40% or more of the cases).

The facial appearance may be quite distinctive (see below).

Supplementary Findings: Apart from a white fore-lock, partial albinism may be manifest as pale blue colouring – or heterochromia – of the iris, as depigmented areas of skin, as pigment-free strands of hair elsewhere on the head, or as pigment anomalies of the retina.

A relatively small cranium, thick heavy hair with low anterior hairline, relative hypoplasia of the alae nasi, protrusion of the lower jaw, and full lower lip may be features. Furthermore, hyperopia; cleft lip, jaw, and/or palate; occasionally associated with Hirschsprung disease (in type I); relatively short stature and diverse skeletal anomalies of the upper extremities (the latter apparently in a further variant or type). Occasional mental retardation.

Manifestation: Birth (for the malformations including hearing impairment). The white forelock may be present at birth and darken later on. Also the scalp hair in some areas or generally may become prematurely grey or white.

Aetiology: Genetically determined disorder, heterogeneity. Autosomal dominant mode of inheritance for both types with considerable variability of penetrance and expressivity. New mutations more likely with advanced paternal age.

Frequency: Estimation for Holland of 1:42000 persons, with congenital deafness in about 4% of cases (1951); the latter figure for Thuringia approximately the same (1965); more than 1300 cases were reported in the literature up to 1977.

Prognosis: Normal life expectancy. Crucial to the prognosis is whether a hearing impairment is present, whether uni- or bilateral, how severe, and whether progressive.

Diagnosis: From appearance (especially type I) and clinical findings including audiogram. Early diagnosis important because of evaluating hearing and instituting early treatment in case of an impairment (to avoid possible deafmutism and pseudo-mental retardation).

Treatment: Symptomatic and as above. Genetic counselling.

Illustrations:

1 and 2 A 9-year-old girl and her mother, both with Waardenburg syndrome (probably type II). Note the striking facies of the child with broad, coarsely formed nose, high nasal root, and white forelock (the latter in the mother and quite marked in her analogously affected twin sister). Further findings in the child: low anterior hairline and very thick hair; bluish sclerae; patchy depigmentation on the trunk; increased lanugo hair on the back; small cranium; somewhat short stature; kyphoscoliosis, asymmetry of the thorax, and slight coxae valgae; steep palate and caries; hyperopia; mild mental retardation; audiogram negative so far; normal female chromosome complement.

References:
Ahrendts H.: Das Waardenburg-Syndrom, dargestellt in fünf Familien. Z. Kinderheilkd. *93*:295 (1965)
De Haas E.B.H., Tan K.E.W.P.: Waardenburg's syndrome. Docum Ophthalmol. *21*:239 (1966)
Hageman M.J., Delleman J.W.: Heterogeneity in Waardenburg syndrome. Am.J.Hum.Genet. *29*:468 (1977)
Meinecke P.: Das Waardenburg-Syndrom Typ I. Klin.Pädiatr. *194*:112 (1982)

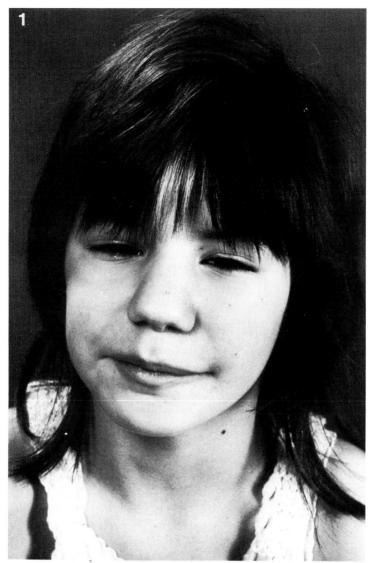

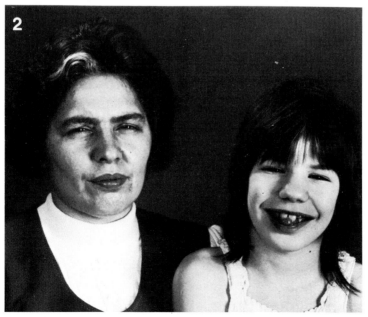

131. Oculocutaneous Albinism with Tyrosinase Negativity

The 'classic' form of albinism, with total absence of pigment in all of the skin, the hair, and the eyes and absent pigment formation in the tyrosinase test (see below).

Main Signs:
1. Generalised absence of visible pigment in the skin and hair (**1–4**). No tanning of the skin. Absence of pigmented naevi and freckles. Light white hair.
2. Total pigment deficiency of the eyes. Unpigmented fundus, 'red pupils', translucent irises appearing blue to grey-blue in an oblique light. Marked nystagmus, pronounced photophobia, and poor vision. Incapable of binocular vision.
3. No formation of pigment by hair roots incubated in L-tyrosine solution.

Supplementary Findings: Possible additional anomalies of the eye.

Manifestation: Birth.

Aetiology: Hereditary defect with autosomal recessive transmission.

Frequency: 1:39000.

Course, Prognosis: No change with regard to the pigment deficiency, nor improvement in visual acuity during the course of life. Average life expectancy probably somewhat shortened due to increased danger of accidents secondary to weak-sightedness and as a result of increased disposition to develop skin cancer.

Differential Diagnosis: Oculocutaneous albinism with tyrosinase-positivity (p.264) and other forms of albinism.

Treatment: Avoidance of exposure to sunlight (clothing, sun-ray filter cream). Tinted spectacles or contact lenses. Genetic counselling.

Illustrations:
1–4 Persons affected with this form of albinism. **4**, two affected brothers and their healthy sister.
(By kind permission of Frau Dr A. Blankenagel, Heidelberg.)

Reference:
Witkop, C.J., jr, et al: Oculocutaneous albinism. In: Nyhan W.L. (Ed): Heritable Disorders of Amino Acid Metabolis, J. Wiley & Sons, New York 1974

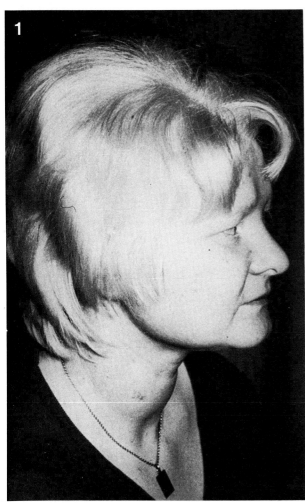

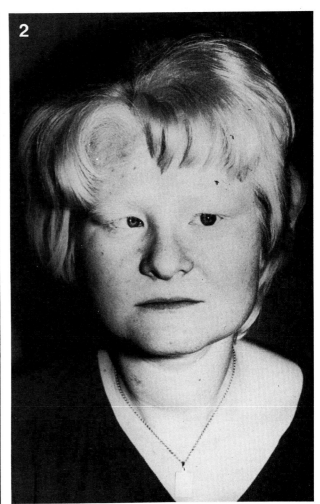

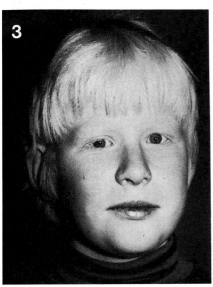

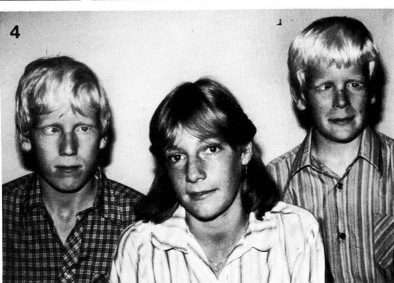

132. Oculocutaneous Albinism with Tyrosinase Positivity

('Albinism II')

Oculocutaneous albinism with decreased pigment in the integument, the hair, and the eyes, and evidence of pigment formation in the tyrosinase test (see below).

Main Signs:
1. Decreased pigment of all skin and all hair (**1** and **2**). However, the severity of pigment deficiency is dependent on age (and race), and the clinical picture of this form varies between that of 'classic' albinism (p.262) and that of a normal pigment-poor complexion. Pigmented naevi and freckles may be present.
2. Pigment deficiency of the eyes. Unpigmented fundus and 'red pupils' in early childhood (possibly improving later). Translucent iris. Distinct nystagmus and photophobia (but both less severe than in classic albinism). Weak-sightedness. Incapable of binocular vision.
3. Formation of pigment by hair roots incubated in L-tyrosine solution.

Supplementary Findings: Possible additional anomalies of the eyes.

Manifestation: Birth.

Aetiology: Hereditary defect with autosomal recessive transmission.

Frequency: About 1:40000 (in American Negroes about 1:15000, in Ibos about 1:1000).

Course, Prognosis: Increasing pigmentation during the course of years, with corresponding darkening and change of the colour of the eyes and hair (in some cases to light brown) and improvement of visual acuity. However, average life expectancy probably shortened as a result of increased danger of accidents due to poor vision and as a result of increased disposition to develop skin cancer.

Differential Diagnosis: Oculocutaneous albinism with tyrosinase negativity (p.262) and other forms of albinism.

Treatment: Avoidance of exposure to sunlight (clothing, sun-ray filter cream). Tinted spectacles or contact lenses. Genetic counselling.

Illustrations:
1 and **2** Carriers of this form of albinism. In **1**, siblings; in **2**, parents with dark complexions and their child.
(By kind permission of Frau Dr A. Blankenagel, Heidelberg.)

Reference:
Witkop C.J., jr, et al: Oculocutaneous albinism. In: Nyhan W.L. (Ed): Heritable Disorders of Amino Acid Metabolism, John Wiley & Sons, New York 1974

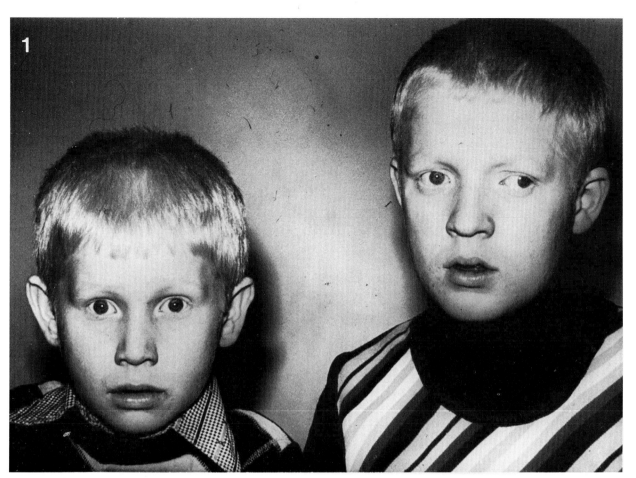

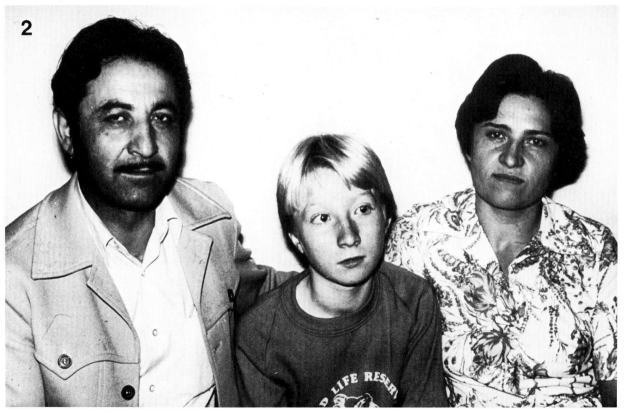

133. Sturge–Weber Syndrome

(Cerebrocutaneous Angiomatosis Syndrome, Angiomatosis Encephalofacialis)

A characteristic syndrome of macular haemangiomas particularly of the face, signs of cerebral foci (due to ipsilateral meningoencephalic angioma) and, usually, mental retardation.

Main Signs:
1. More or less expansive 'port wine coloured' naevus flammeus of the face and cranium most commonly in the trigeminal area, mostly unilateral, often sharply outlined medially (possibly with corresponding involvement of the oral mucosa), less frequently bilateral, and sometimes also of the body (1–5).
2. Focal or generalised cerebro-organic seizures. Spastic hemiparesis (contralateral to the side of the angioma). Secondary mental impairment, more or less severe.

Supplementary Findings: Possible angiomatose changes of the ipsilateral chorioides with or without consequent glaucoma or hydrophthalmos (7). Possible homonymous hemianopsia contralateral to the facial angioma.

Skull X-ray: More or less extensive double-contoured garland-like calcifications, especially over the posterior parietal and occipital regions on the side of the skin angioma (6 and 8).

Occasionally marked asymmetrical development of the cranium.

Manifestation: Naevus flammeus usually present at birth. Possible congenital glaucoma (7). Onset of epileptic activity and of spastic hemiparesis and mental retardation usually in infancy. Dystrophic calcifications of the cerebral cortex as a rule usually not demonstrable by X-ray until the latter half of early childhood; tissue densities detectable much earlier with computer tomography.

Aetiology: In spite of almost invariable sporadic occurrence, a hereditary basis (dominant transmission with variable penetrance) is likely.

Frequency: Not extremely rare; 1 case showing the fully expressed syndrome estimated to occur in about 230 000 of the general population.

Course, Prognosis: Epileptic seizures may be very difficult to control. There are milder and oligosymptomatic cases in some of whom intelligence is unaffected. Although the intensity of colour of the angioma tends to fade with increasing age, the affected area of skin not infrequently becomes thicker and coarser.

Treatment: Essentially conservative except for those cases requiring prompt surgery for glaucoma. Only in cases with very widespread intracranial changes and in which consistent appropriate antiepileptic treatment is ineffective in preventing relentless progressive intellectual and psychic deterioration should a neurosurgical procedure, possibly hemispherectomy, be considered.

Illustrations:
1 Patient 1 at birth. Congenital hydrophthalmos on the right, seizures or epilepsy since birth; early development of left-sided spasticity and of idiocy; intracranial calcifications demonstrable since age 1½ years.
2 and 7 Patient 2 at birth (2). Hydrophthalmos and buphthalmos on the left (7) with subsequent mandatory enucleation; right-sided focal findings on EEG, left-sided seizures.
3–6 and 8 Patients 3, 4, and 5 (6-year-old, 9½-year-old and 14-year-old boys) all mentally retarded and epileptic; hemiparesis in patients 3 and 4; foci of calcification in both patient 4 and (6 and 8) patient 5, who was operated on for glaucoma at age 3 months.

References:
Any neurology, paediatrics, or internal medicine textbook

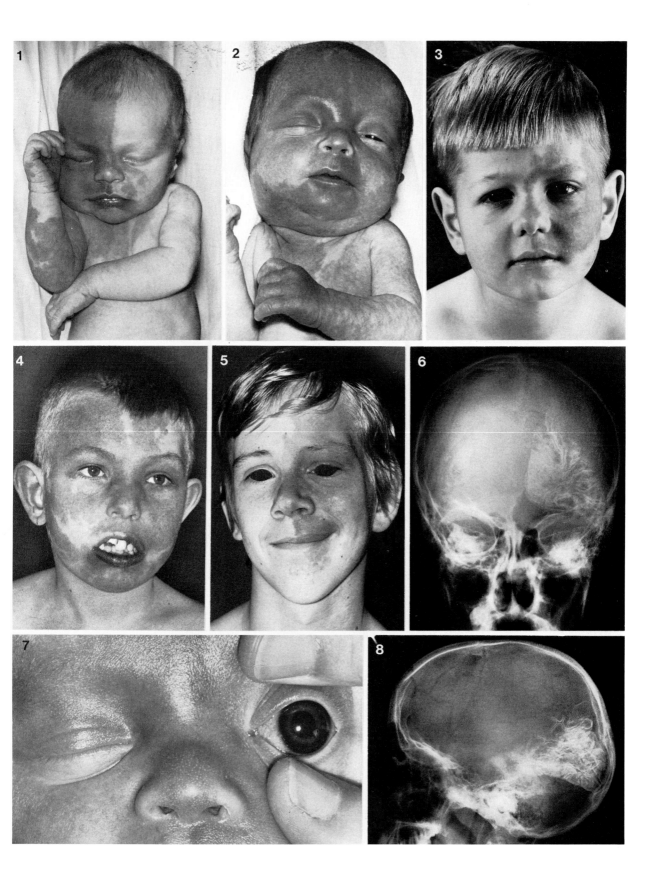

134. Klippel–Trénaunay Syndrome

(Syndrome of Naevi, Varicosities, and Osteohypertrophy)

A dysplasia syndrome of localised, frequently disproportionate macrosomia; naevi; and varicosities.

Main Signs:
1. As a rule, one extremity or a part thereof is affected, much more frequently the lower than the upper.
2. Flat haemangioma of the skin (naevus flammeus), bright red to dark violet, more or less extensive, solitary or multiple, irregular contours, by no means always sharply outlined at the midline when located (also) on the trunk (**1, 3, 4a,** and **6**).
3. Partial macrosomia, with involvement of all tissues, usually in the region of the vascular naevus (**1, 3,** and **4**), but sometimes contralaterally too (**6** and **7**), often disproportionate within itself (**4, 5,** and **7**).
4. Phlebectasias, varices, may be readily apparent (**5**) or detectable only radiologically (phleboliths) or phlebographically (lymphangiectasias exclusively by lymphangiography).

Supplementary Findings: Local anomalies of hair, sweating, etc.

Frequent secondary osteoarticular changes.

Numerous other anomalies optional, e.g., distal vascular dysplasias, macrocrania, changes involving the skin, skeleton, eyes, oral cavity, urinary tract, etc. Thus, a highly variable clinical picture.

Manifestation: Birth and later. Vascular naevi usually congenitally; but postnatal development or expansion also. More or less rapid onset and progression of the development of macrosomia; skeletal involvement only detectable on X-ray in the course of time. In young children, varicosities not (yet) clinically identifiable.

Aetiology: Genetic factors may be assumed; an autosomal dominant pleiotropic gene with relatively low penetrance may be involved. Most cases are sporadic.

Frequency: Not so rare.

Course, Prognosis: Initially definite progression of the 'overgrowth' and handicap in many cases; after the child has stopped growing, the changes may remain stationary. Possible late complication: ulcera cruris which tends to heal poorly.

Diagnosis: Phlebography to rule out obstruction; dysplasia or aplasia of deep leg veins may be found. In some cases arteriography to rule out A-V fistula. Possible lymphangiography. The studies presuppose the child having reached a certain age.

Differential Diagnosis: Possible Sturge–Weber syndrome (p.266), von Recklinghausen neurofibromatosis (p.248), F.P. Weber syndrome (p.300).

Treatment: Symptomatic (compression, positioning, etc.). Orthopaedic care, conservative and/or operative. In some cases extirpation of a section causing venous stenosis. Superficial varices should not be removed.

Illustrations:
1–3 A patient at ages 3 and 14 months. Macrosomia of the right leg with general mild hemihypertrophy. Flat haemangioma on the right, in part with a sharp border at the midline, in part extending onto the left side. Scoliosis.
4 and 5 A 3-year-old patient with an irregular flat angioma. Varicosities and overgrowth of the left leg (tilted pelvis, scoliosis), especially of toes II and III.
6 1¾-year-old patient; angioma especially of the right leg (and the left half of the trunk) with macrosomia of the left leg.
7 Lower extremity of an infant; superficial vascular naevus on the right, disproportionate macrosomia on the left.

References:
Weber J.: Der umschriebener Riesenwuchs, Typ Parkes Weber (Beitrag zur Diskussion des Klippel–Trenaunay–Weber–Syndroms). Fortschr. Röntgenstr. *113*:734 (1970)
Kontras S.B.: The Klippel–Trenaunay Weber syndrome. Birth Defects *10*/7:177 (1974)
Thomas M.L., Macfie G.B.: Phlebography in the Klippel–Trenaunay syndrome. Acta Radiol. (Stockh.) Diagn. *15*:43 (1974)

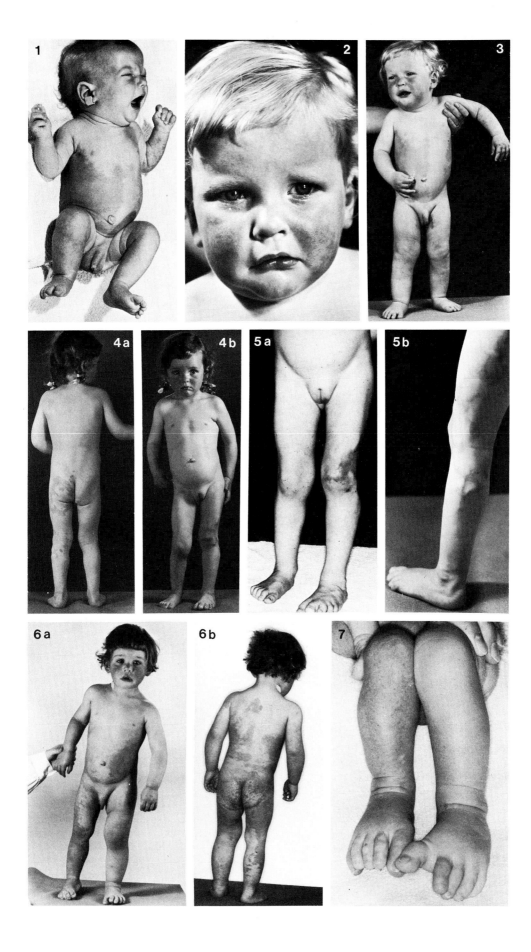

135. Bloom Syndrome

(Congenital Telangiectatic Erythema and Stunted Growth)

A recessively inherited syndrome comprising short stature and telangiectatic erythema.

Main Signs:
1. Marked pre- and postnatal growth deficiency (average birth weight in males about 2100 g, in females about 1850 g; adult height up to 150 cm), with a decidedly gracile body build (**1**).
2. Telangiectatic erythema, more marked after exposure to sun, most commonly in a butterfly distribution on the face, also on the dorsal surface of the forearms. Sometimes blistering and scarring of the lips and lower eyelids. Skin changes more pronounced in males than in females (**1–3**).
3. Long narrow face with prominent nose; hypoplastic zygomatic region; micrognathia; sometimes microcephaly (**1** and **2**).

Supplementary Findings: Small testicles, probably infertility in males (married females unknown).

Frequent infections, especially when younger. Disposition to develop malignant tumours, frequently leukaemia in the younger patients.

Chromosome instability with typical exchange figures in homologous chromosome pairs.

Manifestation: Birth; however, erythema usually first appears during the first summer of life.

Aetiology: Autosomal recessive hereditary disorder. The excess of males probably only apparent and due to their more severe skin involvement facilitating the diagnosis. Basic defect unknown.

Frequency: Rare; since first described in 1954, about 100 cases have been recognised.

Prognosis: Dubious. Early malignant tumours have occurred in about 20% of the patients. The rate must be decidedly greater, since the average age of the known patients was rather low at 16.4 years in 1979, and up to now all patients older than 30 years have become ill with tumours.

Differential Diagnosis: Rothmund–Thomson syndrome (p.244), but the parti-coloured poikiloderma of this syndrome is not present in Bloom syndrome; in the latter, growth deficiency tends to be more marked and the shape of the face is different.

Treatment: Regular check-ups for cancer, restriction of exposure to the sun, genetic counselling. In cases of further pregnancy in the mother, prenatal diagnosis (ultrasonography, amniocentesis and chromosome analysis).

Illustrations:
1–3 A patient at age 7 years, 11 months (**1**) and at 8½ years (**2** and **3**). Birth measurements 2020 g and 45.5 cm. Moderately retarded development in early childhood. Erythema appeared in the first summer of life. Frequent infections during the first year of life. Body measurements at age 7 years: height 116 cm (3rd–10th percentile), weight 16.3 kg (3rd percentile) and head circumference 47.1 cm (about 3rd percentile). Typical chromosome findings.

References:
German J., Bloom D., Passarge E.: Bloom's syndrome. 7th progress report for 1978. Clin. Genet. *15*:361 (1979)
Thomas P.: Das Bloom-Syndrom. Pädiatr. Prax. *24*:283 (1980/81)
Mulcahy M. T., French M.: Pregnancy in Bloom's syndrome. Clin. Genet. *19*:156 (1981)

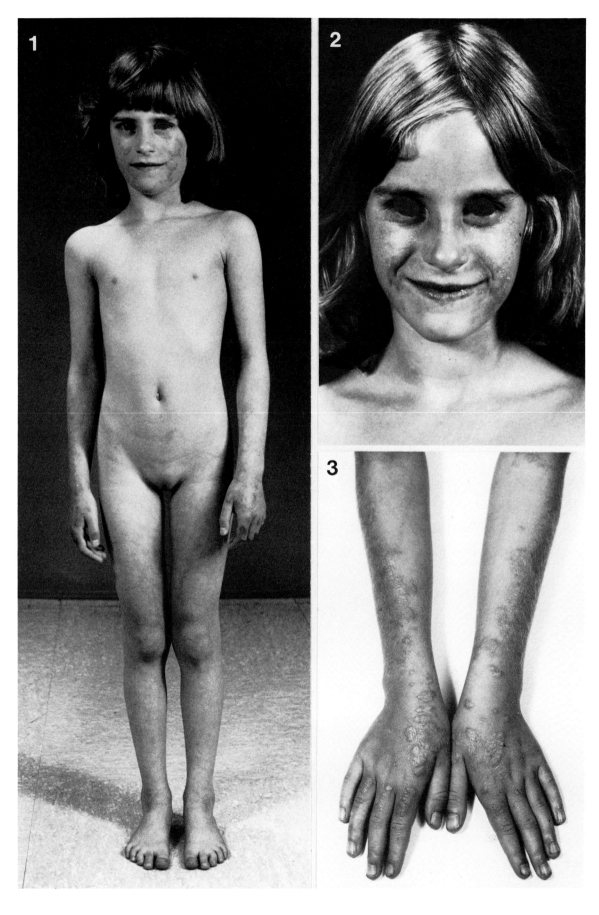

271

136. Ehlers–Danlos Syndrome

A connective tissue disorder characterised by hyperelastic skin, hypermobility of the joints, tissue fragility, eye changes, and a vascular bleeding diathesis.

Main Signs:
1. Hyperelastic, velvety – in childhood strikingly white – very fragile skin, that characteristically gapes 'like a fish mouth' when injured, healing slowly and leaving a cigarette paper-like scar, e.g., on the forehead. Formation of so-called molluscous pseudotumours on exposed areas, e.g., knees, elbows, shins (3–5). Ears very elastic and pliable. Easily damaged blood vessels, thus skin and soft tissue haemorrhages, which may calcify, as do the frequently occurring fatty cysts.
2. Hypermobility of the joints (**2** and **6–8**) with danger of luxation, instability, and bleeding into the joints. Kyphoscoliosis (**1**), spondylolisthesis; pes planus (**2**).
3. Epicanthus, blue sclera, strabismus; myopia; ectopic lenses, retinal detachment, and bulbar tears from light trauma.

Supplementary Findings: Raynaud phenomenon, inguinal hernias, incisional hernias, diaphragmatic hernias.

Occasional short stature.

Rapid physical fatigability.

Possible diverticula and perforations of the gastrointestinal tract.

Haemorrhages from any possible location; dissecting aneurysm; heavy bleeding after dental extractions.

Rumpel–Leede sign frequently present. Varicosities.

Demonstration of specific enzyme defects possible in certain types.

Pregnancy signifies a high risk to the affected mother due to further slackening of the connective tissues and heavy post partum bleeding; also for the affected child, subject to early rupture of the dysplastic fetal membranes and subsequent premature birth.

Manifestation: Birth. The diagnosis is usually made later.

Aetiology: This heterogeneous group of disorders is based on hereditary defects of connective tissue. About 10 forms have been differentiated, based on severity of the clinical picture, variously developed signs in the individual organs, the genetics, and the specific enzyme defects; of the 10, the autosomal dominant type gravis has probably been described the most frequently.

Frequency: Relatively rare.

Course, Prognosis: Average life expectancy decreased due to the above-mentioned possible complications.

Treatment: Avoidance of trauma. Operation only for vital indications. Since sutures do not hold well, tissue clamps are preferable. Caution with angiography. Thorough biochemical–genetic analysis and genetic counselling.

Illustrations:
1–8   A girl at age 12 years, probably affected with the autosomal recessive type 6. Myopia, keratoconus.

References:
McKusick V. A.: Multiple forms of the Ehlers–Danlos syndrome. Arch. Surg. 109:475 (1974)
McEntyre R. L., Raffensperger J. G.: Surgical complications of Ehlers Danlos syndrome in children. J. Pediatr. Surg. 12:531 (1977)

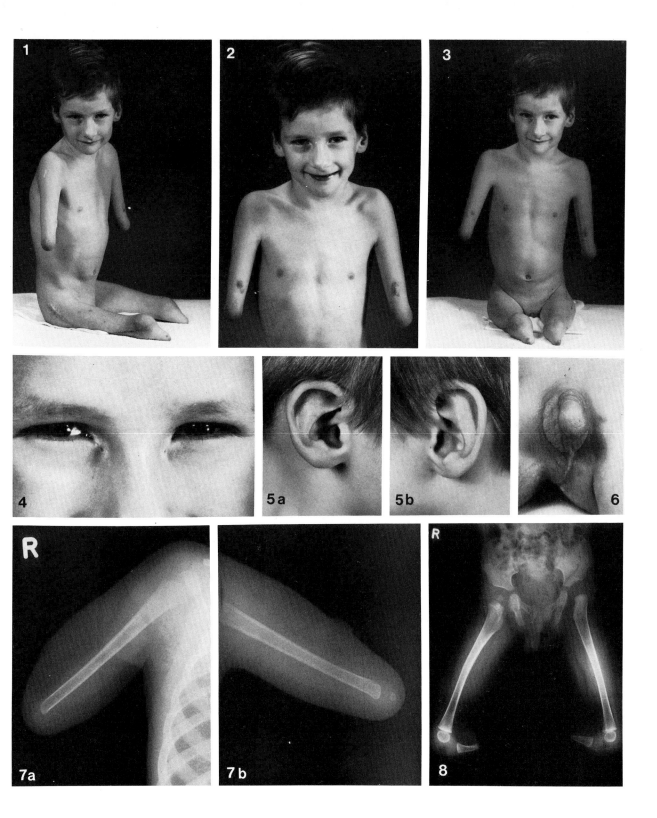

145. 'EEC' Syndrome

(Ectrodactyly–Ectodermal Dysplasia–Clefting Syndrome)

A syndrome of ectrodactyly of the hands and feet (usually cleft), signs of ectodermal dysplasia, and facial clefts (usually of the lips).

Main Signs:
1. More or less severe anomalies of the midportion of the hands and feet, from syndactyly to (usually present) cleft hands and cleft feet (**1, 3–5**).
2. Cleft lip, palate, or both. High palate, hypoplastic upper jaw.
3. Sparse, thin, light hair of the head; meagre brows and lashes (**2b**). Light, thin skin, dry and possibly slightly hyperkeratotic; little sweating. Possible mamillary hypoplasia, anomalies of the nails, small pigmented naevi.
4. Stenosis or atresia of the naso-lacrimal canal, blepharo-(kerato-) conjunctivitis (possible dacryocystitis, corneal scars), blepharophimosis, photophobia (**2b**).
5. Dysodontiasis (small, carious teeth with hypoplastic enamel; also missing teeth). Possible xerostomia.

Supplementary Findings: Conductive hearing impairment may be a feature, also urinary tract and renal anomalies or cryptorchidism.

Mental development probably usually normal; however, developmental retardation, in part with microcephaly, not so infrequent.

Manifestation: Birth.

Aetiology: Genetically determined syndrome. Cases frequently sporadic, probable new mutations. Autosomal dominant mode of inheritance with variable expressivity and penetrance. Heterogeneity or multiple alleles possible. Basic defect unknown.

Frequency: Rare.

Course, Prognosis: Dependent on the degree to which the syndrome is manifest and on the quality of the efforts toward 'rehabilitation' and social adjustment.

Differential Diagnosis: In case of doubt, other known syndromes in which facial clefts are known to occur should be considered.

Treatment: Early correction of stenosis of the naso-lacrimal canal, with some patients requiring continuous ophthalmological supervision for the problem. In addition, care by an orthopaedic surgeon, oral surgeon, and orthodontist. In some cases a wig. Genetic counselling.

Illustrations:
1–6   A child at ages 10 weeks (**2a, 4b**, and **5**), 3 years (**1, 2b, 3a** and **b, 4a**, and **6**), and 4 years (**3c**). Patient shows psychomotor retardation, microcephaly. High palate, slight mamillary hypoplasia, left renal agenesis and right hydronephrosis, cryptorchidism. **3** shows the left, **4** the right hand, **5** the feet. In addition to the familiar signs of EEC, the following are present: bilateral microphthalmos with coloboma of the iris, choroid membrane, retina, and optic nerve (**2a**), bipartite clavicle on the right (**6**) and ventricular septal defect with pulmonary hypertension. Height below the 3rd percentile.

References:
Gehler J., Grosse R.: Fehlbildungs-Retardierungs-Syndrom mit Spalthänden-Spaltfüßen, Iriskoloboma, Nierenagenesie und Ventrikelseptumdefekt. Klin. Pädiatr. *184*:389 (1972)
Pashayan H. M., et al: The EEC syndrome. Birth Defects *10*:105-127 (1974)
Schmidt R., Nitowsky H. M.: Split hand and foot deformity... (EEC). Hum. Genet. *39*:15-25 (1977)

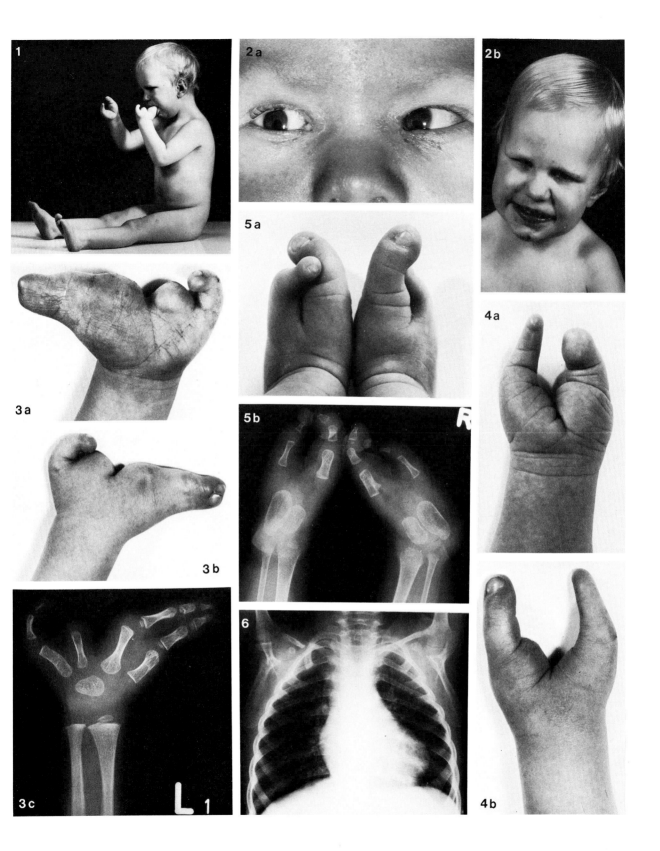

146. Amniotic Bands Syndrome

A syndrome of usually multiple malformations resulting from grooves, constrictions, and adhesions caused by amniotic bands in utero.

Main Signs:
1. Circular grooves – mainly involving the extremities – usually with gross swelling, hypoplasia, or even amputation of the distally lying segment (**3**, **5**, and **6**).
2. Peripheral syndactyly, frequently with grooves from the amniotic bands encircling the fused rays (**2**). Adhesions of the cranium to the placenta. Defects of the cranium with or without encephaloceles or other anomalies of the brain (**1** and **4**).
3. Cheilognathopalatoschisis (or its individual components) as well as facial clefts, which frequently do not correspond with temporal-physiological intrauterine development (**1** and **4**).
4. Clefts and adhesions of the eyelids; microphthalmos ranging to anophthalmos. Anomalies of the nose and auricles (**1** and **4**).
5. Abdominal clefts, focal skin defects (**4**).
6. Remains of amniotic strands not infrequently found in the grooves (**2**, **5**, and **6**).
These anomalies may occur alone or in quite varied combinations.

Supplementary Findings: Scoliosis, subluxation of the hip joints, club feet and club hands have been regarded as the results of the above-mentioned malformations.
   Very rarely 'birth' of an amputated limb.

Manifestation: Birth.

Aetiology: Controversial. Currently, the prevailing theory is that after an amnion rupture, fibrous strands are formed which cause the anomalies by constriction and adhesion. Essentially no risk of recurrence.

Frequency: About 1:10 000 of the population.

Course, Prognosis: Life expectancy limited only in those cases with malformations of the brain or deep facial clefts.

Differential Diagnosis: The multiple deep, benign transverse grooves of the skin, especially of the extremities, that occur in some individuals as an autosomal dominantly transmitted trait should not be confused with those of the amniotic bands syndrome. The same holds true for the congenital scalp defects occurring with amniogenous-like changes of the extremities; here, too, autosomal dominant inheritance has been observed.

Treatment: Symptomatic (possibly plastic surgery, prosthetic aids). Genetic counselling (see above).

Illustrations:
1–3   Case 1 on the first day of life; death on the 2nd day of life due to respiratory failure. External ear dysplasia on the left, internal hydrocephalus, club-foot on the left.
4–6   Case 2 at age 5 days. Death at 3 months from pneumonia. Aplasia of the corpus callosum. In both cases, uneventful pregnancy.

References:
Torpin R.: Amniochorionic mesoblastic fibrous strings and amniotic bands: associated constricting fetal malformations or fetal death. Am. J. Obstet. Gynecol. *91*:65 (1965)
Heege K.: Amniogene Fehlbildungen der Gliedmaßen mit Beteiligung von Kopf und Gesicht. Med. Inaugural-Dissertation. Westfälische Wilhelms-Universität zu Münster, 1971
Keller H., Neuhäuser G., Durkin-Stamm M. V., et al: 'ADAM complex' (*Amniotic Deformity, Adhesions, Mutilations*) – a pattern of craniofacial and limb defects. Am. J. Med. Genet. 2:81 (1978)
Higgenbottom M. C., Jones K. L., Hall Br. D., et al: The amniotic band disruption complex: Timing of amniotic rupture and variable spectra of consequent defects. J. Pediatr. *85*:544 (1979)
Kunze J., Riehm H.: A new genetic disorder: Autosomal dominant multiple benign ring-shaped skin creases. Eur. J. Pediatr. *138*:301 (1982)

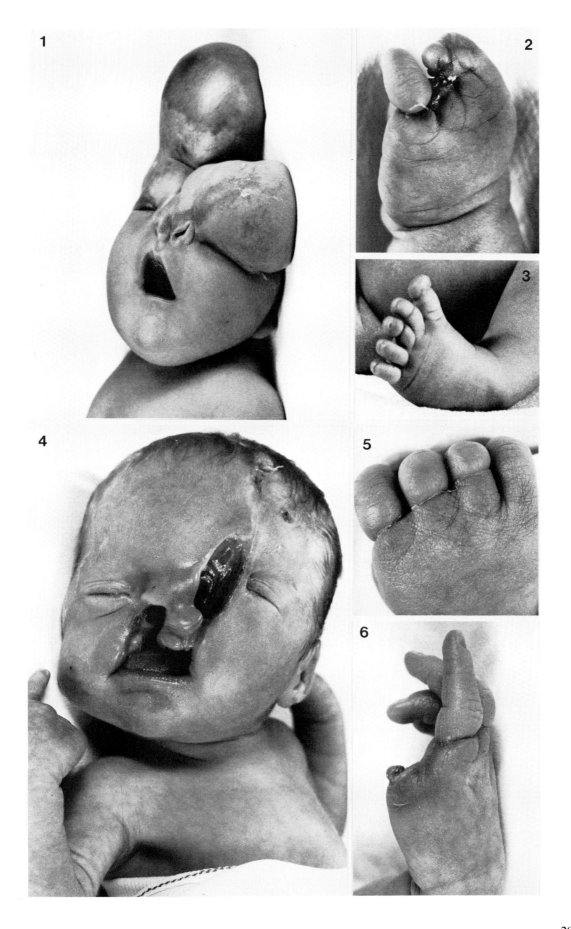

147. Poland Syndrome

(Poland Anomaly, Poland Complex, Poland's Syndactyly)

Unilateral aplasia of the pectoralis muscle and ipsilateral anomalies of the hands.

Main Signs:
1. Aplasia of the pectoralis major and also minor, with frequent ipsilateral hypoplasia and occasionally aplasia of the nipple and mammary glands (1). Not infrequently flattening of the thoracic skeleton on the affected side, rarely bony defects.
2. Ipsilateral anomalies of the upper extremity, predominantly as symbrachydactyly, but also as absence of rays, ankyloses of finger joints, hypoplasia of the forearm and very rarely of the (upper) arm (2–6).

Supplementary Findings: Very rarely unilateral hypoplasia of the kidney and hemivertebrae.
    Defect right-sided in 75% of cases.
    Sex ratio (boys:girls) 3:1.

Manifestation: Birth.

Aetiology: The great majority are sporadic cases; autosomal dominant inheritance has been described occasionally. No increased risk of recurrence for the family if neither parent is affected.

Frequency: About 1:30000 of the population. At least 300 cases in the literature by 1980.

Course, Prognosis: Normal life expectancy.

Differential Diagnosis: The Poland syndrome can occur as a feature of the Möbius syndrome (p.372).

Treatment: If necessary, surgical. Genetic counselling.

Illustrations:
1–3 and 6 Patient 1: Symbrachydactyly, index finger rudimentary.
4 Patient 2: Aplasia of fingers 1–4 on the right, rudimentary 5th finger, absence of the ipsilateral pectoralis major.
5 Patient 3: Symbrachydactyly on the right with hypoplastic middle phalanges, shortening of the right arm, aplasia of the pectoralis major on the right.

References:
Ireland D.C.R., Takayama N., Flatt A.E.: Poland's syndrome. A review of forty-three cases. J.Bone Jt.Surg. *58A*:52 (1976)
Sujansky E., Riccardi V.M., Matthew A.L.: The familial occurrence of Poland syndrome. Birth Defects *13*/3A: 117 (1977)
Castilla E.E., Paz J.E., Orioli I.M.: Pectoralis major muscle defect and Poland complex. Am.J.Med.Genet. *4*:263 (1979)
Parker D.L., Mitchell P.R., Holmes G.L.: Poland-Möbius syndrome. J.Med.Genet. *18*:317 (1981)

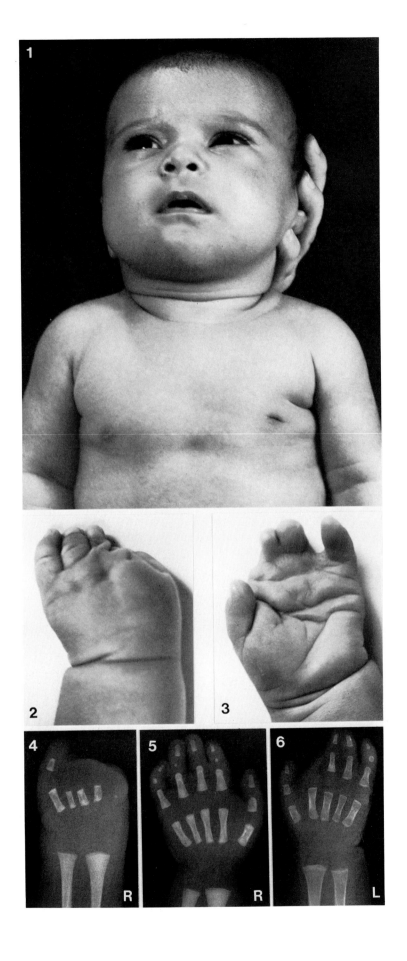

148. An Unfamiliar Syndrome of Dysplastic Extremities– Polydactyly–Dyscrania

A syndrome of partial tibial defect, preaxial polydactyly, general micromelia, and trigonomacrocephaly.

Main Signs:
1. Unilateral partial tibial defect (**1a, 2,** and **5**). Ipsilateral preaxial (on the side of the big toe) polydactyly (clinically nonodactyly, **3**; radiologically octadactyly). General micromelia (**1**).
2. Macrotrigonocephaly with pronounced medial ridge of the forehead (**1a**). Low nasal root. Initially slight antimongoloid slant of the palpebral fissures. Bluish sclera.
3. Short neck. Thickset trunk with low-set umbilicus (**1a**). Luxation of the left hip, impaired extension of the left knee joint. Luxation of the right knee joint.

Supplementary Findings: Unremarkable hands and fingers.

Inguinal hernia on the left, cryptorchidism on the left, retained testicle on the right. Muscular hypotonia.

On X-ray: Large cranium with relatively small facial part of the skull; cranially convex curvature of the base of the skull; delayed closure of fontanelles (anterior fontanelle still open at age 3 years). High, narrow pelvis with steep ischia. Luxatio coxae on the left. Hip dysplasia on the right. Strikingly slender femora, the left being shorter than the right. Halfmoon-like, dysplastic, shortened right tibia with short stubby, dislocated fibula. Short left tibia with relatively long fibula. Seven metatarsals on the right. The four toes on the fibular side correspond to four 3-membered toes; preaxially two additional 3-membered toes (and also the rudimentary third preaxial toe later manifested 3 bony phalanges); abnormally broad proximal phalanx of the large toe, doubled second phalanx (clinically: double nail). Doubling of the talus on the right could also be recognised later. Bilateral ureteral dilatation without evidence of renal malformation.

Manifestation: Birth.

Aetiology: Genetic basis likely. Mother macrocephalic with flat orbits and mild exophthalmos (unusually striking resemblance of the mother's and the patient's facial features); the mother's grandfather had had a congenital malformation of the right foot, perhaps with shortening, since he 'limped' (further medical details not available).

Course, Prognosis: With qualified 'rehabilitation', favourable.

Comment: The typical picture of the tibial defect and the accompanying formation of 7 metatarsals and *pre*axial polydactyly is presented here within the framework of a comprehensive dysplastic clinical picture, which we have not been able to identify as a previously described syndrome.

Illustrations:
1–5 The child under discussion at the age of 3 months. The boy is the 2nd child of healthy young parents (1st child healthy); no parental consanguinity. Birth at term with normal weight and small length (47 cm). Head circumference at 5 months 44.5 cm, at 2½ years 52.5 cm, at 5 years 54 cm. Mental development normal for age.

296

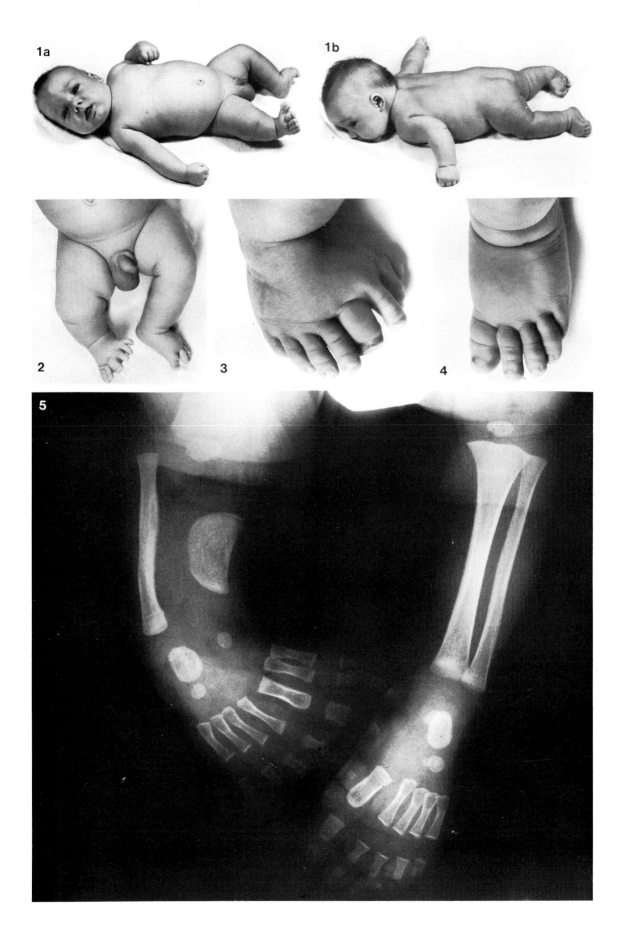

149. Dysplasia Epiphysealis Hemimelica

(Trevor's Disease, 'Tarsomegaly')

Osteochondromatous outgrowth and overgrowth at usually one, but possibly several joints of a lower extremity with consequent disability, deformity, and sometimes pain.

Main Signs:
1. Generally unilateral swelling – more frequently medially than laterally – or limitation of motion of an ankle or knee (less frequently hip or even wrist) joint. In addition, deformity of the affected region in the form of pes valgo-planus or equinus, genu valgum or varum, or occasionally unequal lengths of the legs, more likely due to shortening than to lengthening of the affected extremity (1–4). Pain usually occurs later, at least in the ankle region.
2. Radiologically usually evidence of accelerated development of the ossification centre in the affected area and of an irregular, frequently multicentric opacity adjacent to the affected epiphysis or to the affected carpal or tarsal bone (5), later fusing with it and giving the appearance of irregular enlargement or of a protuberance (5 and 7).

Supplementary Findings: Principally, the dysplasia affects epiphyses of tarsal bones; only exceptionally is an analogous region of an upper extremity affected instead. Usually localised medially, less frequently laterally; again, involvement of the whole epiphysis is the exception (5 and 6). Not infrequently several epiphyses of one extremity affected. Involvement of several extremities is very unusual; systemic involvement (see caption to illustrations) has been reported on only one previous occasion.

Manifestation: The disorder is usually discovered sometime during childhood (or later), exceptionally in the 1st year of life or even at birth.

Aetiology: Unsettled. Sporadic occurrence; boys:girls = about 3:1 (asymmetrical cartilagenous over- and outgrowth of one or several epiphyses (or a carpal or tarsal bone) with subsequent endochondral ossification is the formal pathogenesis).

Frequency: Low; up to 1980, about 85 observations were reported in the literature.

Course, Prognosis: Good, with early adequate orthopaedic treatment.

Differential Diagnosis: Enchondromatosis (p.310), multiple cartilagenous exostoses (p.306), and chondrodysplasia punctata (p.154ff) should not be difficult to exclude.

Treatment: Prompt qualified orthopaedic care of a conservative or, if required, operative nature (excision or partial resection of the osteochondromatous excrescences).

Illustrations: The 1st child of young, healthy, nonconsanguineous parents. Contractures of all large joints of the right lower extremity noted at birth, and increasing overgrowth of the extremity after the 2nd month of life.

1–4 The severely physically handicapped boy as a 3-year-old; on the left side, the lateral malleolus is also enlarged and lower than normal; limitation of pro- and supination of both hands and limitation of motion of the fingers bilaterally.

5 Overgrowth of the right pelvis and proximal femur with epiphyseal dysplasia noted at 10 months.

6 and 7 Correspondingly coarse changes in the right knee and foot regions ('tarsomegaly' with severe deformity of the talus) at the age of 3 years.

Milder epiphyseal changes in the left lower extremity and – even more discrete – in both upper extremities, as in a systemic disorder.

References:
Kettelkamp D. B., Campbell C. J., Benfiglio M.: Dysplasia epiphysealis hemimelica. A report of fifteen cases. J. Bone Jt. Surg. *48A*:746
Spranger J. W., Langer L. O., jr, Wiedemann H.-R.: Bone Dysplasias. An Atlas of Constitutional Disorders of Skeletal Development, Stuttgart and Philadelphia, G. Fischer and W. B. Saunders 1974
Fasting O. J., Bjerkeim I.: Dysplasia epiphysealis hemimelica. Acta Orthop. Scand. *47*:217 (1976)
Carlson D. H., Wilkinson R. H.: Variability of unilateral epiphyseal dysplasia. Radiology *133*:369 (1979)
Wiedemann H.-R., Mann M., Spreter v. Kreudenstein P.: Dysplasia epiphysealis hemimelica. Eur. J. Pediatr. *136*:311 (1981)

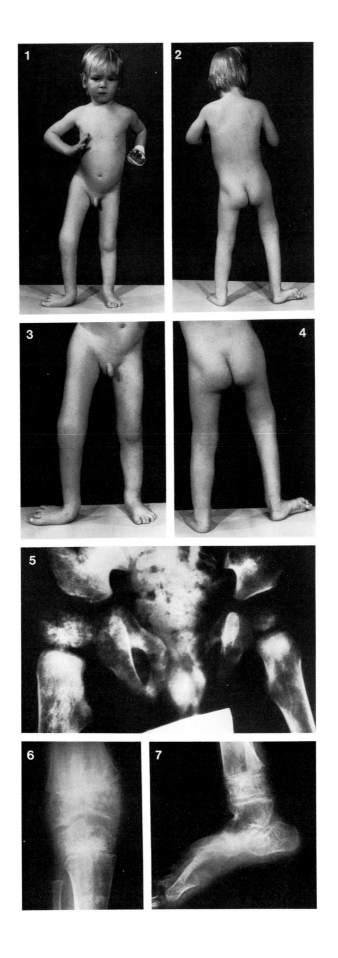

150. F. P. Weber Syndrome

(Syndrome of partial macrosomia of an extremity with haemodynamically effective A-V fistula)

A dysplasia syndrome of partial macrosomia, usually proportional in itself, usually of a lower extremity and due to haemodynamically active, usually multiple, congenital A-V fistulas.

Main Signs:
1. Partial macrosomia of an extremity or a part of it. As a rule, one of the lower extremities is affected, and the changes are more or less in proportion to each other (1–4).
2. Evidence of A-V shunt: dilatation of arteries and veins; prominent vascular pulsations continuing into the veins, vascular thrills, and hyperthermic skin.
3. Congenital A-V fistulas, usually multiple, demonstrated by arteriography in soft tissue or bone.

Supplementary Findings: Large A-V shunts lead to signs of cardiac overload, possibly to severe cardiac insufficiency, with no signs of a cardiac malformation.

Possible secondary osteoarticular changes such as tilted pelvis, scoliosis, etc.

Naevi flammei may occur over the affected region, or in other areas.

Manifestation: Childhood.

Aetiology: Not settled. Genetic factors may be assumed. Mostly sporadic occurrence. Cf. Klippel–Trénaunay syndrome p.268).

Frequency: Relatively rare.

Course, Prognosis: Tendency to progress after the child has finished growing. The affected extremity, even the patient's life, may be seriously threatened.

Diagnosis: Careful angiographic analysis mandatory.

Differential Diagnosis: Simple partial macrosomia without vascular malformations. Klippel–Trénaunay syndrome (p.268); in some cases the two syndromes may be extremely difficult to differentiate.

Treatment: Urgent measures to decrease the shunt volume by vascular surgery if possible. If unsuccessful or impossible, amputation may be considered as a last resort.

Illustrations:
1–4 A 10-year-old girl with 'gigantism' of the entire right lower extremity, especially of the lower leg and foot. Footdrop, flexion contracture of the knee, tilted pelvis, and scoliosis. No naevus flammeus of the skin. Hyperthermia of the affected leg. Dilated veins, pulsations. Multiple A-V fistulas on angiogram.

References:
Vollmar J.: Zur Geschichte und Terminologie der Syndrome nach F.P. Weber und Klippel–Trénaunay. VASA 3:231 (1974)
Vollmar J.: Die Chirurgie kongenitaler arteriovenöser Fisteln der Gliedmaßen. In: Arteriovenöse Fisteln – Dilatierende Arteriopathien. J.F. Vollmar, F.P. Nobbe (eds), Thieme, Stuttgart, 1976, p.66ff

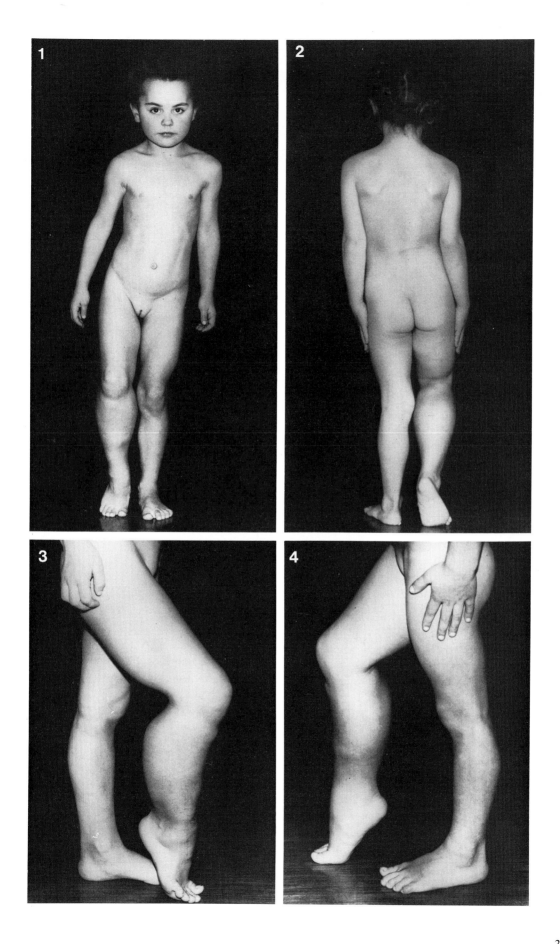

151. Arthrogryposis Multiplex Congenita

([So called] Guérin–Stern Syndrome)

A collective term for a group of clinically and aetiologically heterogeneous congenital, multiple, nonprogressive disorders of joint mobility.

Main Signs:
1. Congenital, nonprogressive contractures (flexion and/or extension) in at least two joints from different regions of the body.
2. Absence of normal flexion creases over the joints; abnormal dimple-like indentations or soft tissue folds at the joints (3–5).

Supplementary Findings: Frequent secondary changes such as, e.g., scoliosis.

Classification: Three categories of arthrogryposis can be differentiated:
(a) 'Primary arthrogenic' clinical pictures. As a rule symmetrical involvement of all extremities with extension or mild flexion contractures; shoulders rotated inward; talipes equinovarus; wrists and fingers flexed; muscular hypoplasias and/or atrophies. Intellect not affected.
(b) Clinical pictures with additional generalised hypotonia and other anomalies of the musculature (clinical, possible biochemical – e.g., elevated CPK – and bioelectric): as a rule flexion contractures of the extremities. Feet in equinovarus or talipes calcaneus position. Musculature abnormal to palpation. Possible cleft palate and other malformations such as scoliosis, etc. (No doubt a heterogeneous category in itself!)
(c) Clinical pictures with additional evidence of central nervous system disorder (considerable mental retardation, possible microcephaly, and others): flexion contractures of the extremities, possibly spasticity.

Manifestation: Birth (frequently breech presentation).

Aetiology: Not uniform. Cases of category (a) are usually sporadic, with a very low risk of recurrence for the parents. Familial cases usually fall into category (b); autosomal dominant, and especially autosomal recessive (exceptionally sex-linked recessive) modes of transmission have been observed.

Frequency: Not extremely rare (about 1–3:10 000).

Course, Prognosis: Retarded motor development as a result of limitation of movements. Otherwise dependent on the type and severity of the disorder, on whether mental retardation is present, and on the quality and intensity of treatment.

Differential Diagnosis: Contractural arachnodactyly (p.90), Freeman–Sheldon syndrome (p.34), and diastrophic dysplasia (p.166) should not be difficult to rule out.

Treatment: Intensive physiotherapeutic and various orthopaedic, sometimes including surgical, measures are required. Genetic counselling.

Illustrations:
1–5 A newborn infant with arthrogryposis.
(By kind permission of Prof. B. Lieber, Frankfurt a.M.)

References:
Hall J. G.: Arthrogryposis. In: Klinische Genetik in der Pädiatrie. J. Spranger & M. Tolksdorf (Eds) Thieme, Stuttgart 1980
Hall J. G., Reed S. D., Scott C. I., et al: Three distinct types of X-linked arthrogryposis... Clin. Genet. 21:81 (1982)

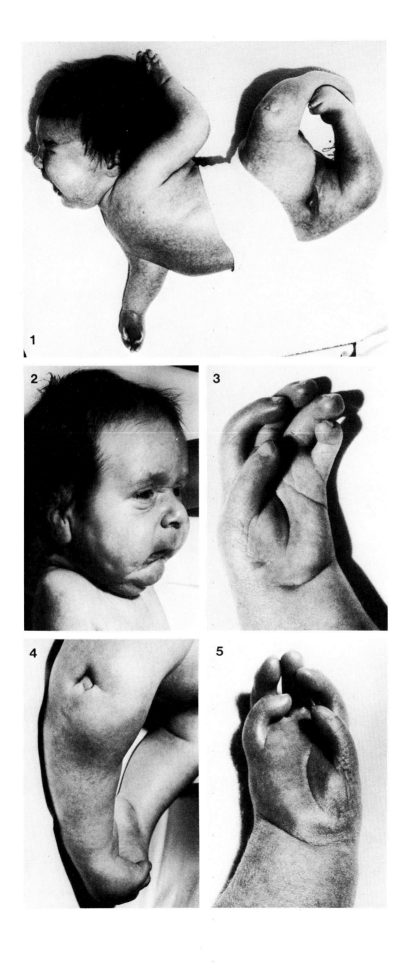

303

152. Larsen Syndrome

A quite characteristic hereditary syndrome of multiple congenital joint dislocations, facial dysmorphism, and hand, finger, and foot anomalies.

Main Signs:
1. Dislocation especially of the hips, knees, and elbows (2). Flat face with low nasal root, prominent forehead, and hypertelorism (1, 2, and 6).
2. 'Spatula-like' thumbs and as a whole, somewhat cylindrical fingers with broad fingertips and short nails (5). Pedes equinovari or -valgi with torsion of the front part of the foot (2 and 4).

Supplementary Findings: Cleft palate not uncommon. Frequent development of progressive curvature of the spine.

Decreased adult height.

On X-ray, distal phalanx of the thumb triangular and remaining distal phalanges short and broad, short metacarpals (especially II), accessory ossification centres in the wrist bones and an extra ossification centre in the calcaneus. Frequent segmentation anomalies especially in the upper region of the vertebral column.

Manifestation: Birth.

Aetiology: Probably monogenic hereditary disorder; heterogeneity; to date, clinical differentiation of an autosomal dominant and, probably less favourable, autosomal recessive form with certainty not yet possible. Girls more frequently affected. Basic defect unknown.

Frequency: Relatively rare; however, many cases are probably not recognised as such; about one hundred case reports in the literature.

Course, Prognosis: Respiration may be endangered in early infancy due to softness of the thoracic cartilage, especially in the laryngotracheal area (and especially in the recessive form?). Variable, frequently severe physical disablement as a result of luxations. Also, without timely preventative measures, the spinal cord may become compressed due to severe deformity of the vertebrae.

Mental development as a rule within normal limits.

Differential Diagnosis: Difficult to differentiate exactly from the oto-palato-digital syndrome (p.16). Numerous dislocated joints, including the knee joints; multiple carpal ossicles; and additional ossification centre in the calcaneus would suggest the Larsen syndrome. The two syndromes may be closely related genetically. Ehlers–Danlos syndrome and the Marfan syndrome (p.272 and 88, respectively) or arthrogryposis (p.302) can be differentiated readily by their characteristic signs.

Treatment: Early application of various orthopaedic measures (feet; hips; the severe, problematic luxations of the knee joints; careful attention to the vertebral column, etc.) and comprehensive, prolonged multidisciplinary care of the physical handicaps. Genetic counselling.

Illustrations:
1–6 A typically affected 6-year-old boy. Height when supported by orthopaedic appliances, at the 3rd percentile. Kyphoscoliosis; spina bifida at two cervicothoracic vertebrae; 13 pairs of ribs. Slight funnel breast. Bifid uvula.
(By kind permission of Prof. W. Blauth, Kiel.)

References:
Spranger J. W., Langer L. O., Wiedemann H.-R.: Bone Dysplasias. An Atlas of Constitutional Disorders of Skeletal Development. G. Fischer and W. B. Saunders, Stuttgart and Philadelphia 1974
Micheli L. J., Hall J. E., Watts H. G.: Spinal instability in Larsen's syndrome. J. Bone Jt. Surg. *58*-A: 562 (1976)
Galanski M., Statz A.: Radiologische Befunde beim Larsen-Syndrom. Fortschr. Röntgenstr. *128*:534 (1978)

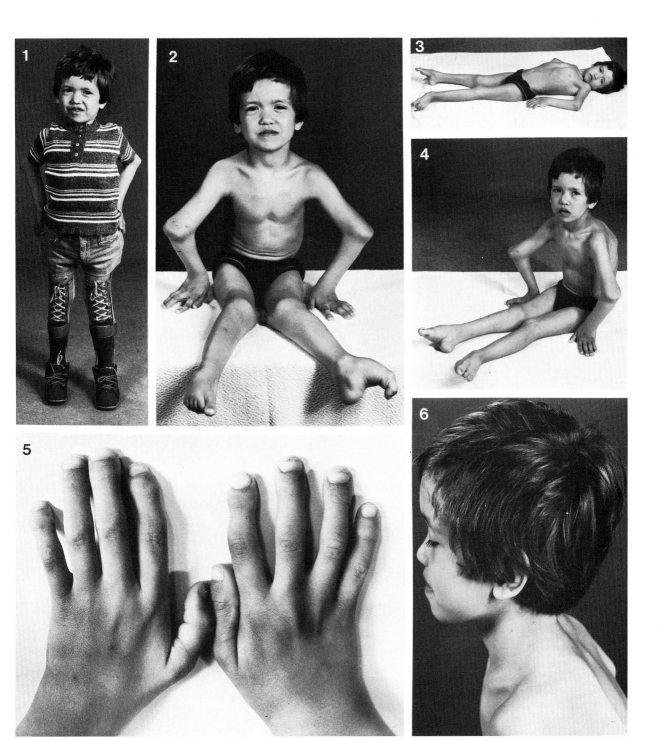

153. Syndrome of Multiple Cartilaginous Exostoses

A hereditary syndrome, very characteristic in its severe form, of more or less numerous bony outgrowths and protuberances, most frequently at the ends of long bones, resulting in deformity and limited motion of the extremities.

Main Signs:
1. Multiple bony excrescences (covered by hyalin cartilage), especially at the ends of the long bones (**1b, 2,** and **3**), most frequently in the knee region, but often on ribs, medial edges of the shoulder blades, iliac crests, and other areas.
2. Secondary deformities of the long bones such as shortening and bowing: most frequently of the ulna, and thus the forearm (**1a** and **b**) with ulnar deviation of the hand; possible radioulnar synostosis. Also shortening of the fibula, tibiofibular synostosis, genu valgum and/or pes valgus.

Supplementary Findings: Possible moderate short stature.

X-rays show exostoses in addition to those palpable.

Manifestation: Variable, usually in early childhood and on into the 1st decade of life. (With growth of the child, exostoses originating in the metaphyseal areas move to the diaphyses.)

Aetiology: Autosomal dominant hereditary disorder with very high penetrance in males, lower in females. Definite sporadic cases may be regarded as new mutations.

Frequency: Not rare (by 1964 over 1000 cases had been reported in the literature).

Course, Prognosis: Slowing of growth of the exostoses during adolescence (with exceptions); thereafter, no further growth of the excrescences. Functional impairment due to the resultant disproportions of parts of the skeleton (see above) and possibly due to pressure on the tendons, vessels, or nervous tissue. Neoplastic degeneration of the exostoses possible in adulthood (in about 10% of cases).

Differential Diagnosis: The Langer-Giedion syndrome (p.308) should not be difficult to rule out.

Treatment: Surgical treatment in case of markedly impaired function or if the development of a malignancy is suspected. Genetic counselling.

Illustrations:
1a and b A 6-year-old boy with deformity of the left forearm, typical X-ray findings (bowing of the radius, which alone articulates with the wrist, and especially of the markedly shortened, distally exostotic ulna pes valgus bilaterally, and multiple further palpable and/ or radiologically demonstrable exostoses.
2 Large, sharply bordered exostosis originating from the proximal humeral metaphysis in a 7-year-old boy with multiple bony excrescences.
3 X-ray of the right knee of a 3½-year-old boy with exostoses on all long bones as well as on several ribs, a scapula, hands, and feet.

References:
Spranger J. W., Langer L. O., jr, Wiedemann H.-R.: Bone Dysplasias. An Atlas of Constitutional Disorders of Skeletal Development. Stuttgart and Philadelphia, G. Fischer and W. B. Saunders 1974
Ochsner P. E.: Zum Problem der neoplastische Entartung bei multiplen kartilaginären Exostosen. Z. Orthopäd. 116:369 (1978)
Shapiro F., Simon S., Glimcher M. J.: Hereditary multiple exostoses. J. Bone Jt. Surg. A 61/6:815 (1979)

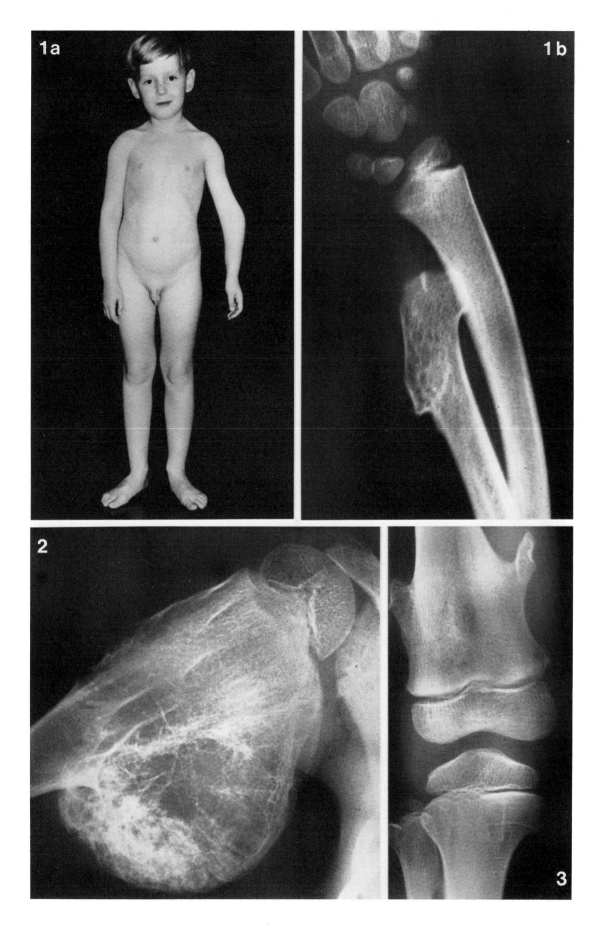

307

154. Langer–Giedion Syndrome

(Giedion–Langer Syndrome, Trichorhinophalangeal Syndrome Type II, Syndrome of Acrodysplasia with Exostoses)

A malformation–retardation syndrome of growth deficiency; peculiar facies; sparse, fragile scalp hair; multiple exostoses; mild microcephaly; and mental retardation.

Main Signs:
1. Typical facial dysmorphism: large, prominent, poorly differentiated ears, broad eyebrows, bulbous nose with broad septum and coarse alae, high philtrum, narrow upper lip, receding chin (**1**).
2. Small stature. Slight microcephaly and slight to moderate mental retardation.
3. Sparse scalp hair (**1**). Frequently lax or lax-wrinkled skin early in life, also muscular hypotonia. Later maculopapular pigmented naevi especially on the upper half of the body.
4. Multiple cartilaginous exostoses of the long bones (sometimes also of the smaller tubular bones, shoulder blades, ribs, and pelvis). On X-ray cone-shaped epiphyses of the hands and feet (**2**).

Supplementary Findings: Optic defects, sensorineural hearing impairment and delayed speech development may occur. Also, winged scapulae, and general hyperextensibility of the joints, Perthes-like dysplasia of the head of the femur, and increased tendency to fractures; clinobrachydactyly. In early childhood possible increased susceptibility to infections.

Manifestation: Birth and infancy. Radiologically, the combination of exostoses/cone-shaped epiphyses tends to become apparent in the 3rd–4th year of life.

Aetiology: Initially all reported cases were sporadic, with both sexes affected; not long ago, the first reports of father to daughter inheritance. Thus, autosomal dominant inheritance, the majority of reported cases having been new mutations. On the other hand, a chromosomal abnormality (8q− deletion) of still unsettled significance has been observed recently in several cases.

Frequency: Extremely rare (up to 1981, only 15 cases reports in the literature).

Course, Prognosis: Laxity and wrinkling of the skin tend to regress during infancy, the susceptibility to infections disappears by about school age. The extent to which the patient is handicapped depends principally on the severity of a mental and/or hearing impairment, then on the exostoses and their effect on joint mobility and local growth. General vitality and life expectancy are not necessarily reduced.

Differential Diagnosis: The syndrome of multiple cartilaginous exostoses shows only exostoses and possibly short stature (p.306). The trichorhinophalangeal syndrome type I (p.318) lacks the exostoses, the microcephalic mental retardation, often the short stature, and other features.

Treatment: Symptomatic. Genetic counselling.

Illustrations:
1a and b A 15-year-old with the typical syndrome, but unimpaired mental development. Exostoses noted on both ends of the long bones toward the end of the first year of life. Head circumference 48.5 cm; height below the 3rd percentile at 133.5 cm. Delayed speech development; considerable hearing impairment (noted at 4 years). Normal sexual development.
2a and b From the same child at different ages.
(By kind permission of Drs J. W. E. Oorthuys and F. A. Beemer, Amsterdam.)

References:
Spranger J. W., Langer L. O., jr, Wiedemann H.-R.: Bone Dysplasias. An Atlas of Constitutional Disorders of Skeletal Development, Stuttgart and Philadelphia, G. Fischer and W. B. Saunders 1974
Oorthuys J. W. E., Beemer F. A.: The Langer–Giedion syndrome or trichorhino-phalangeal syndrome, type II. Eur. J. Pediatr. *132*:55 (1979)
Bühler E. M., Bühler U. K., Stalder, G. R., et al: Chromosome deletion and multiple cartilaginous exostoses. Eur. J. Pediatr. *133*:163 (1980)
Murachi S., Nogami H., Oki T., et al: Familial tricho-rhino-phalangeal syndrome type II. Clin. Med. *19*:149 (1981)
Fryns J. P., Logghe N., van Eggen M., et al: Langer–Giedion syndrome and deletion of the long arm of chromosome 8. Hum. Genet. *58*:231 (1981)
Zabel B. U., Baumann W. A.: Langer–Giedion syndrome with interstitial 8q-deletion. Am. J. Med. Genet. *11*:353 (1982)
Bühler E. M.: Editorial comment: Langer–Giedion syndrome and 8q-deletion. Am. J. Med. Genet. *11*:359 (1982)

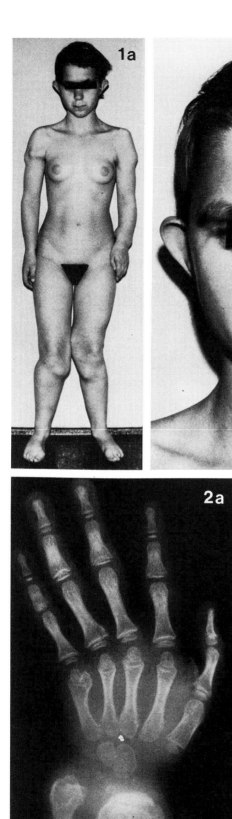

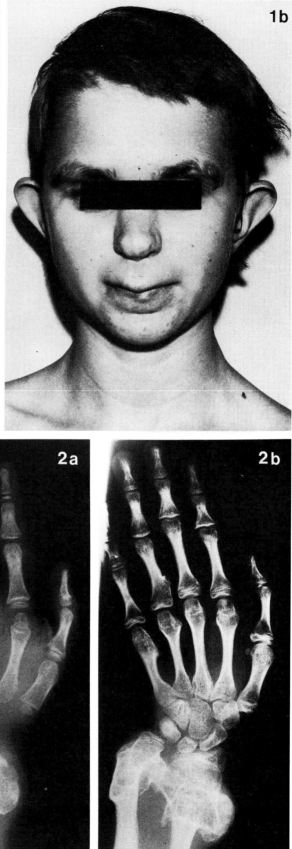

155. Syndrome of Enchondromatosis

(Dyschondroplasia, Multiple Enchondromas, Ollier Syndrome)

A syndrome of localised hard asymmetrical swellings of the fingers and/or toes in combination with asymmetrical shortening of the extremities.

Main Signs:
1. Taut-elastic, firm, indolent, rounded swellings or distensions continuous with the bone on one or more fingers or toes (**1** and **2**).
2. Shortening and possibly bowing of parts of the extremities, most frequently the forearm and/or lower leg (**1** and **4**).
3. Marked asymmetry of the swellings (to possible unilateral involvement).

Supplementary Findings: Possible secondary impairment of mobility of one or several joints; less frequently compression effects.

Occasional 'spontaneous' fractures in an affected area.

On X-ray, characteristic ovoid, pyramid-shaped, and linear translucent defects in the metaphyses of the affected long bones and in flat bones (with sparing of the calvarium), frequently with considerable swelling of the affected area and disappearance of the cortex (**3** and **4**).

Manifestation: Usually after the 2nd year of life.

Aetiology: Uncertain. Sporadic occurrence. Risk of recurrence for the affected family not increased.

Frequency: Relatively rare.

Course, Prognosis: Guarded. Appearance and growth of further foci up to sexual maturity; localised impairment of growth and mobility of extremities or parts of extremities may be considerable and thus an important handicap for the patient. As a rule, no new foci appear after adolescence; rather, old foci become replaced by bony substance. Malignant degeneration of enchondromas may occur in adulthood (perhaps in about 5% of cases); renewed growth of a focus should suggest this possibility.

Treatment: Extirpative surgery in cases of marked impairment of function, considerable disfigurement, or suspected malignant transformation. Orthopaedic regulation, conservative or surgical, of differences in lengths of the legs.

Illustrations:
1–4 A 6½-year-old boy, normally developed for his age; enchondromatosis manifest since his 3rd year of life. Limited to unilateral involvement. Left extremities, especially the leg, shorter than the right. Secondary tilting of the pelvis. Considerable impairment and disfiguration of the left hand. Also enchondromatous changes of the carpal bones, radius and humerus, ilium and os pubis, and tarsal bones and toes.

References:
Spranger J. W., Langer L. O., jr, Wiedemann H.-R.: Bone Dysplasias. An Atlas of Constitutional Disorders of Skeletal Development, Stuttgart and Philadelphia, G. Fischer and W. B. Saunders 1974
Shapiro F.: Ollier's disease. J. Bone Jt. Surg. 64A:95 (1982)

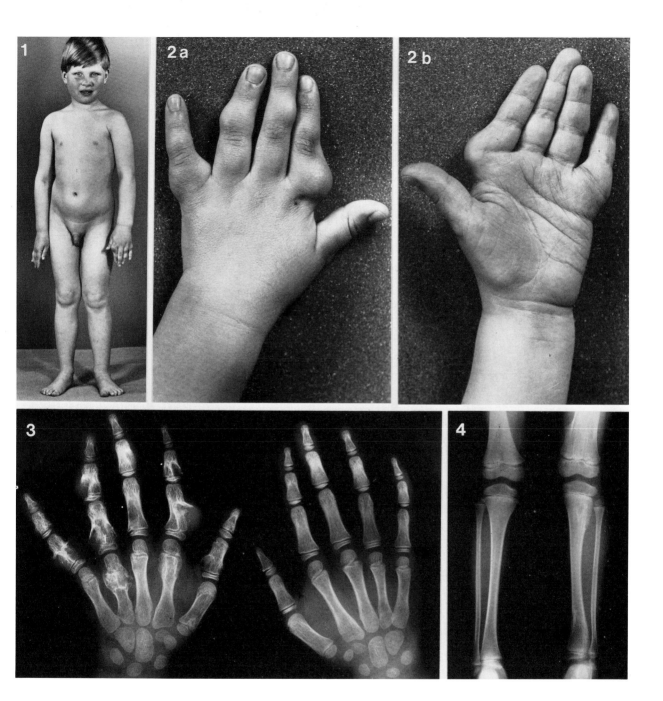

156. Greig's Polysyndactyly–Dyscrania Syndrome

A hereditary syndrome of polydactyly and syndactyly of the hands and feet, and dyscrania.

Main Signs:
1. Broad thumbs and halluces or preaxial polydactyly of the hands and feet as well as postaxial polydactyly of the hands, less frequently of the feet. More or less pronounced syndactyly of fingers II–IV (V) and of various toes (**3–6**).
2. Brachycephaly with high sinciput and protruding forehead with a medial ridge (**1** and **2**). Broad nasal root, hypertelorism, possible slight antimongoloid slant of the palpebral fissures and wide nares (**2**).

Supplementary Findings: Radiological picture of the thumbs and big toes variable, from mere broadening to complete doubling of the ray.

Manifestation: At birth.

Aetiology: Autosomal dominant hereditary disorder with variable expressivity.

Frequency: Rare.

Course, Prognosis: Favourable.

Diagnosis, Differential Diagnosis: Exclusion of the Carpenter syndrome (p.12) should not pose any difficulties.

Treatment: Surgical correction of the extremities should be begun sufficiently early, at a time determined with the hand surgeon and suited to the individual case. Genetic counselling.

Illustrations:
1 and 3–5 A 4-month-old boy; clinical and radiological polysyndactyly of the right hand (**3** and **5**); **4**, the fore part of the right foot of the same child.
2 and 6 Twin brother of boy in **1** and **3–5**; unusually severe polysyndactyly of the right foot (**6**).
(By kind permission of Dr J. P. Fryns, Leuven.)

References:
Hoostnick D., Holmes L.B.: Familial polysyndactyly and craniofacial anomalies. Clin. Genet. *3*:124 (1972)
Fryns J.P., van Noyen G., van den Berghe H.: The Greig polysyndactyly craniofacial dysmorphism syndrome. Eur. J. Pediatr. *136*:217 (1981)

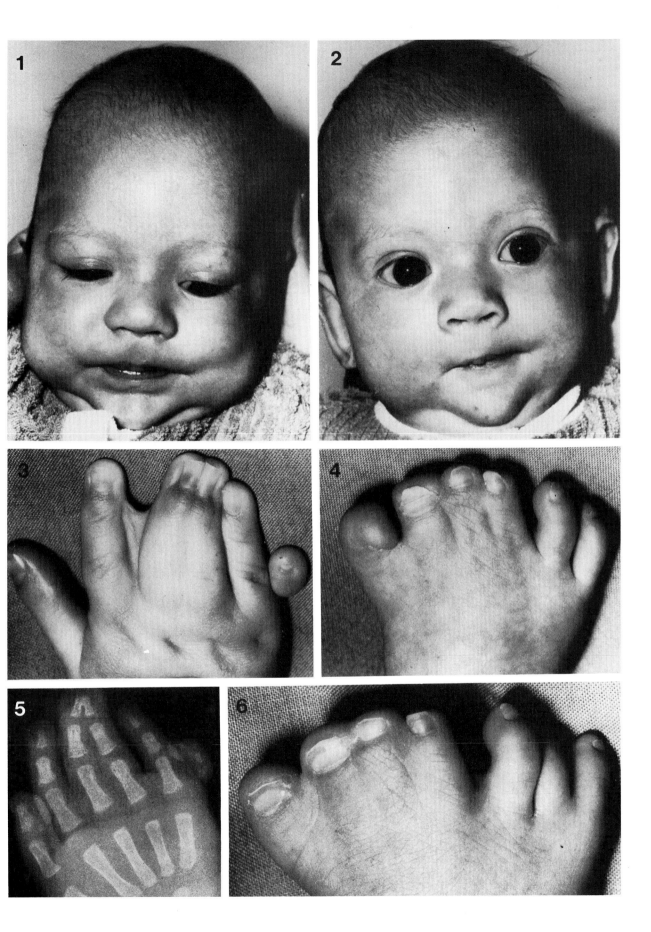

157. Oro-Facio-Digital Syndrome II

(OFD Syndrome II, Mohr Syndrome)

A hereditary syndrome occurring in both sexes and comprising bilateral polysyndactyly of the big toes, lobulation of the tongue and hyperplastic frenula, peculiar facies, and anomalies of the hands.

Main Signs:
1. Polysyndactyly of both big toes (**2**).
2. Brachy-, syn-, clino-, or polydactyly of the hands (**1**).
3. Clefting or lobulation of the tongue (into 2 or more lobules) with nodules at the base of the lobular clefts; hyperplastic oral frenula.
4. Peculiar facies; Broad nasal root and wide tip of the nose, which may show a median groove; possible median cleft lip; hypoplasias within the jaw area; frequent absence of the central incisors; high palate or cleft palate.

Supplementary Findings: X-rays of the feet show broad, short (or more or less duplicated) metatarsals I, cuneiforms, and naviculars. Possible conductive hearing impairment with malformation of the incus.

Manifestation: At birth.

Aetiology: Autosomal recessive hereditary disorder.

Frequency: Rare.

Course, Prognosis: Life expectancy usually unaffected.

Differential Diagnosis: The oro-facio-digital syndrome I occurs only in females (X chromosomal dominant inheritance); differentiating characteristics, see p.46.

Treatment: Operative correction of clefts and hypertrophic frenula; early evaluation of hearing, adequate treatment if needed; orthodontic and dental care; removal of the extra hallaces and possible corrective surgery of the hands. Genetic counselling.

Illustrations:
1 and 2 A girl with Mohr syndrome, the 2nd child of healthy parents. Broad nasal root, medial notch of the upper lip, cleft tip of the tongue with small fibromas bilaterally; high palate, indentation of the alveolar ridges, and thick frenula. Polydactyly of the hands and feet with duplication of the rays of the big toes.
(By kind permission of Prof. F. Majewski, Düsseldorf.)

References:
Pfeiffer R. A., Majewski F., Mannkopf H.: Das Syndrom von Mohr und Claussen. Klin. Pädiatr. *184*:224 (1972)
Levy E. P., Fletcher B. D., Fraser C1.: Mohr syndrome with subclinical expression of the bifid great toe. Am. J. Dis. Child. *128*:531 (1974)

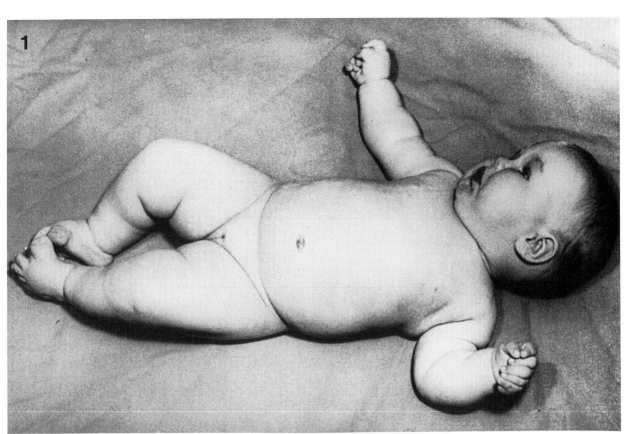

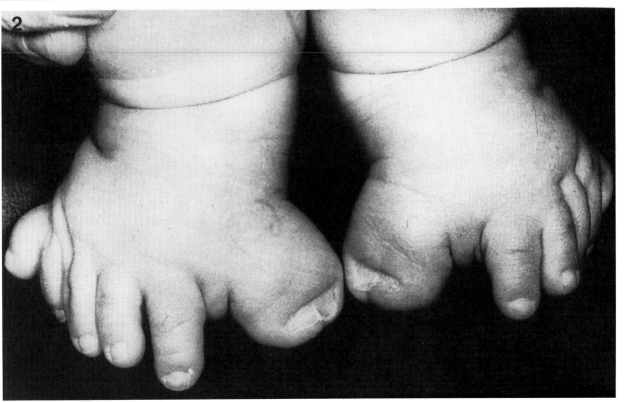

158. Syndrome of Absent 5th Ray of the Hands and Feet, Cleft Lip and Palate, and Dysplastic Ears and Eyelids

(Postaxial Acrofacial Dysostosis Syndrome)

A hereditary syndrome in which the principal sign is oligodactyly due to absence of the 5th rays, and which includes cleft palate and/or lip, dysplastic ears and eyelids, characteristic large-eyed appearance, and occasionally, psychomotor retardation.

Main Signs:
1. Bilateral absence (in isolated cases also rudimentary anlagen) of the 5th fingers and toes with abnormally short forearms (especially the ulnae) with tendency to ulnar clubhand position (1–3 and 5–7).
2. Cleft lip and/or palate; dysplasia of the external ear (4); anomalies involving the eyelids (antimongoloid slant, short palpebral fissures; more or less distinct coloboma of the lower lids laterally; deficient hair on the eyelids; inability to close the eyes completely, and abnormally large-appearing eyes).
3. Peculiar appearance (compounded by hypertelorism, simply formed nose, and receding chin).

Supplementary Findings: Accessory nipples in some patients. Psychomotor retardation and impaired hearing, each in 2 of the 14 cases known to date.

X-rays show anomalies of the carpals and possible radioulnar synostosis, in addition to absence of the 5th rays.

In some cases further diverse clinical and/or radiological anomalies of the skeleton or of internal organs (heart, kidneys, genitalia).

Manifestation: At birth.

Aetiology: Probably monogenic hereditary disorder, autosomal recessive.

Frequency: Rare.

Differential Diagnosis: Nager's dysostosis acrofacialis (p.38) presents something of a 'counterpart', with preaxial involvement of the extremities (in addition it is limited to the upper extremities), and is thus easily excluded. Mandibulofacial dysostosis is also easily ruled out (p.36), in spite of diverse similarities in the facial region.

Treatment: Symptomatic. Closure of clefts. Possible orthopaedic or surgical correction of limb defects, in some cases also cosmetic surgery and orthodontic treatment. Early evaluation of hearing. Genetic counselling.

Illustrations:
1–7 An affected child as an infant (1 and 4), at barely 3 (5 and 7), and at 4½ years (2, 3, and 6). Brachycephaly. Dysplasias of the eyelids with notching of the lateral lower eyelids, inability to close the eyes completely, large-appearing eyes. Cleft palate. Microgenia. Congenital heart defect. Cryptorchidism. Pedes plani. Mental retardation. Radiologically, hypoplasia of the poorly formed ulna, especially proximally, in addition to absence of the 5th rays (5 and 7); at this time only one ossification centre in the wrists; anomalies of the metacarpals and phalanges as well as of the metatarsal and toe bones.

References:
Wiedemann H.-R.: Mißbildungs-Retardierungs-Syndrom mit Fehlen des 5. Strahls an Händen und Füßen, Gaumenspalte, dysplastischen Ohren und Augenlidern und radioulnarer Synostose. Klin. Pädiatr. *185*:181 (1973)
Miller M., Fineman R. M., Smith D. W.: Postaxial acrofacial dysostosis syndrome. J. Pediatr. *95*:970 (1979)
Fineman R. M.: Recurrence of the postaxial acrofacial dysostosis syndrome in a sibship: Implications for genetic counselling. J. Pediatr. *98*:87 (1981)
Meinecke P., Rauskolb R.: Autosomal rezessive mandibulo-faziale Dysostose mit Aplasie des 5. Strahls an Händen und Füßen. In: Klinische Genetik in der Pädiatrie. M. Tolksdorf, J. Spranger (eds) Milupa AG, Friedrichsdorf 1982 (445-450)

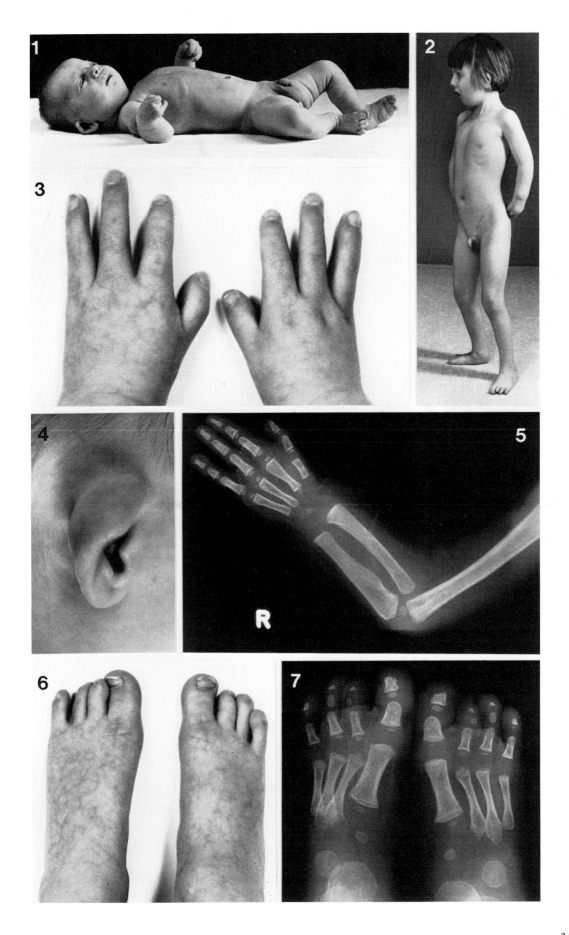

159. Trichorhinophalangeal Syndrome Type I

A hereditary syndrome with unusual facies, sparse and fragile scalp hair, clinical and radiological peculiarities of the hands, and not infrequently small stature.

Main Signs:
1. Facial dysmorphism due to more or less 'bulbous', 'pear-shaped' nose, large and sometimes prominent ears, long and wide philtrum, and thin upper lip. Eyebrows poorly developed laterally (**1**).
2. Sparse, fine, brittle, usually light-coloured scalp hair (**1**).
3. Short hands and feet, the fingers deformed due to broadening of the middle phalangeal joints and possible deviation of the phalangeal axes with no or little limitation of motion. Thumbs and big toes short and stubby (**2** and **3**). 'Cone-shaped' epiphyses on X-ray; shortening of some of the metacarpal and metatarsal bones (**5** and **6**).

Supplementary Findings: Not infrequently growth deficiency, often only moderately severe.

Fragile, brittle finger- and toenails. Possible dysodontiasis.

Possible Perthes-type dysplasia of the head of the femur, kyphosis, scoliosis, scapulae alatae, deformities of the thorax, or cardiovascular anomalies.

Manifestation: Facial characteristics and sparse hair growth may be apparent from birth; as a rule the affected are first brought to medical attention later in childhood because of 'swelling' over the middle phalangeal joints.

Aetiology: Hereditary defect. Usually autosomal dominant mode of transmission; variable penetrance, very variable expression. Apparent occurrence of an autosomal recessive form also. Thus, probable heterogeneity.

Frequency: Rare; by 1981, about 160 cases reported in the literature.

Course, Prognosis: Normal life expectancy. The osteoarticular changes are more or less distinctly progressive; in some cases relatively early arthroses in the hands, the vertebral column, and other areas. The sparse hair and consciousness of an unsightly nose, deformed hands, and possible growth deficiency may cause problems especially in women and girls.

Differential Diagnosis: Trichorhinophalangeal syndrome type II (Langer–Giedion syndrome, p.308).

Treatment: Orthopaedic and orthodontic care, possible cosmetic surgery (nose), and a wig may be indicated. Psychological guidance. Genetic counselling.

Illustrations:
1–6 An almost 15-year-old, 167.5 cm tall (= ± 0) school boy showing the typical syndrome, apparently inherited from his father. Scalp hair, lateral eyebrows and body hair sparse. Relatively small lower jaw with narrowly spaced teeth. Nails thin and extremely brittle, skin of the fingertips very fragile and sensitive. Ingrown nails of the big toes with inflammation. Painless swelling and slight deflection of the interphalangeal joints, but good mobility. Thumbs and halluces especially short and stubby.

References:
Spranger J. W., Langer L. O., jr, Wiedemann H.-R.: Bone Dysplasias. An Atlas of Constitutional Disorders of Skeletal Development. Stuttgart and Philadelphia, G. Fischer and W. B., Saunders 1974
Frias J. L., Felman A. H., Garnica A. D., et al: Variable expressivity in the trichorhinophalangeal syndrome type I. Birth Defects 15/5B:36 (1979)
Ranke M. B., Heitkamp H-Ch.: Tricho-rhino-phalangeales Syndrom. Monatschr. Kinderheilkd. 128:208 (1980)
Goodman R. M., Trilling R., Hertz M., et al: New clinical observations in the trichorhinophalangeal syndrome. J. Craniofacial Genet. Develop. Biol. 1:15 (1981)
Gaarsted Ch., Madsen E. H., Friedrich U.: A Danish kindred with tricho-rhino-phalangeal syndrome type I. Eur. J. Pediatr. 139:84 (1982)

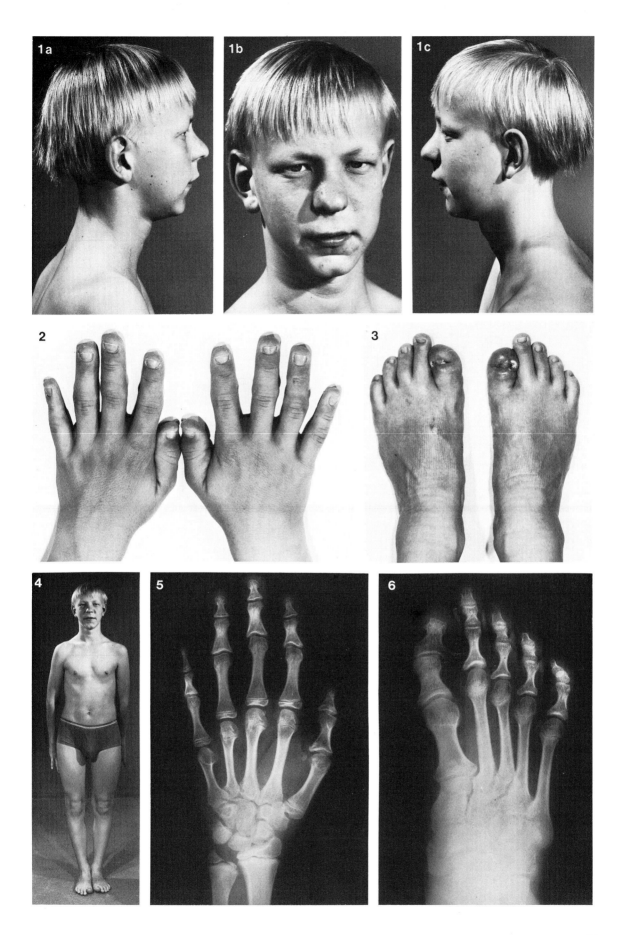

319

160. Symphalangism–Brachydactyly Syndrome with Conductive Hearing Impairment

(Syndrome of Multiple Synostoses with Conductive Hearing Impairment)

A hereditary syndrome of malformations of the hands and feet, characteristic facies, and defective hearing.

Main Signs:
1. Congenitally impaired mobility of the proximal interphalangeal joints of fingers II-V (radiologically, fusion of these phalanges may not be apparent until later) with absence of the normal articular folds, possible limitation of motion at the elbow joints, and eventual limited motion at the wrist and ankle joints, in some cases associated with abnormalities of gait.
2. Brachydactyly, possible absence of the distal segments of fingers (and/or toes), cutaneous syndactyly (**1** and **2**).
3. Characteristic facies: long and narrow face with long, quite prominent nose, broad nasal bridge, and thin upper lip (**1**).
4. Conductive hearing impairment, possibly beginning after adolescence (ankylosis of the auditory ossicles).

Supplementary Findings: Normal development of height with possible abnormal proportions due to shortness of the arms.

Radiologically, abnormally short metacarpals/metatarsals I; (development of) symphalangism of proximal phalanges of fingers II-V (**3** and **4**); later, ankylosis also of the carpals (**4**) and tarsals; possible diverse anomalies of the elbow region, including radiohumeral synostosis (**5**).

Manifestation: At birth and thereafter.

Aetiology: Hereditary defect, autosomal dominant. Considerable intrafamilial variability.

Frequency: Rare.

Course, Prognosis: Symphalangism, ankylosis in the wrist and ankle regions, and conductive hearing impairment tend to be progressive.

Treatment: Corrective surgical measures for the extremities usually not indicated. Early evaluation of hearing; adequate treatment as required. Genetic counselling.

Illustrations:
1–3 and 5 A 2-year-old boy.
4 An X-ray of one of his father's hands.
(By kind permission of Dr P. Maroteaux, Paris.)

References:
Maroteaux P.: Les maladies osseuses de l'enfant. Flammarion, Paris 1974
Königsmark B.W., Gorlin R.J.: Dominant symphalangism and conduction deafness. In: Genetic and metabolic deafness. W.B. Saunders Co., Philadelphia 1976

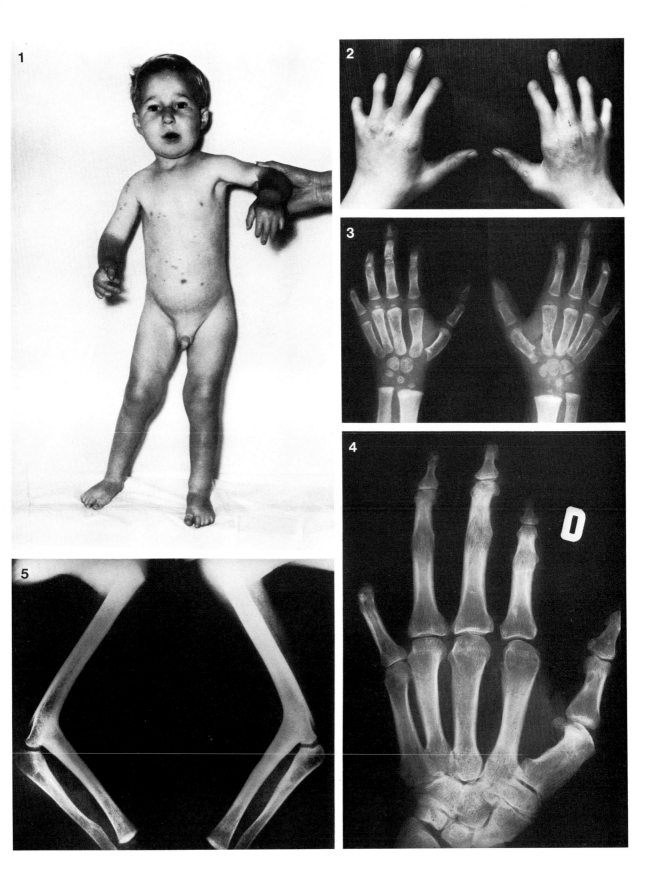

161. A Malformation–Retardation Syndrome of Unknown Aetiology

A syndrome of psychomotor retardation with microcephaly, peculiar facies, and other diverse anomalies.

Main Signs:
1. Primary psychomotor retardation; (brachy-)-microcephaly.
2. Facies: Slight antimongoloid slant of the palpebral fissures, left more than right, right epicanthus, relatively narrow palpebral fissures, narrow alae nasi and large mouth. Low-set, prominent, simply modelled ears (1 and 2). Microretrognathia. High-arched palate.
3. Broad wrist, barely delimited from the forearm (3) as well as undifferentiated, pillar-like lower legs (1). Short hands with proximal cutaneous syndactyly between fingers II-V bilaterally, clinodactyly of the left index finger, and short, tapering fingers with hypoplastic terminal phalanges (3). Limited motion at the ankles. Short feet in clubfoot position with dysdactyly; big toes relatively too long (5 and 6).

Supplementary Findings: Slightly short stature. Suggestion of pterygium colli. Relatively sparse growth of hair. Undescended testicles bilaterally (at 4 years) and left-sided cryptorchidism (at 12¾ years); small penis. Possible small ventricular septal defect.

Radiologically: crudely formed clavicles, high narrow pelvis, pronounced coxae valgae. Clubbing of the proximal ends of the metacarpals, especially V, bilaterally. Fingers slender with unusually short distal phalanges (4). Dysdactyly of the feet (6).

Manifestation: Birth and later.

Aetiology: Unknown.

Treatment: Symptomatic.

Illustrations:
1–6 A 12¾-year-old boy, the 3rd child of healthy nonconsanguineous parents (father 43, mother 33 years at the patient's birth). Normal birth after an unremarkable pregnancy 3 weeks before term with 2500 g and 49 cm. Endocrinological, clinical, and blood chemistry investigations negative; repeated chromosome analyses unremarkable (incl. banded preparations).
(In part, by kind permission of Prof. Dr H. Doose, Kiel.)

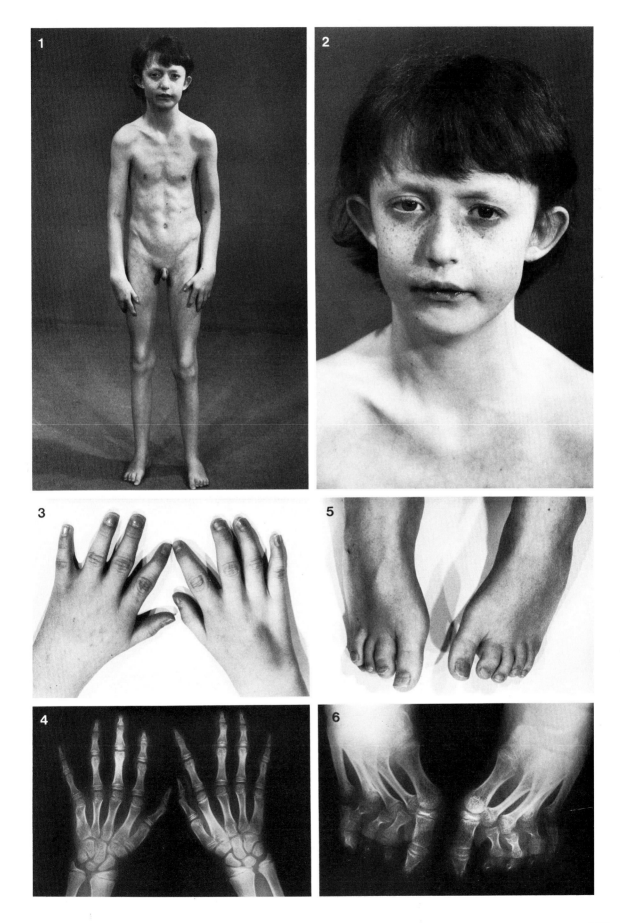

162. Syndrome of Autosomal Dominant Hereditary Carpotarsal Osteolysis with Nephropathy

A characteristic hereditary syndrome with progressive carpotarsal osteolysis and chronic progressive nephropathy.

Main Signs:
1. Gradual shortening of wrists and ankles, metacarpus, and metatarsus bilaterally – usually more or less symmetrically – as a result of progressive carpotarsal osteolysis (1, 3, 5–10). Possibly preceded or accompanied by soft-tissue swelling, sensitivity, limited mobility, and warming of the affected region. Increasing deformity in the form of ulnar deviation or volar subluxation of the shortened hands and eventually formation of claw hands or short pes cavus with overlapping toes (7).
2. Progressive nephropathy (proteinuria, possible erythrocyturia; development of arterial hypertension, etc.).

Supplementary Findings: Not infrequently kyphoscoliosis; development of muscular atrophy, especially in the distal extremities, as well as flexion contractures of the large joints.

Distinctive facies including slight exophthalmos, hypoplasia of the upper jaw, and micrognathia have been noted; furthermore, mental retardation and short stature in isolated cases.

Manifestation: Osteolysis in the 1st decade of life, generally in the toddler, seldom as early as the first year of life. Nephropathy toward the end of the 1st decade or during the 2nd.

Aetiology: Autosomal dominant hereditary disorder, basic defect unknown.

Frequency: Rare.

Course, Prognosis: Osteolysis usually slowly progressive, eventually with complete dissolution of the carpal and tarsal bones and 'popsicle-stick-like' narrowing and shortening of the ends of the neighbouring long bones (9). Thus, the distal forearms and possibly lower legs slowly become shortened; elbow region similarly affected and in some cases further, more remote joint regions may show corresponding limitation of mobility. The skeletal involvement may stabilise toward the end of the 2nd decade of life. However, the nephropathy may run a protracted course, with dubious prognosis.

Differential Diagnosis: Other osteolysis syndromes (see also pp.326, 328). Rheumatoid arthritis may be suspected at the onset of the illness, but can be easily ruled out.

Treatment: Symptomatic. Counselling with regard to choice of an appropriate vocation. Genetic counselling.

Illustrations:
1 and 2, 5, 7 and 9   A 39-year-old woman.
3 and 4, 6, 8, and 10   Her 9-year-old slightly mentally retarded son.

Two older children healthy. Mother and son of normal height; in both, a slightly receding chin; the mother finds her son's broad nasal bridge quite conspicuous ('not at all in the family'). Onset of symptoms in the left hand in both mother and son as young school children, subsequently less severe involvement of the right also; feet more severely affected (left > right). The mother's narrowed, shortened, left hand, with markedly impaired mobility – as in the son – yields a Dupuytren-like picture; analogous development of connective tissue nodules and cords in the plantar fascia bilaterally. Proteinuria in both mother and son (in the former with fluctuating hypertension) varying between 1 and 3 g/day.

References:
Erickson Chr. M., Hirschberger M., Stickler G. B.: Carpal-tarsal osteolysis. J. Pediatr. 93:779 (1978)
Fryns J. P., Pedersen J. C., Hauglustaine D., et al: Carpal and tarsal osteolysis. Ann. Génét. 23:123 (1980)

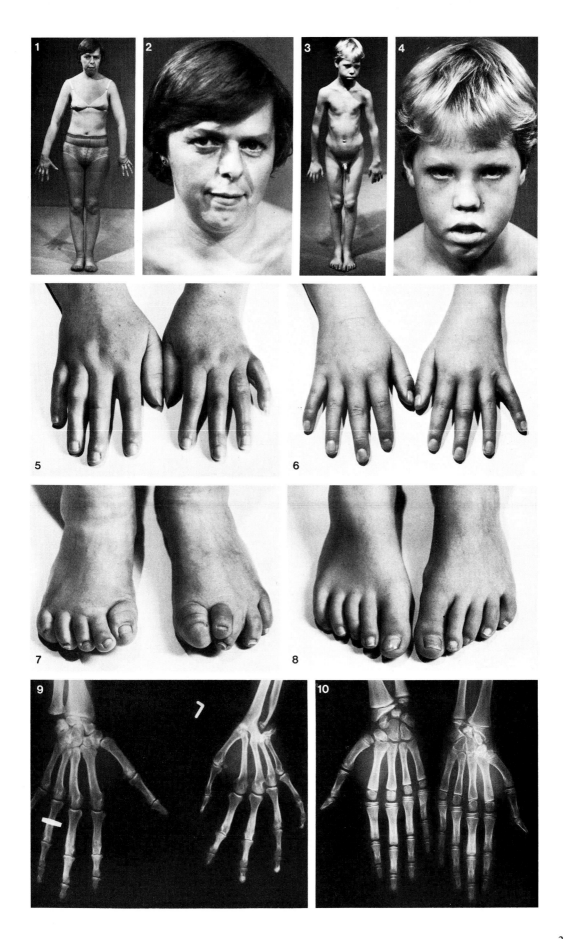

325

163. Syndrome of Idiopathic Carpotarsal Osteolysis Type François

(Familial Dermo-Chondro-Corneal Dystrophy)

A characteristic hereditary syndrome comprising progressive carpotarsal osteolysis with skin and corneal changes.

Main Signs:
1. Gradual shortening of the wrist, ankle, metatarsus and metacarpus bilaterally (accompanying or following sensitivity, warming, and soft tissue swelling) as a result of the onset of progressive carpotarsal osteolysis (3–5). Increasing deformity (ulnar deviation of the shortened hands, eventual claw-hand (1 and 2); short pes cavus).
2. In some cases decreased visual acuity beginning in the school child.
3. Xanthomatous nodules occurring on, e.g., the hands, the elbows, the face.

Supplementary Findings: Corneal clouding (subepithelial and central [possibly seen only on split lamp examination]).

In some cases idiopathic nephropathy with proteinuria.

Manifestation: Usually at a pre-school or school age.

Aetiology: Monogenic hereditary disorder, autosomal recessive.

Frequency: Very rare.

Course, Prognosis: Slow progression of the osteolysis with resulting physical handicap. Life expectancy without nephropathy, probably unaffected; with nephropathy, dubious to unfavourable.

Differential Diagnosis: Other osteolysis syndromes (see also pp.324, 328). Rheumatoid arthritis may be suspected early in the disease, but is easy to rule out.

Treatment: Symptomatic. Genetic counselling.

Illustrations:
1–5 A 16-year-old girl; bone involvement manifest in early childhood; xanthoma-like nodules; corneal clouding determined by slit lamp examination at age 14 years; nephropathy since an early school age; death due to nephrosclerosis at 22 years.

References:
Wiedemann H.-R.: Zur François'schen Krankheit. Ärztl. Wochenschr. *13*:905 (1958)
Spranger J. W., Langer L. O., jr, Weidemann H.-R.: Bone Dysplasias. An Atlas of Constitutional Disorders of Skeletal Development. Stuttgart and Philadelphia, G. Fischer and W. B. Saunders 1974

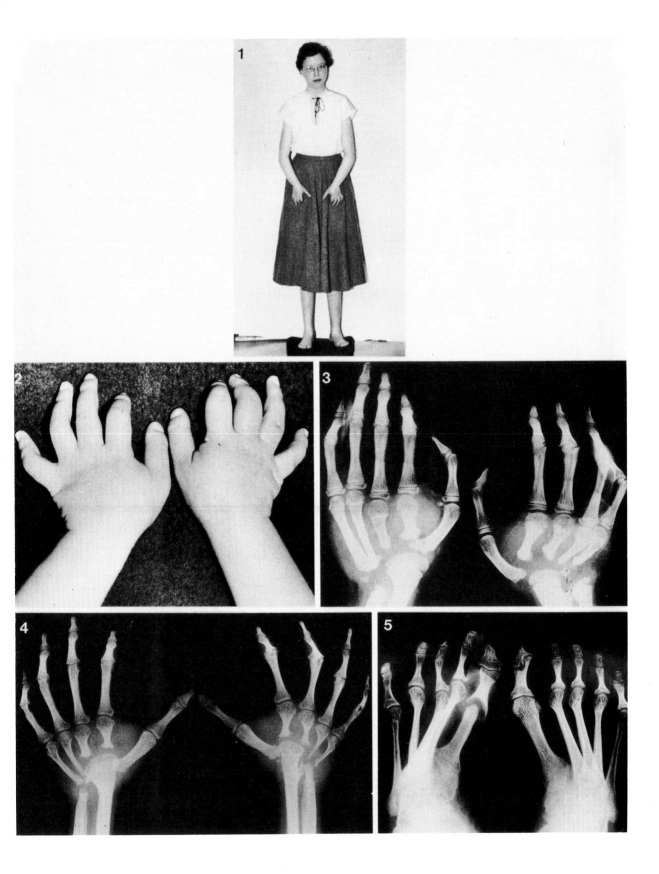

164. Hajdu–Cheney Syndrome

(Idiopathic Osteolysis Type Hajdu–Cheney)

A hereditary syndrome comprising peculiar facies, persistence of cranial sutures and fontanelles, hyperextensible joints, growth deficiency, increased tendency to fractures, premature loss of teeth, and – radiologically – osteolysis.

Main Signs:
1. Distinctive facies: broad with very prominent eyebrows, hypoplasia of both jaws, wide philtrum and broad, thin-lipped mouth (1). Strong, coarse scalp hair.
2. Cranial anomalies: Persistence of sutures and fontanelles; eventual development of dolichocephaly with protrusion of the occiput.
3. Laxity of the joints; short stature more or less apparent with short neck; tendency to 'spontaneous fractures'; premature dental caries and loss of teeth.
4. Shortening and broadening of the tips of the fingers and possibly also the toes, which may be sensitive or painful and may show nail deformities (2).

Supplementary Findings: Possibly coarse external integument, often with hypertrichosis. Frequently hoarse voice. Possible conductive hearing impairment and in some cases also anomalies of the eyes or visual acuity.

Radiologically: Persistence of fontanelles and sutures with numerous wormian bones especially in the lambdoid suture (5 and 6); later dolichocephaly with prominent occiput, platybasia, elongation of the sella (latter, 6); small jaw, deficient pneumatisation of the sinuses.

Osteolysis, in particular acroosteolysis with formation of typical transverse clefts of the distal phalanges of the fingers (3 and 4).

Possible generalised osteoporosis with corresponding changes in the form of the vertebral bodies (in some cases secondary kyphoscoliosis); multiple fractures; also anomalies of form and deformity of the long bones.

Manifestation: Distinctive facies, hirsutism, and hoarse voice may be apparent from birth. Changes of the finger tips with radiologically apparent osteolysis and generalised osteoporosis, sometimes with 'spontaneous fractures' may be apparent from early childhood but possibly also much later; in many cases the diagnosis has been made in an adolescent or adult patient.

Aetiology: An autosomal dominant gene seems to be responsible. Most cases occur sporadically (representing new mutations).

Frequency: Rare; by 1979 barely 20 cases had been described in the literature.

Course, Prognosis: Progression and expansion of the processes, including the inevitable secondary changes.

Differential Diagnosis: Other osteolysis syndromes (see also pp.324, 326) as well as pyknodysostosis (p.136) and cleidocranial dysplasia (p.22) are usually not difficult to rule out. The normal mental development immediately excludes Cornelia de Lange syndrome (p.118), which may be suggested by the similarity of facies during childhood.

Treatment: Early evaluation of hearing and sight; adequate care as needed. Dental care. Orthopaedic care and attention to secondary changes. Genetic counselling.

Illustrations:
1–6 A girl, the 3rd child of non-consanguineous parents, at ages 7 years (1, 2, and 4) and 2¼ years (3, 5, and 6). At 7 years: short stature (around the 3rd percentile), short neck, funnel chest and scoliosis; general laxity of the joints as well as myohypotonia. Coarse skin with abundant hair, bristly scalp hair; defective dentition; impaired hearing, hoarse voice; normal intellect. On X-ray beginning of dolichocephaly, widened sutures with wormian bones; general osteoporosis, platyspondyly; multiple fractures (since age 4); short distal phalanges of the feet, acroosteolysis of the distal phalanges of fingers I, II, and V now more pronounced.
(By kind permission of Doz. U. Wendel and Doz. H. Kemperdick, both of Düsseldorf.)

References:
Weleber R. G., Beals R. K.: The Hajdu-Cheney syndrome. J. Pediatr. 88:243 (1976)
Wendel U., Kemperdick H.: Idiopathische Osteolyse vom Typ Hajdu-Cheney. Monatschr. Kinderheilkd. 127:581 (1979)

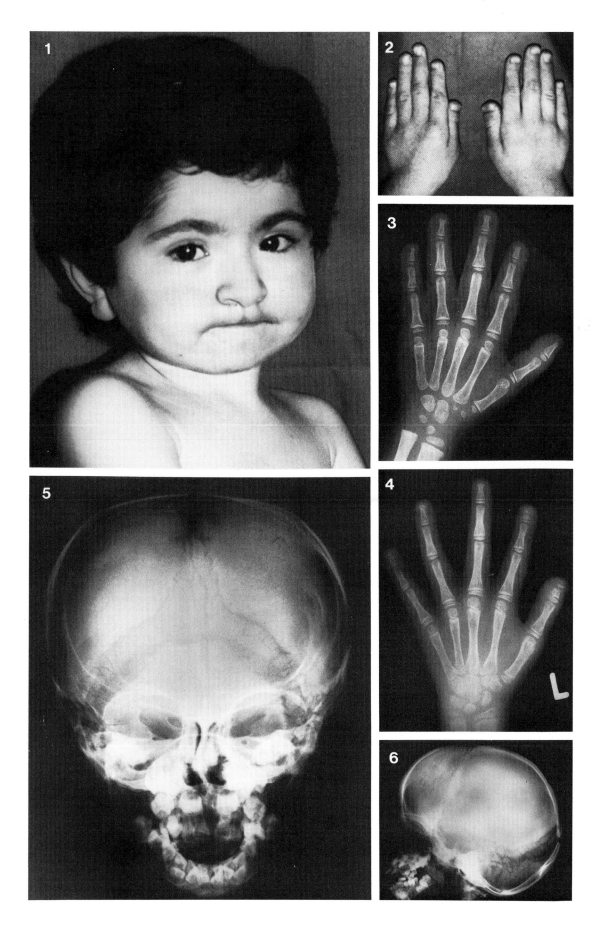

329

165. Syndrome of Partial Gigantism with Macrocrania, Subcutaneous Haemangiomas and Lymphangiomas, and Pigment Anomalies

A syndrome of congenital macrodactyly of the feet, abnormal asymmetry of the face and arms, macrocranium, systemic pigmented naevus, and further, postnatal appearance of subcutaneous haemangiomas and lymphangiomas.

Main Signs:
1. Congenital, somewhat symmetrical overgrowth of the 3rd, 5th, and especially 4th toes bilaterally (1–3).
2. Distinctly greater development of the left side of the face and the left arm, especially the forearm, the left hand being short and stubby. (1).
3. Most of the right side of the neck, the right half of the trunk, and the right arm affected by epidermal naevoid dysplasia (grey-brown discoloration of varied intensity with a rough, coarsened surface) sharply delimited at the midline, including the right half of the penis and scrotum. On the right arm, within this pigmented naevus, several stripe-like areas spared (1).
4. In part congenital, in part postnatally appearing subcutaneous 'tumours': venous angioma on the right side of the neck; thick swelling of the left thenar and hypothenar with coarsening of the hand; soft movable cystic lymphangiomas (or lymphohaemangiomas; lipomatous components not ruled out) on both sides of the thorax, on the left epigastrium, and the right paraumbilical area (1).
5. Macrocranium (51 cm at 2 years).

Supplementary Findings:
Normal height and mental development.

Slight residual of a congenital left facial paresis (1b); neurological examination otherwise negative.

Ophthalmological examination: Marked amblyopia on the left and ipsilateral convergent strabismus (no paresis of the eye muscles); otherwise negative.

Low-set, dysplastic right pinna. (No naevus flammeus; no enchondroma).

Manifestation: Birth and – some of the subcutaneous masses – early childhood.

Aetiology: Uncertain; genetic factors likely.

Course, Prognosis: Apparently not unfavourable. Spontaneous involution of the mass on the right side of the neck (however, with the appearance of a new soft-tissue mass in the right axilla in the 5th year of life). Cranial circumference developing toward the norm.

Comment: The patient shows neither Klippel–Trénaunay (p.268), Schimmelpenning–Feuerstein–Mims syndrome (p.230), nor von Recklinghausen neurofibromatosis (p.248). Rather, this observation probably fits with the sibling cases described by Zonana et al and the 'new syndrome' described by Tentamy and Rogers.

Treatment: Symptomatic (amputation of toes 3–5 bilaterally in the 4th year of life).

Illustrations:
1–3 The proband at age 2 years. The first child of healthy, young, nonconsanguineous parents. The boy, who appears older than his actual years (chromosome analysis negative), has three younger brothers, the second of whom has hydrocephaly–macrocephaly and facial characteristics strongly resembling those of the patient.

References:
Tentamy S.A., Rogers J.G.: Macrodactyly, hemihypertrophy, and connective tissue nevi: Report of a new syndrome and review of the literature. J.Pediatr. 89:924 (1976)
Zonana J., Rimoin D.L., Davis D.C.: Macrocephaly with multiple lipomas and hemangiomas. J.Pediatr. 89:600 (1976)

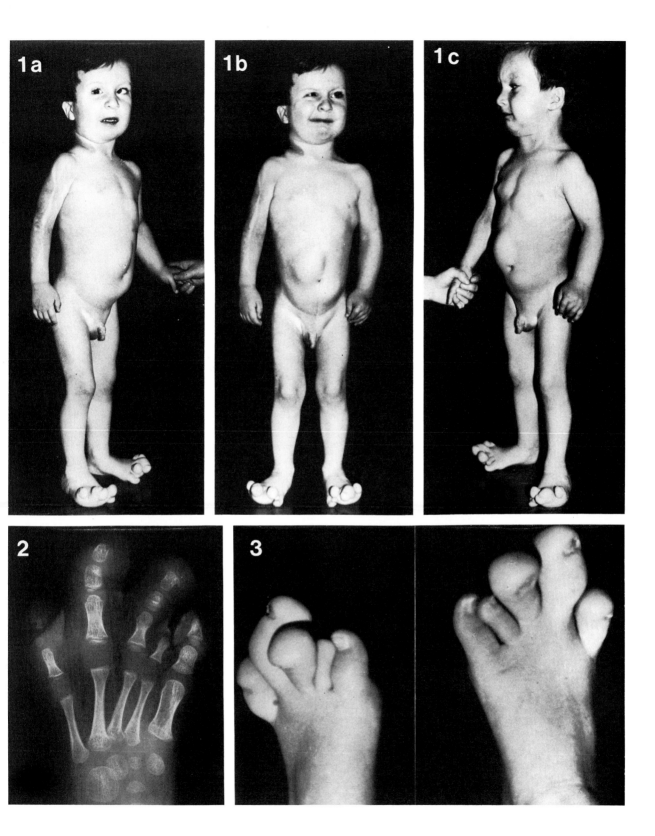

166. Syndrome of Triphalangism of the First Ray of the Hands, Thrombocytopathy, and Inner Ear Hearing Impairment

A syndrome with three-membered fingers instead of thumbs, thrombocytopathic bleeding disorder, and inner ear hearing impairment.

Main Signs:
1. Three-membered, well-developed or hypoplastic fingers instead of thumbs (4–6), possibly with hypoplasia of the forearms (1a and b) or of the radii and with radiological anomalies of the wrists.
2. Bleeding disorder, with episodic bleeding from the skin and mucous membranes.
3. Inner ear hearing impairment.

Supplementary Findings: Normal thrombocyte count. Pathologically prolonged bleeding time. Negative Rumpel–Leede phenomenon.

Manifestation: Birth and early life.

Aetiology: Probably monogenic hereditary disorder. Mode of inheritance not determined.

Frequency: Probably very rare.

Course, Prognosis: As far as can be determined, favourable.

Differential Diagnosis: Fanconi anaemia syndrome (see also under Differential Diagnosis): p.338.

Treatment: Symptomatic (transfusions of fresh blood or thrombocyte concentrate for severe haemorrhages).

Illustrations:
1–6 A 13¼-year-old girl, normal birth, robust development and normal height, with recurrent bleeding from the skin and mucous membranes since the end of the first year of life. Repeated hospital admissions and transfusions necessary. No bleeding into the joints; heavy menstrual flow. Probably congenital inner ear hearing impairment. Three-membered, strong, non-opposable finger in the thumb position on the right with a thenar-like broad bridge of soft tissue to the 2nd ray; hypoplastic, flexed, contracted three-membered finger in the thumb position of the (as a whole also somewhat smaller) left hand. Diverse anomalies of the wrist, differing on the two sides (4–6). Relatively coarse facies with hypertelorism, broad nose, and prognathism (1a and c). Large area of alopecia on the head (2). Pigmented naevus on the right side of the back (1b and 3). Multiple haematomas (e.g., on the left arm and left lower leg, both on the inner surfaces, 1a). Normal thrombocyte count, markedly prolonged bleeding time, moderate decrease of factor X. Chromosome analysis: unremarkable.

References: Not known.

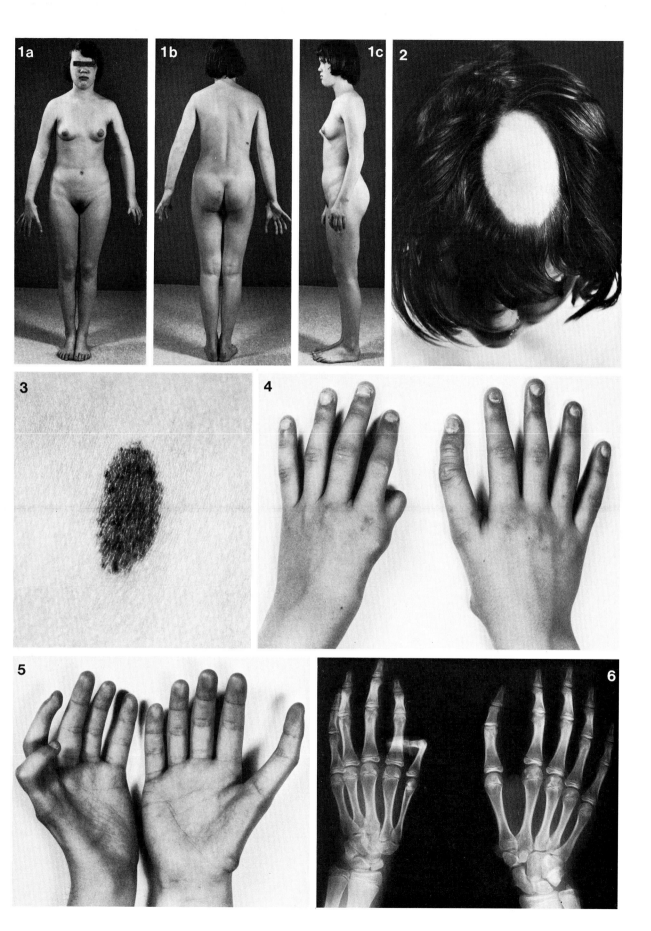

167. Syndrome of Hypoplastic Anaemia with Triphalangeal Thumbs

(Aase and Smith)

A characteristic syndrome comprising three-membered thumbs, early manifested hypoplastic anaemia, and growth deficiency.

Main Signs:
1. Prenatal dystrophy and decreased postnatal growth (possible tendency to eventual partial compensation).
2. Triphalangism of the thumbs (possibly with hypoplasia of the thenar eminence and the radius).
3. From infancy, hypoplastic (thus, normochromic, normocytic) anaemia manifest (low reticulocyte count; hypoplastic erythropoiesis in the marrow).
4. Optional mild mental retardation.

Supplementary Findings: An unusual appearance, antimongoloid slant of the palpebral fissures, cleft lip or palate, low posterior hairline, unusual skin pigmentation, and ventricular septal defect have been noted in individual cases.

Normal values regarding leucocytes and thrombocytes and their precursors.

Fetal haemoglobin increased. No increased chromosome breakage.

Manifestation: At birth (anaemia also manifest in the 1st year of life, usually in its first half).

Aetiology: Probably monogenic hereditary disorder with recessive transmission.

Frequency: Very rare.

Course, Prognosis: Favourable as a whole.

Differential Diagnosis: Fanconi anaemia syndrome (p.338), in which the haematological disorder usually is manifest much later, initially with thrombocytopenia, then pancytopenia; the great majority of patients with hypoplasia or aplasia of the thumbs; chromosomal breakage.

Treatment: Administration of corticosteroids as soon as the diagnosis is established. (Iron therapy contraindicated.) Possible operative correction of the hands. Genetic counselling.

Comment: This syndrome has been considered by some investigators to fall within the framework of Diamond–Blackfan hypoplastic anaemia. However, in the latter the dysmorphisms are absent (especially triphalangeal thumbs) in the vast majority of cases. And the disorder does not appear to be genetically uniform.

Illustrations:
1–4 A 12½-year-old boy. Hypoplastic anaemia since early infancy. On admission to hospital, 8.3 g% Hb; 2.5 mill RBCs; 6% reticulocytes; leuco- and thrombopoiesis normal. Shortly after increasing corticosteroids: 10.3 g% Hb; 2.8 mill RBCs; 78% reticulocytes. Growth deficiency (height of a 9½-year-old boy), triphalangeal thumbs, low posterior hairline, pigmented spots. IQ 77. Ocular fundi negative, no cleft formation, no organomegaly, normally descended testicles. Hb electrophoretogram unremarkable. X-ray: no radial dysplasia; absence of the navicular in the right carpus, fusion of the multangular bones (3).

References:
Aase J. M., Smith D. W.: Congenital anaemia and triphalangeal thumbs: A new syndrome. J. Pediatr. *74*:471 (1969)
Terheggen F. G.: Hypoplastische Anämie mit dreigliedrigem Daumen. Z. Kinderheilkd. *118*:71 (1974)
Wood V. E.: Treatment of the triphalangeal thumb. Clin. Orthoped. *120*:188 (1976)
Alter B. P.: Thumbs and anaemia. Pediatrics 62:613 (1978)

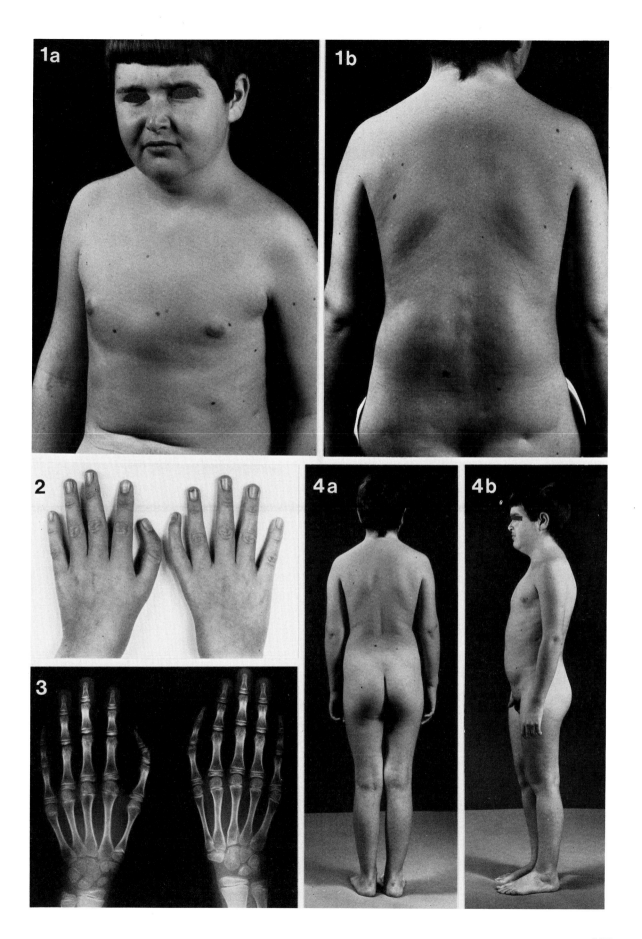

335

168. Holt–Oram Syndrome

(Cardio-digital Syndrome)

A specific hereditary syndrome of malformations of the heart and upper extremities.

Main Signs:
1. Malformation of the upper extremities which may be symmetrical or asymmetrical. Three-membered (**3a**; **2c** *left*), hypoplastic (**1a** und **b**), or even aplastic thumbs; more extensive defects of the 1st ray also possible (dys- or aplasia of the radius; dysplasia of the [upper] arm).
2. Congenital heart disease (**2d** and **3**) in the form of septal defects (frequently atrial septal defect, secundum type, possibly with disturbance of rhythm) or other dysplasias.

Supplementary Findings: Possible dysplasias of the little fingers (see clinodactyly **1**, **1a** and **b**), of the wrist (**3a**, *right*), of the elbow joint, and of the shoulder girdle (clavicles, shoulder blades, among others; **3**). On X-ray, spur formation on the lateral ends of the clavicles as a characteristic (but unspecific) phenomenon.

Manifestation: At birth (malformations of the upper extremities) and later, depending on the severity of the cardiac malformation.

Aetiology: Monogenic hereditary disorder, autosomal dominant. Variable expressivity, often more severe in females.

Frequency: Relatively rare; however, a whole series of affected sibships have been observed.

Course, Prognosis: Dependent from case to case on the severity of the cardiac defect and on the possibility for operative correction.

Differential Diagnosis: TAR syndrome (p.282), Fanconi anaemia (p.338), thalidomide syndrome (p.278).

Treatment: Adequate care for the specific anomalies. Genetic counselling.

Illustrations:
1 and 2 Mother and daughter.
1a and b Hands of the mother.
2a, b, and c Hands of the daughter. X-ray of the daughter's hands (**2c**) shows three-membered thumb on the left with hypoplasia of the metacarpal I, the wrist, and the radius. **2d:** Chest X-ray of the daughter.
3, 3a X-rays from another girl; note shoulder anomalies (among others, os acromiale on the left) and the almost symmetrical triphalangeal thumbs with asymmetry of the wrists.

References:
Holt M., Oram S.: Familial heart disease with skeletal malformations. Br. Heart. J. 22:236 (1960)
Kaufmann R.L., Rimoin D.L., McAlister W.H., Hartmann A.F.: Variable expression of the Holt-Oram syndrome. Am. J. Dis. Child. 127:21 (1974)
Capek-Schachner E., May L., Schwarzbach E.: Holt-Oram-Syndrom. Pädiatr. Prax. 21:607 (1979)
Smith A.T., Sack G.H., Taylor G.J.: Holt-Oram syndrome. J. Pediatr. 95:538 (1979)

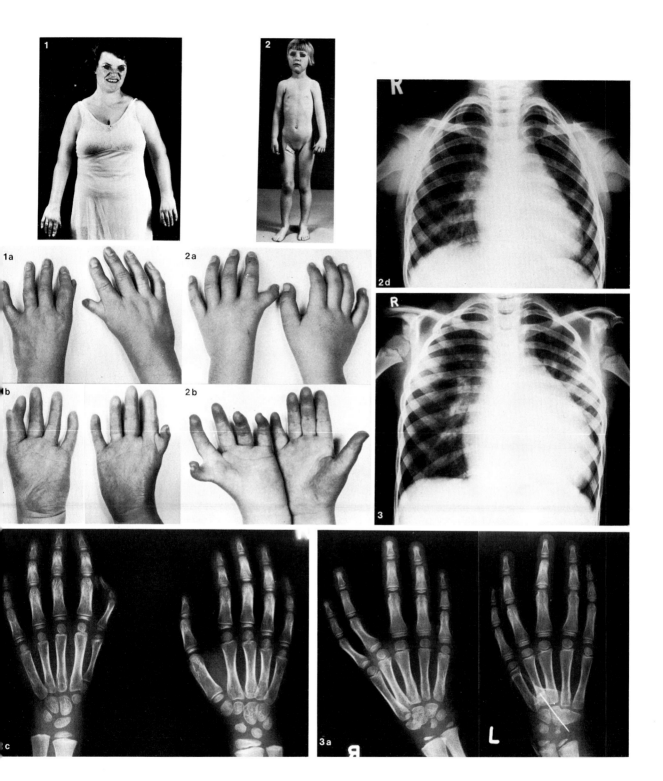

337

169. Fanconi Anaemia Syndrome

(Fanconi-Panmyelophthisis Syndrome)

A characteristic syndrome of reduction malformations of the thumbs and radii, growth deficiency, hyperpigmentation, and signs of panmyelophthisis.

Main Signs:
1. Pronounced pre- and postnatal growth deficiency; hypo- or aplasia of the thumbs (also doubling or triphalangism), short or absent radii (4, 5, 7, and 8). Dirty-brown hyperpigmentation of the skin, spotty or affecting target areas, especially of the trunk and the articular folds of the large joints.
2. Peculiar facies (3 and 6). Possible microphthalmos, strabismus, nystagmus, coloboma.
3. Microcephaly, usually also in relation to body size; mild mental retardation in ca. 20% of cases.

Supplementary Findings: Hypoplastic genitalia in males, undescended testes, hypospadias.

Malformations of the ears, possible deafness. Hyperreflexia.

Kidney malformations. Occasional cardiac anomaly. Frequent infections.

Pancytopenia (including lymphocytopenia); panmyelophthisis. Fetal haemoglobin elevated.

Increased chromosome breakage with exchange figures in heterologous chromosome pairs.

Disposition to malignant tumours, especially to leukaemia.

Retarded bone age (5 and 7).

Manifestation: Malformations and chromosome breakage at birth. Hyperpigmentation from birth or apparent later (increasing). Signs of myelophthisis usually between the 5th and 10th years of life, as an exception as early as infancy or as late as the 3rd decade of life. At first, decrease of thrombocytes, then leucocytes and erythrocytes. Since other signs may be only weakly expressed, chromosome findings are of particular importance.

Aetiology: Autosomal recessive hereditary disorder with extremely variable picture; heterogeneity. Increased chromosomal breakage, small stature, thrombocytopenia, and other signs may also occur in heterozygotes.

Frequency: Not so rare.

Course, Prognosis: Chronic progression. Untreated patients survive about 2 years after the onset of haematological signs; since therapy has been introduced, survival has increased significantly. Death due to bone marrow failure or malignancy, especially leukaemia (ca. 10%).

Treatment: Testosterone, sometimes corticosteroids; attempts at bone marrow transplantation. Genetic counselling. Prenatal diagnosis has recently become possible.

Differential Diagnosis:
1. Holt–Oram syndrome (p.336): Here, only similar thumb and arm malformations and cardiac anomalies, the latter occurring only occasionally in Fanconi syndrome.
2. Thrombocytopenia–radial aplasia syndrome (p.282), which always involves radial aplasia but with thumbs being present; only thrombocytopenia which occurs in the 1st year of life; prognosis good after this is surmounted.
3. Syndrome of hypoplastic anaemia with triphalangism of the thumbs (p.334): here, only the signs in the name.
4. Syndrome of triphalangism of the 1st rays of the hands, thrombocytopathy, and inner ear hearing impairment (p.332): normal thrombocyte count.

Illustrations:
1–5 A 3¼-year-old patient; mother only 1.52 m. Birth measurements 2250 g, 45 cm. Actual measurements 79 cm (= ~ 17 months), 8.8 kg (= ~ 8 months), head circumference 48 cm (= normal for body size). Bone age 4-5 months. Intelligence age 2½ years. Isolated patches of hyperpigmentation. Bilateral microphthalmos with coloboma on the right. Hypo-

References:
Gmyrek D., Syllm-Rapoport I.: Zur Fanconi-Anämie (FA). Analyse von 129 beschriebenen Fällen. Z. Kinderheilkd. 91:297 (1964)
Prindull G., Stubbe P., Kratzer W.: Fanconi's anaemia, I. Case histories, clinical and laboratory findings in six affected siblings. Z. Kinderheilkd. 120:37 (1975)
Schroeder T. M., Tilgen D., Krüger J., et al: Formal genetics of Fanconi's anaemia. Hum. Genet. 32:257 (1976)
Aynsley-Green A., Zachmann M., Werder E. A., et al: Endocrine studies in Fanconi's anaemia. Arch. Dis. Child. 53:126 (1978)
Schroeder T. M., Pöhler E., Hufnagl H.D., et al: Fanconi's anaemia: Terminal leukemia and 'forme fruste' in one family. Clin. Genet. 16:260 (1979)
Auerbach A.D., Adler B., Chaganti R.S.K.: Prenatal and postnatal diagnosis and carrier detection of Fanconi anaemia by a cytogenetic method. Pediatrics 67:128 (1981)
Voss R., Kohn G., Shaham M., et al: Prenatal diagnosis of Fanconi anaemia. Clin. Genet. 20:185 (1981)

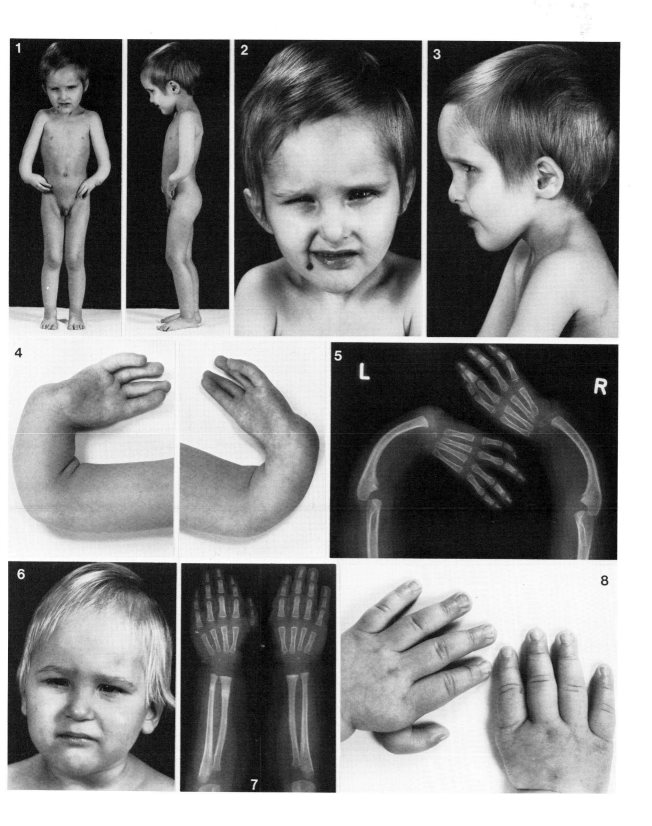

plastic genitalia. Haematologically only mild thrombocytopenia to date.

6–8 A 2-year-old patient. Birth measurements 2640 g, 48 cm. Actual height 80 cm (= ~ 17 months), 8.8 kg (= ~ 8 months), head circumference 43 cm (= 5 months). Bone age 3 months. Psychomotor development about normal for age. Generalised hyperpigmentation. Persistent foramen ovale. Genital hypoplasia. Elevated HbF. Evidence of thrombocytopenia and anaemia since age 13 months.

170. Münchmeyer Syndrome

(Fibrodysplasia ['Myositis'] Ossificans Progressiva)

A specific hereditary syndrome of congenital micro-dactyly of the big toes, also often of the thumbs, and – usually developing later – dysplastic connective tissue swellings with subsequent ossification in muscle and other tissues.

Main Signs:
1. Congenital short halluces in valgus position (**8, 11,** and **12**) due to dysplasia especially of metatarsal I; less regularly, analogous shortening of the thumbs also (**5, 6, 9,** and **10**) and clinodactyly of the little fingers (**5, 6,** and **9**).
2. Soft-tissue swellings (occasionally with pain and fever) which may be noted perinatally, but usually first appear during the first two years of life and on into the first decade of life; preferentially located in the occipi-tonuchal region, neck, and shoulder girdle ('torticol-lis'; **1** and **2**). Danger of subsequent ossification. Inter-mittent progressive course with new episodes of ossification affecting further body and muscle regions in a craniocaudal direction and causing increasing limitation of motion (**3** and **4**), in some cases on to almost complete mechanical 'freezing'.

Supplementary Findings: Frequent dental anomalies. Delayed sexual maturity.

Aetiology: Monogenic hereditary disorder, autosomal dominant. Most cases represent new mutations, often associated with increased paternal age.

Frequency: Not extremely rare. By 1958, more than 300 cases had been reported in the literature; the great majority of subsequent cases have not come to pub-lication.

Prognosis: For patients with the typical dysplastic connective tissue swellings from infancy or early child-hood and marked progression: unfavourable life ex-pectancy; not infrequently death from pulmonary dis-ease or heart-failure after the thorax has become im-mobile, before the end of the second decade of life.

Slowing or standstill of the ossification process after the patient has finished growing.

Differential Diagnosis: Soft-tissue swellings appearing in an individual with anomalies of the extremities should signal the diagnosis and thus the avoidance of active procedures. Minimal trauma may provoke new swelling and ossification. Thus, incisions (for sus-pected phlegmon) or biopsies (because of suspected tumour) are contraindicated!

Treatment: In recent trials, 'diphosphonate' (EHDP) administered during exacerbations seems to have li-mited further calcification and ossification in a few cases. Genetic counselling.

Illustrations:
1 and 2 Two-year-old boy with an acute attack of occipito-nucho-dorsal soft-tissue swelling with torti-collis and extensively limited mobility – still no cal-cifications.
3 and 4 A 6½-year-old boy with typical forced atti-tude, numerous sites of ossification in the musculature of the back, bizarre, clasplike periostosis on X-ray.
5 and 7 X-rays of the hands and feet of the child in **2**.
6 and 9, 8 and 11 Hands and feet of the boy in **4**.
10 and 12 Hands and feet of a 13-year-old girl with Münchmeyer syndrome.

References:
Becker P. E., v. Knorre G.: Myositis ossificans progressiva. Ergeb. Inn. Med. Kinderheilkd. N. F. 27:1 (1968)
v. Schnakenburg K., Groß-Selbeck G., Wiedemann H.-R.: Zur Behandlung der Fibrodysplasia ossificans progressiva mit 'Diphosphonat' (EHDP). Dtsch. Med. Wochenschr. 97:1873 (1972)
Amzy A., Bensted J. P. M., Eckstein H. B.: Myositis ossificans progressiva. Z. Kinderchir. 26:252 (1979)
Holmsen H., Ljunghall S., Hierton T.: Myositis ossificans progressiva. Acta Orthop. Scand. 50:33 (1979)

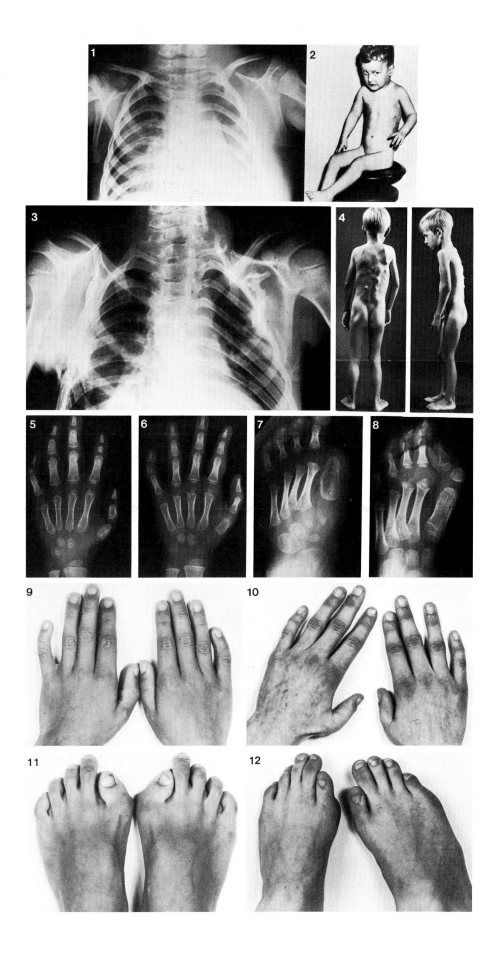

341

171. Syndrome of Osteo-Onycho-Dysostosis

(Nail–Patella–Elbow Syndrome with Pelvic Horns – [Österreicher–] Turner–Kieser Syndrome)

A characteristic hereditary syndrome of skeletal anomalies, dysplasia of the nails, and, frequently, a renal disorder.

Main Signs:
1. Hypo- and dysplasia of the nails (softening, discoloration, longitudinal rippling, abnormal splitting), most frequently affecting thumbs and index fingers (**1** and **2**).
2. Patellar hypoplasia (**5**) with frequent lateral luxation; less frequently aplasia.
3. Hypoplasia of the head of the radius with frequent dorsal luxation and limited motion (**6**).
4. 'Pelvic horns' (symmetrical pyramid-shaped outgrowths from the dorsal surfaces of the wings of the ilia) (**4**) – usually readily palpable.

Supplementary Findings: Hypoplasia of the scapulae; radiologically, hypoplasia of the lateral femoral condyle, coxae valgae, and other findings.

Dark, poorly delimited rims of pigment in the irises surrounding the pupils.

In some cases proteinuria/nephropathy, not infrequently beginning in childhood.

Possible development of cords or pterygia over the elbow joints (**3**); also muscle aplasias.

Manifestation: Actually possible to recognise in the newborn, but usually the child first comes to attention because of difficulty in walking related to the patellar abnormality.

Aetiology: Monogenic hereditary disorder, autosomal dominant, with quite varied expressivity.

Frequency: Not so rare. Well over 500 cases in the literature; estimation (1965) of 22 gene carriers in 1 million of the population.

Prognosis: Dependent on the development (in more than half of the cases) and course of a renal involvement (nephropathy of undetermined nature with slow but, in about 30%, unfavourable course).

Treatment: Orthopaedic care; renal follow-up. Genetic counselling.

Illustrations:
1 and 2 Dysplasia of the nails (fingers >> toes).
3 A 14-year-old boy (shown in all photographs) with firm pterygium-like formations on both elbow joints; nephropathy.
4 Pelvic horns.
5 Hypoplasia of the patellas; angular appearance of the flexed knees.
6 Elbow joint with distinct dorsal luxation of the head of the radius.

References:
Caliebe M.-R., Rohwedder H.-J., Wiedemann H.-R.: Über das Mißbildungs-Erbsyndrom Osteo-Oncho-Dysplasie mit Nierenbeteiligung. Arch. Kinderheilkd: *169*:149 (1963)
Spranger J. W., Langer L. O., jr, Wiedemann H.-R.: Bone Dysplasias. An Atlas of Constitutional Disorders of Skeletal Development. Stuttgart and Philadelphia, G. Fischer and W. B. Saunders 1974

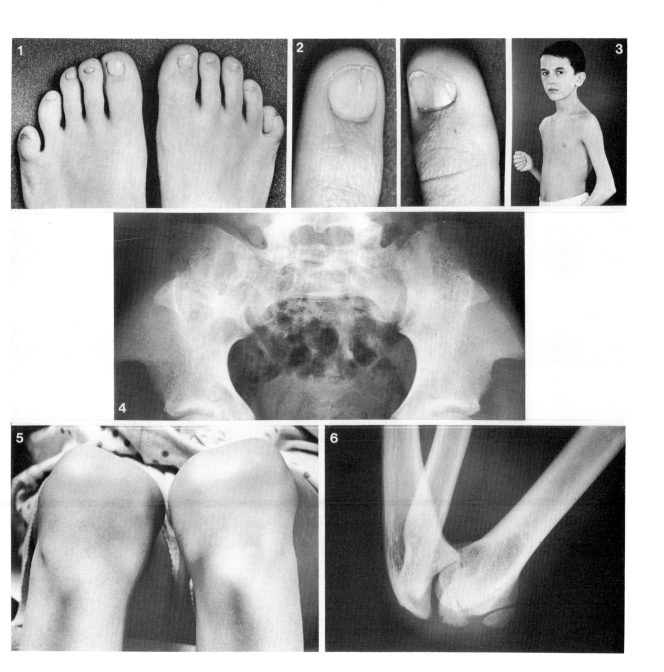

172. Antiepileptic Embryopathy

(Fetal Embryo Hydantoin Syndrome and Fetal Embryo Damage Due to Various Other Anticonvulsives)

A syndrome of minor malformations regarded as resulting from maternal antiepileptic medication.

Main Signs:
1. Facial dysplasia in the form of an unusual midface: short, broad, more or less turned-up nose; broad, low nasal bridge; hypertelorism (**1–4**).
2. Hypoplasia of the end segments of the fingers: shortened distal phalanges and hypo- to aplasia of the nails (**5** and **6**).
3. History of anticonvulsant treatment of the mother in early pregnancy (e.g., hydantoin; phenobarbital; carbamazepin).

Supplementary Findings: Possibly also epicanthi and low-set ears, simian creases.

Not infrequently small size (length, weight) at birth and/or postnatally.

Comment: Independent of the anticonvulsive medication, children of epileptic mothers have a higher risk of major malformations, primarily cleft lip or palate, then congenital heart disease.

Manifestation: Birth.

Frequency: Not so rare.

Illustrations:
1–6 A series of typically affected children of various ages.
(By kind permission of Priv. Doz. Dr Dietrich, Kiel.)

References:
Dieterich E.: Antiepileptika-Embryopathien. Ergeb. Inn. Med. Kinderheilkd. N. F. 43:93 (1979)
Dieterich E., Lukas A., Steveling A., et al: Art und Ausmaß von Fehlbildungen bzw. Fehlbildungsmustern bei Kindern antiepileptisch behandelter Väkter und Mütter. In: Epilepsie 1979, H. Doose et al (eds) G. Thieme, Stuttgart, New York 1980, p.47

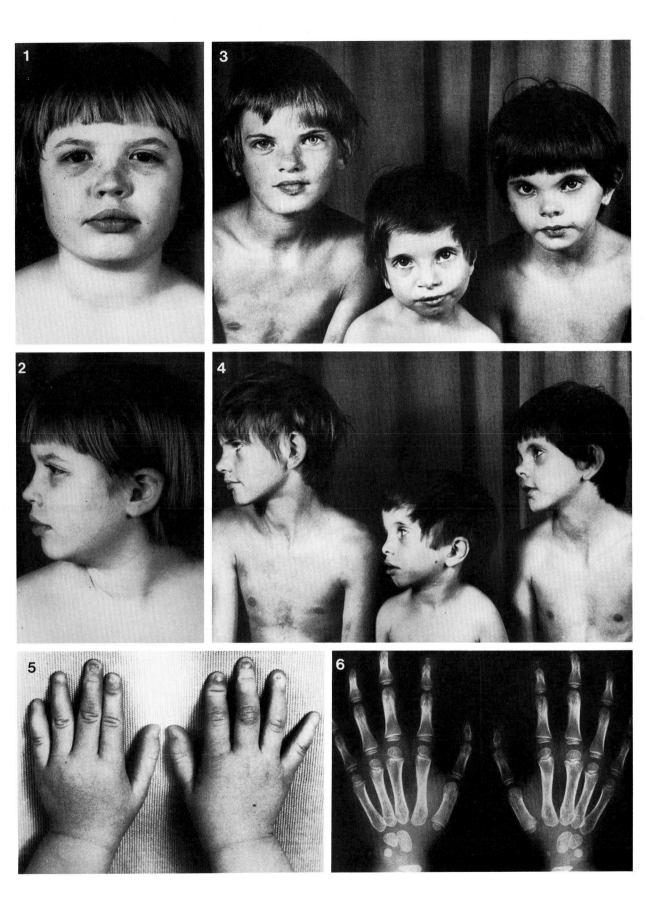

173. Zinsser–Cole–Engman Syndrome

(Dyskeratosis Congenita Type Zinsser–Cole–Engman)

A hereditary syndrome of poikiloderma, nail dystrophy, leucoplakia, and possible pancytopenia.

Main Signs:
1. *Skin:* Formation of blisters (subepidermal, and clinically usually not very prominent), reticular hyper- and depigmentation, atrophy, and telangiectasia which result in a 'mottled skin' appearance (poikiloderma) (**1**).
2. *Mucous Membranes* (especially those adjacent to the external integument): blisters, ulcers, scars, stenoses, and strictures, and otherwise hyperkeratoses and leucoplakia or leucokeratoses (**3**).
3. *Nails:* Dystrophies (longitudinal ridges, splitting, shortness, thinning) (**2, 4–6**).
4. *Eyes:* Blepharitis, lacrimal conjunctivitis with obliteration of the lacrimal points and disturbing flow of tears, possible ectropion and loss of the eyelashes.

Supplementary Findings: Development of pancytopenia (panmyelophthisis) (in about half of the cases).

'Connective tissue weakness' with hyperextensibility of the joints (**2**), tendency to hernias, etc. Thin, sparse hair or alopecia. Dental anomalies.

Manifestation: Usually between the 3rd and 10th years of life (pancytopenia more likely in the 2nd or 3rd decade).

Aetiology: Hereditary disease; definite preponderance of males. Indications for both autosomal recessive and X-linked recessive transmission. Basic defect unknown.

Frequency: Low; by 1977 about 50 cases had been described.

Course, Prognosis: Decreased life expectancy in case of panmyelophthisis or possible malignant transformation at the base of precancerous hyperkeratoses of the mucous membranes.

Diagnosis: Apart from the facial poikiloderma, the lacrimal conjunctivitis and nail changes are the most important signs.

Treatment: Symptomatic. Careful haematological and oncological follow-up; extirpation of leucoplakia patches. Genetic counselling.

Illustrations:
1, 3, 5, and 6 A 10-year-old affected boy. Hyperpigmented areas of skin on the lower eyelids, reticular at the nasogenal folds; lacrimal conjunctivitis, blepharitis, obliteration of the lacrimal points. Pancytopenia.
2 and 4 A 13-year-old-boy.
(By kind permission of Prof. Dr H. Reich, Münster i. W.)

References:
Reich H.: Zinsser-Cole-Engman-Syndrom. Med. Klin. 68:283 (1973)
Trowbridge A. A., Sirinavin C. H., Linman J. W.: Dyskeratosis congenita: Hematologic evaluation of a sibship and review of the literature. Am. J. Hematol. 3:143 (1977)
Rodermund O. E., Hausmann G., Hausmann D.: Zinsser-Cole-Engman-Syndrom. Z. Hautkr. 54:273 (1979)
DeBoeck Kr., Degreef H., Verwilghen R., et al: Thrombocytopenia: First symptom in a patient with dyskeratosis congenita. Pediatrics 67:898 (1981)
Kelly T. E., Stelling C. B.: Dyskeratosis congenita: Radiologic features. Pediatr. Radiol. 12:31 (1982)

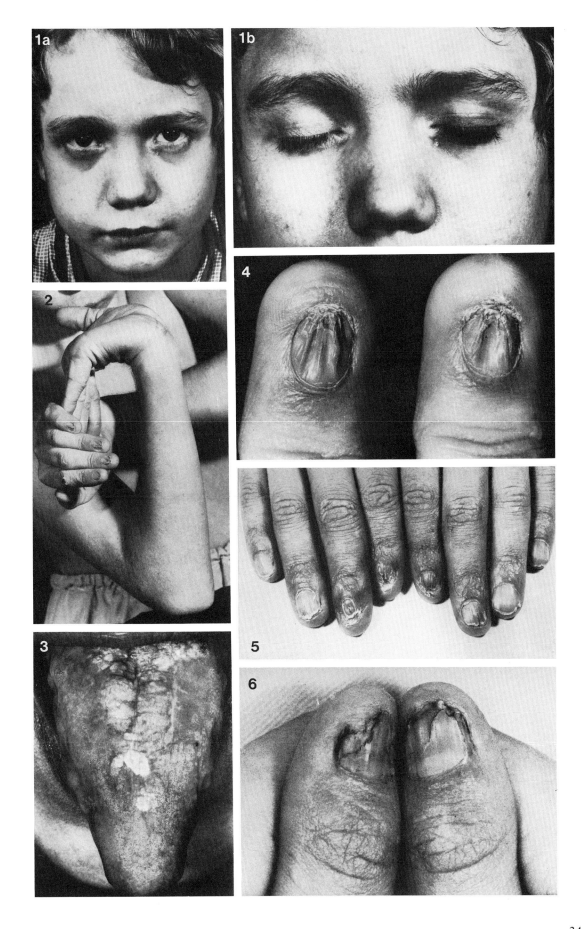

174. Syndrome of Hypohidrotic Ectodermal Dysplasia

A highly characteristic syndrome comprising 'anhidrosis' with the danger of recurring hyperthermia, hypotrichosis, hypo- or anodontia, and typical facies.

Main Signs:
1. Characteristic facies with bulging forehead; prominent supraorbital ridges; hypertelorism; deep-set nasal root; short nose with hypoplastic alae; hypoplasia of the upper jaw; full, pouting lips; protruding chin; and possible prominent ears coming to a point at the top ('satyr ears') (1, 2, and 6).
2. Sparse, light scalp hair; short, fine, and dry. Eyebrows and eyelashes absent or merely suggested. Fine wrinkling of the periocular and sometimes perioral skin, often heavily pigmented (1–4). Premature baldness.
3. Hypoplastic alveolar ridges with anodontia or hypodontia (5).
4. External integument hypoplastic, translucent, soft and also very dry, no sweat formation. Possible papular changes of the face and axilla; frequent depigmentation at the back of the neck and the genital region. Possible hyperkeratosis of the palms and soles. No lanugo hair on the neonate. Later, little or no body hair.
5. Rise in body temperature sometimes with minimal physical exertion (especially in the young) or increased environmental temperature; heat intolerance.

Supplementary Findings: Dry, irritated mucous membranes with tendency to atrophy. Possible deficiency of tears, conjunctivitis. Frequent photophobia. Tendency to chronic atrophic rhinitis. Possible hyposmia; hoarseness. Not infrequently eczema. Possible mild dystrophy of the nails. Possible hypo- or aplasia of the mammary glands and/or nipples.

Sometimes mental retardation, probably as a result of cerebral damage from repeated severe hyperthermia. Possible inner ear hearing impairment.

On biopsy, hypo- or aplasia of the exocrine sweat glands and sebaceous glands of the skin, and hypoplasia or absence of the mucous glands of the mucous membranes.

Manifestation: At birth.

Aetiology: Hereditary defect. Heterogeneity. Sex-linked recessive type by far the most prominent: males affected; females show only microsigns (see below); identification of female gene-carriers important. An autosomal recessive type occurs much less frequently.

Frequency: Relatively rare; (somewhat more than 300 cases reported in the literature up to 1975).

Course, Prognosis: Initially, life or cerebral function endangered by episodes of hyperthermia. In adults, performance and life expectancy usually are no longer appreciably limited.

Diagnosis: Ectodermal syndrome should be ruled out in all cases of unexplained fever in small infants, even when other signs are few. Caution with sweat tests in suspected cases. Female carriers of the X-linked recessive form may show mild dental dysplasia, decreased ability to sweat (regional aplasia of the sweat glands), little breast development.

Differential Diagnosis: Other ectodermal dysplasia syndromes.

Treatment: Immediate cooling of the hyperthermic patient; prevention of convulsions/brain damage. Protection against heat and sunshine; possible change of climate. Eyedrops may be required. Otological care. Dental prostheses, possibly from early childhood! Wigs in some cases. Skin care. Genetic counselling.

Illustrations:
1 Infant with hypotrichosis, 'satyr ears', prominent forehead, wrinkled eyelids, full lips. Deficient tears; rhinitis sicca; dysphonia and hoarseness. Aplasia of the dental germs. Dry scaly skin. History of life-threatening episodes of hyperthermia.
2–6 A 2-year-old cousin of the patient in 1, also with the full clinical picture. Mamillary aplasia. Skin biopsy showed aplasia of sweat and sebaceous glands.

Reference:
Reed W. B., Lopez D. A., Landing B.: Clinical spectrum of anhydrotic ectodermal dysplasia. Arch. Dermatol. *102*:134 (1970)

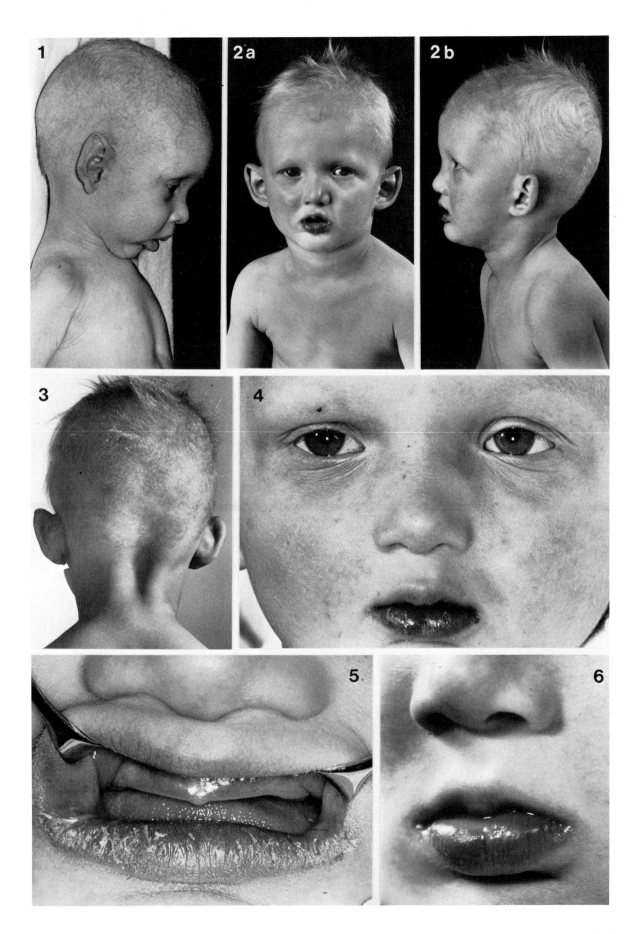

175. Ectodermal Dysplasia Syndrome with Anomalies of the Hair and Syndactyly

A hereditary syndrome comprising hypotrichosis with pili torti, hypoplasia of the teeth, ichthyosiform skin changes, and cutaneous syndactyly of the hands and feet.

Main Signs:
1. Hypotrichosis involving the scalp, eyebrows, and eyelashes (**1, 4–9**). Helical twisting of the hair: pili torti.
2. Generalised dryness of the skin, with hyperkeratoses occurring especially on the lower trunk, lower extremities, palms and soles, with sparing of the axillae and elbows (**10c** and **d**).
3. Various grades of cutaneous syndactyly of the hands (III/IV>II/III; **10a–d** and **12**) and feet (II/III>III/IV; **11a–c**).
4. Marked hypoplasia of the crowns of the teeth with normal number of teeth and dental germs. (Slight delay in change of dentitions and atypical order of eruption.)

Hyperlordosis of the vertebral column.

Supplementary Findings: No hyperthermia. A dermatological sweat test – 1, 4–dehydroxy anthrachinon (Chinizarin) powder, electric cradle – positive (axillae, elbows, soles of the feet, anterior sweat grooves, genito-anal area, thighs, popliteal areas).

In part, thickening and yellow discoloration of the toenails.

Bilateral simian creases.

Absence of hypertelorism, of low nasal root and short nose, of full lips, of periocular or perioral wrinkling of the skin, and of (superiorly pointed) 'satyr ears'.

High palate, normal alveolar processes. Unremarkable mucous membranes.

Very fine opacities of the lenses on ophthalmoscopy. No photophobia. Slight hypermetropia.

Normal mental development. Normal range of hearing on audiometry. Normal height and skeletal maturity. Normally formed mamillae.

Unusual familial resemblance of the affected persons.

Manifestation: At birth.

Aetiology: Hereditary defect; probably autosomal recessive transmission as a result of close parental consanguinity.

Frequency: Unknown; may be assumed rare.

Course, Prognosis: Favourable.

Differential Diagnosis: Other ectodermal dysplasias.

Treatment: Dental care. A wig may be necessary for cosmetic and, no less important, psychological considerations. Genetic counselling.

Illustrations:
1–12 Three siblings of 12, 6, and 3 years (2 further siblings healthy). Hair twisted on itself; in part also smooth or wavy; for the most part white-blond, fine, and soft, in part also dark, strong, and hard; very varied lengths (in part broken off). Eyebrows merely suggested; varied very scanty eyelashes. Simian crease bilaterally in all three children.

Patient 1 (**1** and **2, 4** and **7, 10a** and **11c**) shows additionally a blind fistula below the tragus of each ear. On ophthalmoscopic examination, very tiny peripheral punctiform opacities of the lenses.

Patient 2 (**3, 5,** and **8, 10b** and **11b**) has had surgical correction of syndactyly on the left hand. Ophthalmologically, small subcapsular opacities of the right lens at the dorsal pole.

Patient 3 (**3, 6,** and **9, 10d, 11a,** and **12**) was reputedly 'hairless' at birth. Both hands have been operated on for syndactyly.

(By kind permission of Prof. A. Proppe and Dr H. Hauss, Kiel.)

References:
None known concerning this particular form.

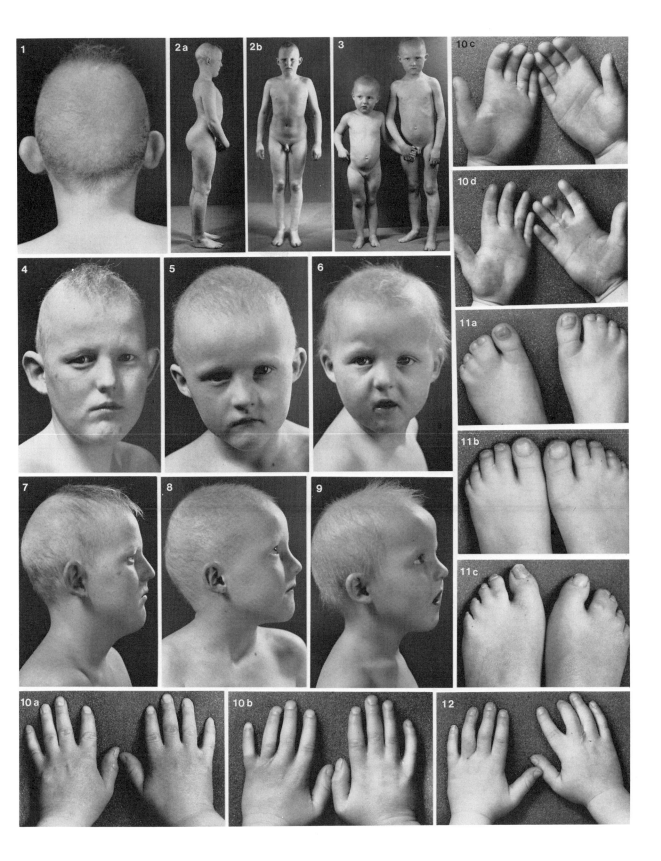

176. Lymphoedema–Distichiasis Syndrome

A hereditary syndrome of late-onset lymphoedema of the lower extremities, double rows of eyelashes (distichiasis), and other anomalies.

Main Signs:
1. Lymphoedema of the legs (2), especially from the knee downwards, in men possibly accompanied by considerable scrotal swelling.
2. Double row of eyelashes on the upper and lower lids (3).

Supplementary Findings: Ectropion of the lower eyelids, uni- or bilateral ptosis, pterygium colli (1), enlargement of the spinal canal due to arachnoidal and extradural cyst formation there, in some cases with neurological signs, and diverse anomalies of the vertebral column have been observed repeatedly.

Manifestation: Lymphoedema beginning in the 2nd half of the 1st decade of life or during the 2nd decade and later. One lower extremity may be affected many years before the other.

Aetiology: Autosomal dominant hereditary disorder with high penetrance and variable expressivity.

Frequency: Rare; up to 1980 about 75 cases were known.

Course, Prognosis: For the most part dependent on the extent and severity of oedema and on the possible development of cysts in the spinal column region.

Differential Diagnosis: Other forms of late-onset lymphoedema type Meige.

Treatment: Symptomatic. Depilation of symptomatic (irritation of conjunctiva or even cornea) lid hair. Surgical treatment of oedematous regions promises little improvement. Genetic counselling.

Illustrations:
1 and 2 A 1.60 m tall 31-year-old woman with extensive oedema of both lower legs, of the right since age 13 years, of the left increasing since her third pregnancy. Double row of eyelashes on all four eyelids; ptosis of the right upper eyelid. (Post) operative correction of the dysplastic left auricle and of pterygium colli. Aneurysm of the ascending aorta, tilted kidneys. Two sons of the proband, 11 and 9½ years, also show distichiasis.
3 Lower lid of one of the sons with a double row of eyelashes and partial depilations); to date no oedema. Further affected persons in the family.
(By kind permission of Frau Dr A. Fuhrmann-Rieger and Prof. W. Fuhrmann, both Gießen a. d. Lahn.)

References:
Holmes L. B., Fields J. P., Zabriskie J. B.: Hereditary late-onset lymphedema. Pediatrics 61:575 (1978)
Fuhrmann–Rieger A.: Familiäres Distichiasis-Lymphödem-Syndrom. In: Klinische Genetik in der Pädiatrie. I. Symposion in Kiel. M. Tolksdorf, J. Spranger (eds), Gg. Thieme, Stuttgart 1979
Schwartz J. F., O'Brien M. S., Hoffmann J. C., jr: Hereditary spinal arachnoid cysts, distichiasis, and lymphedema. Ann. Neurol. 7:340 (1980)

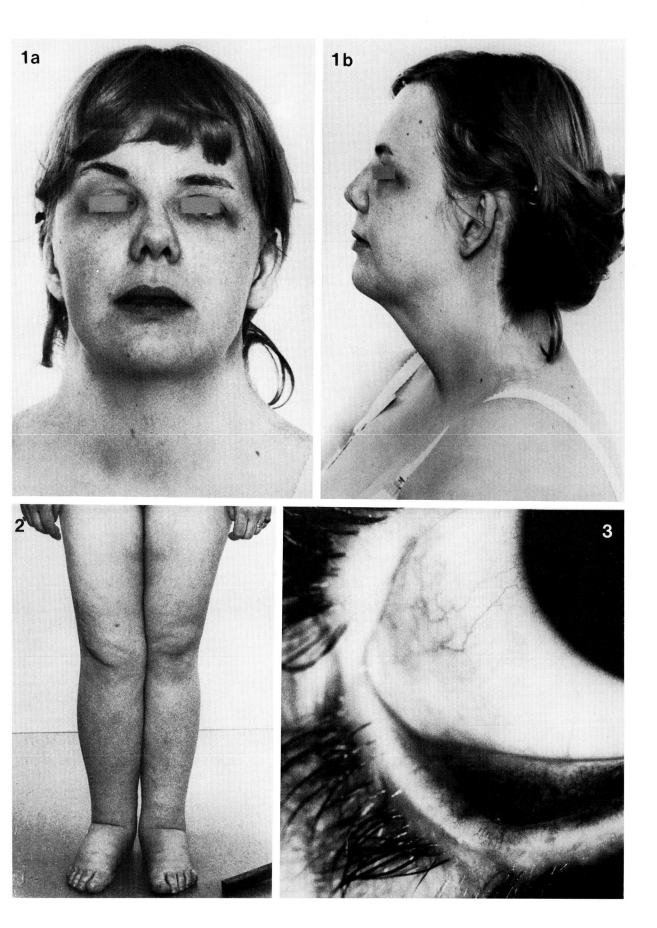

177. Acrodermatitis Enteropathica

A hereditary disorder, frequently with an intermittent course, of periorificial and acral skin changes, alopecia, and diarrhoea, due to a disorder of zinc metabolism.

Main Signs:
1. A distinctive skin disorder with the initial efflorescences usually being vesicobullous, later dry crusted and lamellar-scaly (to psoriasoid), at first distributed symmetrically around the body orifices (especially the genito-anal region) and eyes (1), then also the back of the head, back of the neck, elbows, knees, hands, and feet. Nails and interdigital spaces of the fingers and toes are often impressively involved (3 and 4). Frequent secondary bacterial or parasitic infection.
2. Alopecia (to total loss of scalp hair, eyebrows, and eyelashes) (1).
3. Possible diarrhoea (various grades of severity).

Supplementary Findings: Apart from failure to thrive, deficient growth, and severe psychological problems – frequent secondary glossitis (2) and stomatitis, conjunctivitis, blepharitis, and photophobia (1) as well as severe nail dystrophies (3b) to loss of nails.

Increased susceptibility to infections.

Low serum and urinary zinc levels (and decreased alkaline phosphatase).

Manifestation: Usually sometime during the 1st year of life; typically and frequently, after being weaned from breast milk; sometimes not until later.

Aetiology: Hereditary disease, autosomal recessive; (disorder of zinc metabolism with malabsorption of zinc, and its sequelae).

Frequency: Rare.

Course, Prognosis: Without treatment, intermittent but relentlessly progressive course to usually early death. Adequately treated, a decrease in life expectancy need no longer be feared.

Treatment: Oral zinc substitution (as a rule with zinc sulphate) effects dramatic improvement and healing of all manifestations within a few weeks. Follow-up and in given cases specific treatment of secondary infections. Genetic counselling.

Illustrations:
1 and 3a   An 8-year-old boy with the full clinical picture.
2, 3b and 4   A 3-year-old-girl.
(By kind permission of Prof. Dr H. Reich. Münster i. W.)

References:
Lombeck I., Schnippering H. G., Kasperek K., et al: Akrodermatitis enteropathica – eine Zinkstoffwechselstörung mit Zinkmalabsorption. Z. Kinderheilkd. *120*:181 (1975)
Chandra R. K.: Acrodermatitis enteropathica: Zinc levels and cell-mediated immunity. Pediatrics 66:789 (1980)

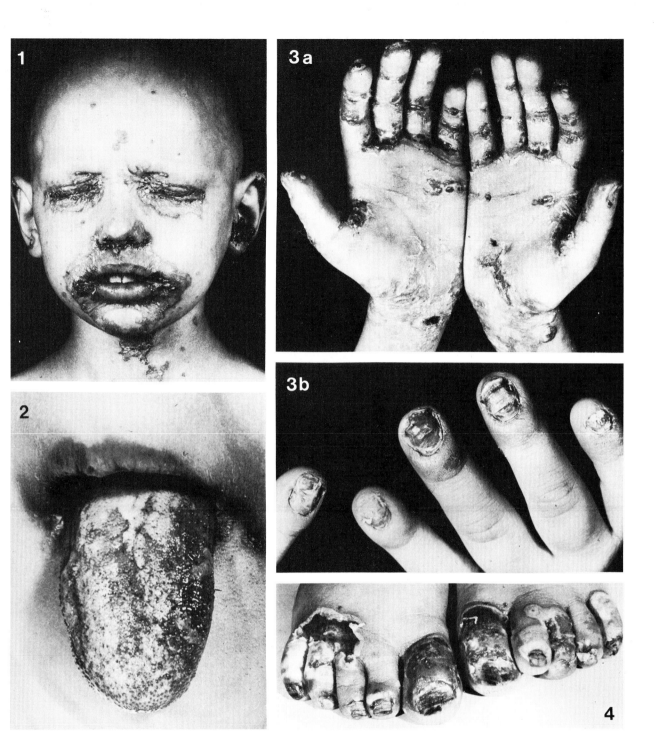

178. Sjögren–Larsson Syndrome

A hereditary syndrome of congenital ichthyosis, spastic paraparesis, mental retardation, and short stature.

Main Signs:
1. Ichthyosis, especially of the nuchal, axillary, and other flexor surfaces; the face may be spared. Hands and feet may show hyperkeratoses.
2. Spastic para- (to tetra-)plegia.
3. Considerable mental retardation (IQ usually between 30 and 60); usually more or less severe speech defect.
4. Short stature (often below the 10th percentile).

Supplementary Findings: Seizures in about one-third of cases.

Pigmentary degeneration of the retina, possibly involving the macula (here, small reflecting spots), in about a quarter to a third of cases.

Decreased ability to sweat. Hypoplasia of teeth and enamel. Possibly sparse scalp hair.

Manifestation: Ichthyosis, scaling, and hyperkeratosis from birth. The central nervous manifestations occur later. Length at birth may be below average.

Aetiology: Hereditary disorder, autosomal recessive.

Frequency: In certain areas with increased inbreeding, frequent; otherwise rare.

Course, Prognosis: Very dependent on the severity of mental deficiency, diplegia, and possible visual impairment.

Differential Diagnosis: Ichthyosis–oligophrenia–epilepsy syndrome, p.358.

Treatment: Symptomatic. Genetic counselling.

Illustrations:
1 and 2 A mentally retarded boy who shows spastic diplegia and congenital ichthyosis with hyperkeratoses.
(By kind permission of Prof. E. Passarge, Essen and of Urban und Schwarzenberg Verlag, Munich.)

References:
Theile U.: Sjögren–Larsson syndrome. Oligophrenia-Ichthyosis–Di/Tetraplegia. Humangenetik *22*:91 (1974)
Jagell S., Lidén S.: Ichthyosis in the Sjögren–Larsson syndrome. Clin. Genet. *21*:243 (1982)

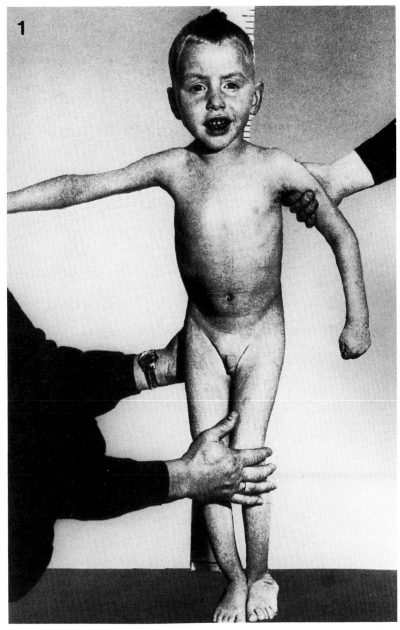

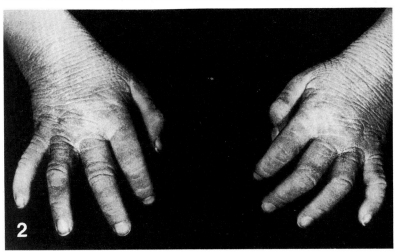

179. Ichthyosis–Oligophrenia–Epilepsy Syndrome

A hereditary syndrome of ichthyosis, mental deficiency, epilepsy, and – more or less constant – hypogonadism.

Main Signs:
1. Ichthyosis, usually present from early infancy.
2. Psychomotor retardation of various grades of severity (IQ between about 30 and 80).
3. Seizure disorder with variable age of onset.

Supplementary Findings: Hypogonadism with eunuchoid appearance and, in some patients, more or less distinct sexual infantilism.

Manifestation: At birth and/or later.

Aetiology: Uniformity of this syndrome questionable. No doubt of a genetic basis. Autosomal recessive transmission has been presumed. Occurrence of an X-linked recessive type also possible.

Frequency: Rare.

Course, Prognosis: Very dependent on the severity of mental retardation and of the epilepsy.

Differential Diagnosis: Sjögren–Larsson syndrome p.356.

Treatment: Symptomatic. Genetic counselling.

Illustrations: Three brothers, the children of healthy parents; ichthyosis congenita in a brother of the mother.

5 and 8 The 16¼-year-old, oldest boy: moderate ichthyosis since birth; delayed development and limited abilities; (to date) no seizures; genitalia shown in **8**.

1–4 and 7 The 'middle' brother at 10 years (**4**), and at 13½ years (**1–3**). Ichthyosis (see in **7**) since birth; oligophrenia; seizure disorder; hypogenitalism (**7**).

6 and 9 The youngest brother at 10 years: moderate ichthyosis since birth; mental development in low-normal range; (to date) no seizures; genitalia shown in **9** (undescended testis on the right). Chromosome analyses of the three brothers negative (banding).

A 14½-year-old sister healthy and normally developed for her age.

(By kind permission of Prof. H. Doose, Kiel.)

References:
Maldonaldo R. R. et al: Neuroichthyosis with hypogonadism (Rud's syndrome). Int. J. Dermatol. *14*:347 (1975)
Larbrisseau A., Carpenter St: Rud syndrome...Neuropediatrics *13*:95 (1982)

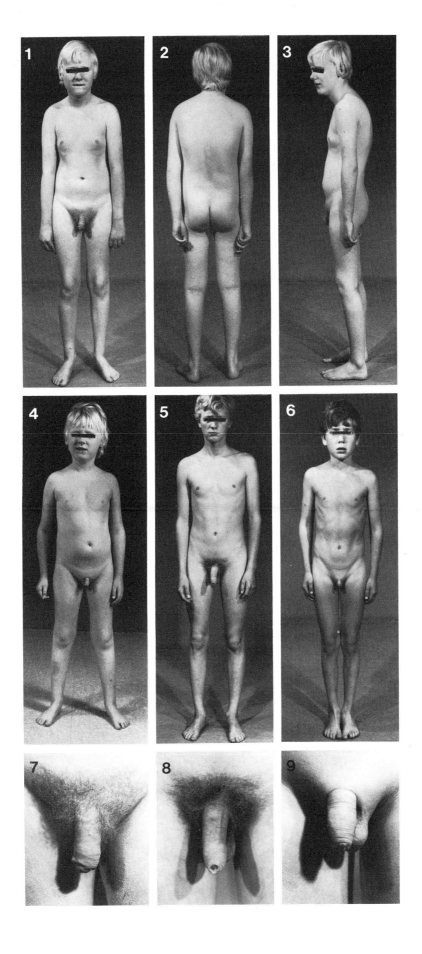

180. Syndrome of Hyperkeratosis Palmoplantaris with Periodontosis

(Papillon–Lefèvre Syndrome)

A hereditary syndrome of plantopalmar hyperkeratosis, periodontopathy, and loss of teeth.

Main Signs:
1. Hyperkeratosis of the soles of the feet and the palms of the hands, usually much milder on the latter (**2** and **3**).
2. Severe periodontosis of the deciduous teeth as well as of the secondary dentition, with loosening and loss of all teeth (**1**).

Supplementary Findings: Severe secondary periodontitis and gingivostomatitis.

Manifestation: Redness and/or hyperkeratosis of the palms and soles may be apparent from birth and, if a previous sibling has shown the typical syndrome, allows an early diagnosis. Otherwise the diagnosis cannot be made until the primary dentition appears and is promptly followed by the first dental problems.

Aetiology: Hereditary disorder, autosomal recessive.

Frequency: Rare; estimation 1:1 million population.

Course, Prognosis: Severe periodontosis (and – secondary – periodontitis) affects the primary dentition and subsequently the 'permanent' dentition with loss of all teeth. The deciduous teeth are lost at about age 5–6 years; the secondary, at about 13–14 years. No occupational handicap from the skin disorder of the palms of the hands.

Treatment: Highly qualified oral hygiene. Dental care. Dental plates for the upper and lower jaws at an appropriate time. Genetic counselling.

Illustrations:
1–4 A 3¾-year-old Turkish boy for whom family history was not available. Dyskeratotic–hyperkeratotic changes of the palms and soles with garland-like sharp-edged borders to the healthy skin at the level of the malleoli and heels. Redness of the skin of the palms and soles. Hyperkeratoses of the patellar regions bilaterally. Premature, extensive loss of the deciduous teeth in both jaws; a few remaining loose teeth with their necks extensively exposed, periodontosis.
(By kind permission of Dr Kl. Heyne, Kiel.)

Reference:
Giasanti J. S., et al: Palmar-plantar hyperkeratosis and concomitant periodontal destruction (Papillon–Lefèvre syndrome). Oral Surg. 36:40 (1973)

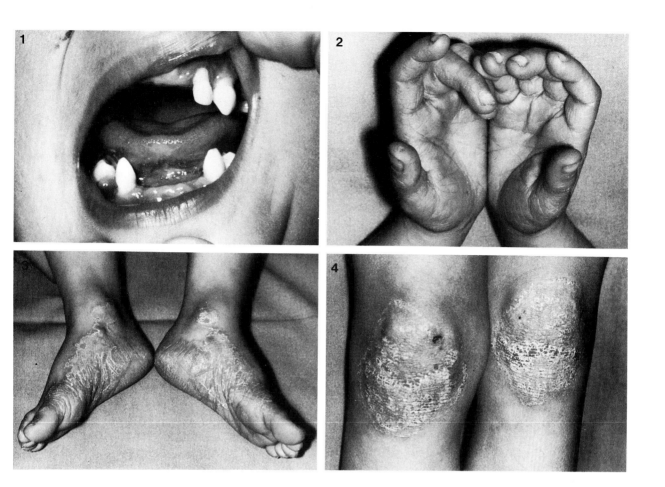

181. Syndrome of Epidermolysis Bullosa Hereditaria

A collective term for a group of hereditary dermatoses in which very minimal trauma or mechanical or other factors lead to blistering of the skin.

Main Signs:
1. Dependent on the particular genotype (see below), blisters are formed on body areas subject to pressure or rubbing, or on other areas, and possibly 'spontaneously'. More precise characteristics of the blisters also depend on the type of this disorder, as do positive or negative Nikolsky phenomenon, healing with or without scarring (in extreme cases, adhesions – 'mutilation' – on the hands and feet, oesophageal stenosis, and danger of carcinoma in scar tissue), involvement or noninvolvement of the mucous membranes, presence of palmoplantar hyperhidrosis and development of hyperkeratoses, nail dystrophies and defective tooth enamel or other dental disorders, dystrophy of the hair and alopecia, and others.

Manifestation: Often from birth or in the first year of life, rarely later.

Aetiology: Monogenic hereditary disorder. At present 16 types have been differentiated, with about equal numbers of autosomal dominant and autosomal recessive genotypes, in addition to an X-linked recessive type. The basic defects are unknown.

Frequency: Taken as a group of diseases, epidermolysis hereditaria is not very rare. Many hundreds of cases in the literature alone.

Course, Prognosis: Dependent on the type. There are early lethal and potentially early lethal courses (especially with the recessive hereditary types), but also types with a tendency for improvement during or around puberty, and types with no effect on life expectancy.

Differential Diagnosis: Exogenous acute conditions such as staphylogenic pemphigoid of infants and newborns, exfoliative dermatitis of Ritter, toxic or allergic combustiform epidermolysis of Lyell, erythema multiforma bullosum, or even blisters from scalding are readily excluded. In addition, acrodermatitis enteropathica (p.354), congenital porphyria, herpetiform dermatitis, and pemphigus usually are not difficult to rule out.

Treatment: Depending on the severity of the case, intensive care may be required, or essentially mere avoidance of precipitating trauma. Vocational counselling in some cases. Genetic family counselling. Possible prenatal diagnosis.

Illustrations:
1a and b A 2-day-old newborn infant.
2a–d A 3-year-old girl with alopecia, damage of the lips and teeth, and nail dystrophy. Both **1** and **2** show autosomal recessive forms of the disorder.
3a and b The lower leg of a newborn infant and the hand of his father with an autosomal dominant form of the disease.

References:
Voigtländer V., Schnyder U. W., Anton-Lamprecht I.: Hereditäre Epidermolysen. In: Korting G. W. (ed) Dermatologie in Praxis und Klinik, Bd III, Thieme, Stuttgart 1979
Rodeck C. H., Eady R. A. J., Gosden C. M.: Prenatal diagnosis of epidermolysis bullosa letalis. Lancet *I*:979 (1980)
Anton-Lamprecht I., Rauskolb R., et al: Prenatal diagnosis of epidermolysis bullosa dystrophica...Lancet *II*:1077 (1981)

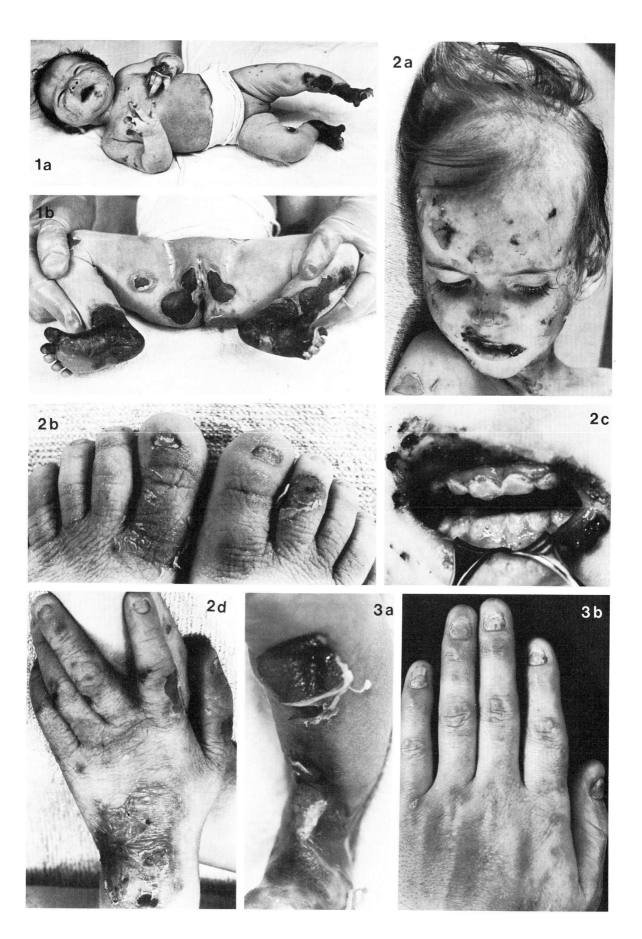

363

182. Fetal Alcohol Syndrome

(Alcohol Embryopathy, Embryofetal Alcohol Syndrome)

Primordial growth deficiency, mental retardation and behaviour disorders with frequent microcephaly, characteristic facies, as well as multiple further anomalies in children of alcoholic mothers.

Main Signs:
1. Marked pre- and postnatal growth deficiency with dystrophy (birth weight almost always less than 2500 g).
2. Mental deficiency of all grades of severity, usually moderate to mild. Microcephaly very common. Not infrequently signs of cerebral defect. Increased irritability and hyperactivity during the first years of life.
3. Typical facies: short palpebral fissures (possible epicanthus, ptosis, microphthalmos), short nasal bridge (sometimes anteverted nostrils), frequently hypoplastic philtrum, thin upper lip with narrow prolabium, retrogenia, and possible dysplastic ears (1–5).

Supplementary Findings: Not infrequently cleft palate, funnel breast (3), limited motion at the joints (especially elbows and interphalangeal joints, also hip dysplasia), abnormally short metacarpals, clinodactyly of the little fingers, and other skeletal anomalies.

Anomalies of the palmar creases, coccygeal foveola, hernias.

Occasional cardiac anomaly (usually septal defects), urinary tract or genital anomalies (e.g., hypoplastic labia; hypospadias).

Low Apgar score, weak feeding, hypotonia; increased susceptibility to infections.

History of maternal alcoholism.

Manifestation: At birth (increased incidence of breech presentations).

Aetiology: This embryofetopathy has been observed only in children of alcoholic mothers. Whether pathogeneticaly attributable to ethyl alcohol, acetaldehyde, or secondary deficiencies is still unsettled.

Frequency: From the time of the first description in 1968 until 1977, about 500 cases became known. In two series of investigations, over 40% of the offspring of chronic alcoholic mothers proved to have the syndrome. When children with milder manifestations are included, the frequency is approximately 2 cases in 1000 births.

Course, Prognosis: The perinatal mortality does not appear to be increased. Frequent infections, failure to thrive, and necessary operations account for numerous hospital admissions. Owing to the mental retardation, the majority of patients are only able to attend a special school for the mentally handicapped.

Differential Diagnosis: Trisomy 18 syndrome (p.58); here severe mental retardation, death almost always within the first year of life, characteristic chromosomal findings. Dubowitz syndrome (p.112) and Noonan syndrome (p.132) also should not be difficult to rule out (especially in the absence of the appropriate social history).

Treatment: Symptomatic. Special feeding frequently necessary initially. In some cases operative correction of cleft palate, hernias, cardiac defects. All appropriate aids for the handicapped. Preventative measures imperative for women with chronic alcohol addiction.

Illustrations:

1–3 A 3-month-old child. Mother a chronic alcoholic. Birth weight 1590 g after unclear length of gestation. Measurements at age 9 months: 68.5 cm; 5700 g; 42 cm (head circumference). Typical facies. Premature synostosis of the frontal suture, cardiac defect, psychomotor retardation.

4 and 5 Two further typically affected young children.

References:
Hanson J. W., Jones K. L., Smith D. W.: Fetal alcohol syndrome. Experience with 41 patients. JAMA 235:1458 (1976)
Majewski F., Bierich J. R., Löser H., et al: Zur Klinik und Pathogenese der Alkohol-Embryopathie. Bericht über 68 Fälle. Münch. Med. Wochenschr. 118:1635 (1976)
Dehaene Ph., Titran M., Samaille-Vilette Ch., et al: Fréquence du syndrome d'alcoolisme foetal. Nouv. Presse Méd. 6:1763 (1977)
Clarren S. K., Smith D. W.: The fetal alcohol syndrome. N. Engl. J. Med. 298:1063 (1978)
Hanson J. W., Streissguth A. P., Smith D. W.: The effects of moderate alcohol consumption during pregnancy on fetal growth and morphogenesis. J. Pediatr. 92:457 (1978); thorough review: Deutsch. Med. Wochenschr. 103:1319 (1978)
Majewski F., Fischbach H., Peiffer J., et al: Zur Frage der Interruptio bei alkoholkranken Frauen. Deutsch. Med. Wochenschr. 103:895 (1978)
Véghelyi P. V., Osztovics M., Kardos G., et al: The fetal alcohol syndrome: Symptoms and pathogenesis. Acta. Paed. Acad. Sci. Hung. 19:171 (1978)
Majewski F.: Die Alkoholembryopathie: Fakten und Hypothesen. Ergeb. Inn. Med. Kinderheilkd. N. F. 43: (1979)
Little R. E., Streissguth A. P., Barr H. M.: Decreased birth weight in infants of alcoholic women who abstained during pregnancy. J. Pediatr. 96:974 (1980)

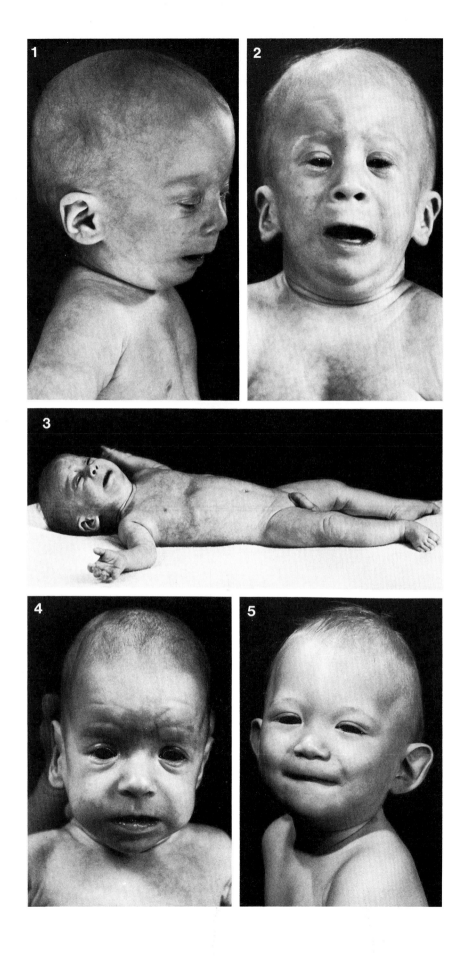

183. Williams–Beuren Syndrome

(Williams Syndrome, Fanconi–Schlesinger Syndrome, Williams' Elfin Face Syndrome)

A malformation-retardation syndrome with characteristic facial dysmorphism, short stature, mental retardation, vascular stenoses, and – infrequently – hypercalcaemia.

Main Signs:
1. So-called elfin facies, essentially characterised by short palpebral fissures, hypotelorism, epicanthus, low nasal root, hypoplasia of the midface, slightly anteverted nostrils, long philtrum, full cheeks, and full, sometimes drooping lips (1, 2, 6–8).
2. Internal strabismus (6). Slight microcephaly.
3. Hypoplastic teeth (5), occasionally hypodontia.
4. Pre- and especially postnatal growth retardation.
5. Moderate to severe mental retardation, with a friendly, lively disposition; deep voice.

Supplementary Findings: Vascular stenoses, especially supravalvular aortic stenosis; peripheral pulmonary stenoses; stenoses of the renal, mesenteric, and other arteries.

Ventricular and atrial septal defects.

Hypercalcaemia infrequent, usually limited to early infancy and when present, associated with the related clinical signs (anorexia, obstipation, etc.), metastatic calcifications, especially of the kidneys. Osteosclerosis (in particular of the skull, metaphyses; 3 and 4).

Craniosynostosis.

Short, hypoplastic nails; hallux valgus; radial deviation of the 5th fingers.

Unusual structure of the iris.

Manifestation: From birth; the typical facies often cannot be recognised until the 2nd year of life.

Aetiology: A disorder of vitamin D metabolism with hypersensitivity to vitamin D assumed. As a rule, sporadic occurrence; no increased risk of recurrence for the affected familiy.

Frequency: Not rare.

Prognosis: Infrequently fatal outcome as a result of hypercalcaemia or – later – of nephrocalcinosis. Course otherwise dependent on the significance of the stenosed vessel(s), the degree of stenosis, and the operability.

Treatment: Operative relief of vascular stenoses. In some cases treatment of hypercalcaemia.

Comment: Presumably isolated aortic stenosis could also be due to a disturbance of vitamin D metabolism. Williams–Beuren syndrome, like isolated supravalvular aortic stenosis, has been observed in siblings on rare occasions.

Illustrations:
1–5 Patient 1 at 2¾ years (1 and 3), at 4¾ years (2, 4 and 5). Severe primary psychomotor retardation. At her initial examination at age 2¾ years, height 79 cm (corresponding to the 50th percentile for a 14-month-old girl); underweight of 1 kg in relation to height; head circumference 46 cm (normal for height); persistent hypercalcaemia, up to 15 mg% (!). At 4¾ years, Ca still as high as 13.2 mg%. Death from uraemia at 5¼ years. At autopsy nephrocalcinosis, calcium metastases in the heart muscle, thyroid gland, and bronchial cartilages; left ventricular hypertrophy; stenosis of the aortic isthmus.
6–8 Patient 2 at 15 months (6 and 7), and at 9 years (8). Since the 2nd half-year of life, anorexia and insufficient weight gain. At the initial examination at age 15 months, height within normal limits, underweight of 1.5 kg in relation to height, head circumference within normal limits. Ca values as high as 17.4%; supravalvular aortic stenosis with hypoplastic aorta; hypoplastic pulmonary vascular trunk, two superior caval veins. Mental deficiency first recognised at age 9 years. Height at this time (124 cm) in the low normal range.

References:
Beuren A. J.: Supravalvular aortic stenosis: a complex syndrome with and without mental retardation. Birth Defects VIII/5:45 (1972)
Jones K L., Smith D. W.: The Williams elfin facies syndrome. J. Pediatr. 86:718 (1975)
Taylor A. B., Stern P. H., Bell N. M.: Abnormal regulation of circulating 25-hydroxy vitamin D in the Williams syndrome. N. Engl. J. Med. 972 (1982)

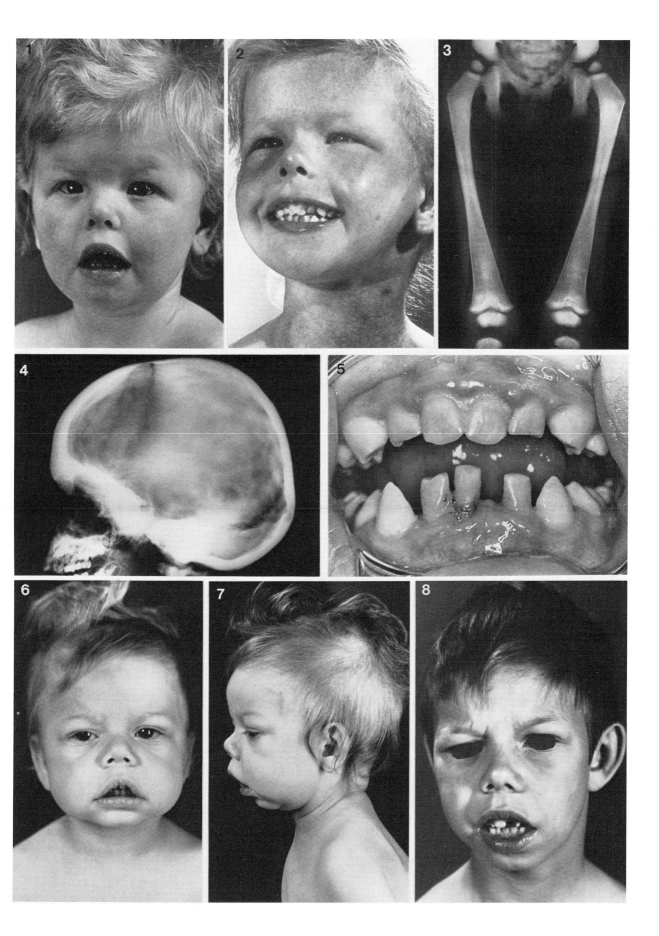

184. A Dysplasia Syndrome of Unusual Appearance and Cardiovascular Anomalies

A syndrome comprising a somewhat unusual appearance, goitre (familial), peculiarities of the hands, unusual proportions, and cardiovascular anomalies.

Main Signs:
1. Facies: Pronounced supraorbital ridges; almond-shaped eyes; small nose with narrow root; hypoplasia of the zygomatic arches; large, prominent, poorly modelled ears; macrostomia; prognathism of the lower jaw (**1** and **2**). Whorl of hair at the back of the neck.
2. Goitre (familial).
3. Short, unusual hands with approximately equal length of digits II and IV bilaterally and clinodactyly of digits II and V bilaterally (**3**). Short toes (**5**).
4. Lanky figure (about the 75th percentile) with excessively long extremities and an almost feminine-appearing pelvic region. Scapulae alatae with elevated left shoulder (**7–9**).
5. Cardiovascular anomalies including partial transposition of the pulmonary veins with drainage into the brachiocephalic vein; small atrial septal defect.

Supplementary Findings: Radiologically, brachy-mesophalangia of the little finger and of toes II–V bilaterally (**4** and **6**).

Manifestation: Birth and later.

Aetiology: Unknown.

Treatment: Symptomatic.

Illustrations:
1–9 An 11-year-old boy with normal mental development, the 2nd child of nonconsanguineous parents. Father 46 years, mother 36 at the patient's birth. (Patient has shown diffuse euthyrotic goitre since age 5 years. His mother and 5 of her siblings are similarly affected, as is the proband's older sister.)
(By kind permission of Prof. P. Heintzen and Frau Dr E. Stephan.)

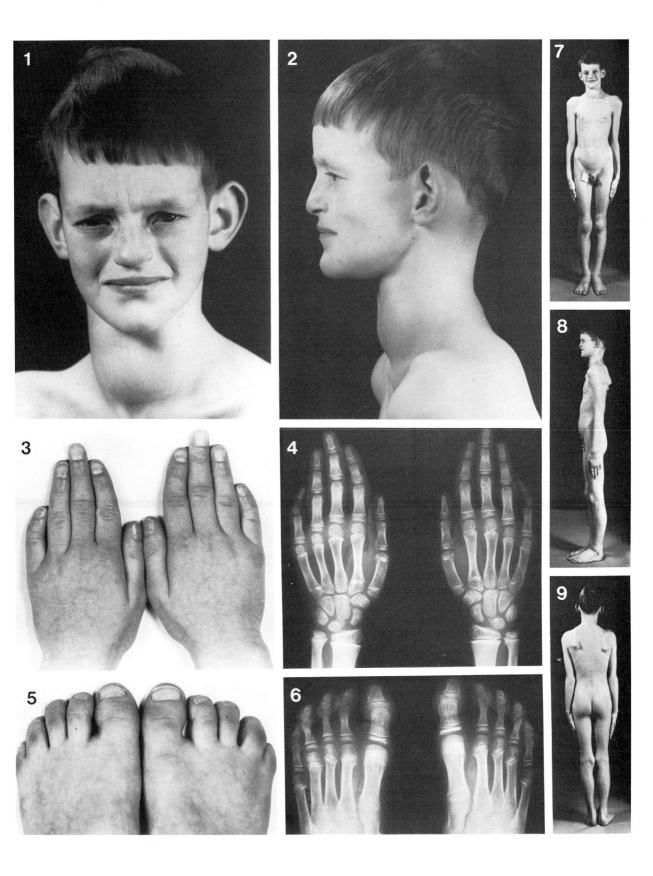

369

185. Rabenhorst Syndrome

A syndrome of typical facial dysmorphism, cardiac defect, and multiple minor anomalies.

Main Signs:
1. Narrow face with high narrow nose, slight mongoloid slant of the palpebral fissures, microstomia, prognathism, adherent ear lobes. High palate. Dolichocephaly (**1** and **2**).
2. Asthenic physique (**3**).
3. Limited mobility at the distal interphalangeal joints with hypoplasia of the corresponding articular folds. Simian crease. Syndactyly of the 2nd and 3rd toes.

Supplementary Findings: Ventricular septal defect with pulmonary stenosis.

Manifestation: At birth.

Aetiology: Probably autosomal dominant hereditary disorder.

Frequency: Two cases described to date.

Prognosis: As far as can be judged from the low number of cases, relatively good.

Treatment: Correction of the cardiac defect.

Illustrations:
1–4 A father (**1**) and his 4-year-old daughter (**2–4**). Both had ventricular septal defect with pulmonary stenosis. In the meantime the girl has undergone successful surgery.

Reference:
Grosse F.R.: The Rabenhorst-syndrome. A cardio-acro-facial-syndrome. Z. Kinderheilkd. *117*:109 (1974)

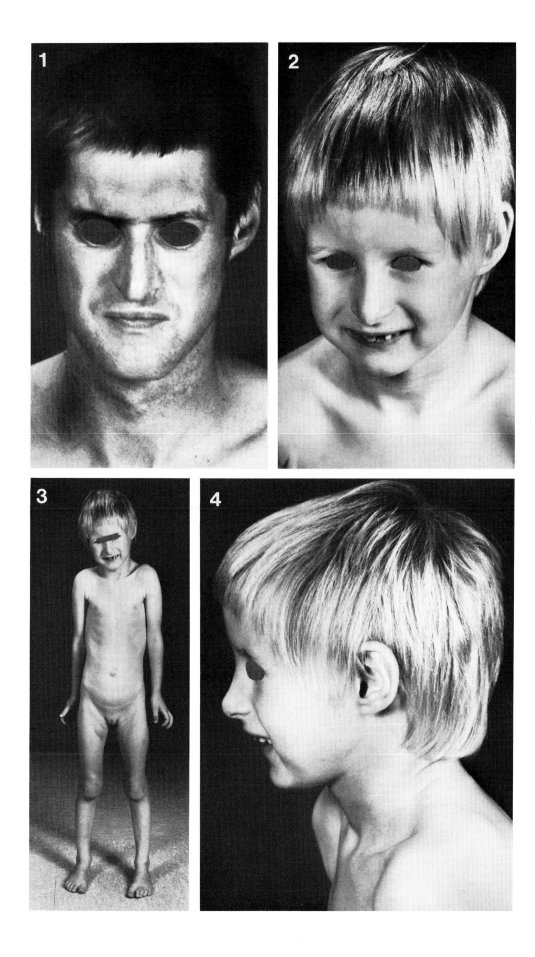

371

186. Möbius Syndrome

A syndrome of congenital, generally bilateral cranial nerve (usually facial-abducens) paralysis with other anomalies.

Main Signs:

1. Expressionless face; difficulties with drinking, swallowing, and speaking; strabismus; and ptosis of the eyelids (1–3) associated with congenital defect of the following cranial nerves: most frequently the facial (not infrequently with preservation of the oral branch) and the abducens; less frequently the oculomotor (usually partial defect, no internal paralysis) and the hypoglossal; very rarely the trochlear nerve or the motor portion of the trigeminal.
2. Nerve involvement usually bilateral.
3. Club feet in about one-fifth of cases (1).

Supplementary Findings: Various hand anomalies, usually symbrachydactyly, also with ipsilateral aplasia of m. pectoralis.

Ear anomalies; occasional deafness.

Aplasia of the lacrimal points.

Infrequent mental retardation, usually mild if present.

Manifestation: At birth.

Aetiology: Usually sporadic cases of uncertain aetiology. Risk of recurrence low. However, hereditary cases showing autosomal dominant or autosomal recessive transmission have been described.

Frequency: Rare (from 1888 to 1970, about 160 cases were reported in the literature).

Course, Prognosis: Feeding problems and danger of aspiration in the newborn and infant. Tendency for the paralysis to improve in isolated cases.

Differential Diagnosis: Oro-acral syndrome (p.286), Poland syndrome (p.294).

Treatment: Prone position and tube feedings for the young infant. Timely initiation of speech therapy. Multidisciplinary care and fosterage. Genetic counselling.

Illustrations:

1–3 A 10-year-old girl with paralysis of the facial and abducens nerves; after bilateral club foot surgery (1).

References:

Henderson J.L.: The congenital facial diplegia syndrome: clinical features, pathology, and aetiology. A review of 61 cases. Brain 62:381 (1939)
Szabo L.: Möbius-Syndrom und Polandsche Anomalie. Z. Orthop. Grenzgeb. 114:211 (1976)
Herrmann J., Pallister P.D., Gilbert E.F., et al: Nosologic studies in the Hanhart and the Möbius syndrome. Eur. J. Pediatr. 122:19 (1976)
Meyerson M.D., Foushee D.R.: Speech, language and hearing in Moebius syndrome: A study of 22 patients. Develop. Med. Child Neurol. 20:357 (1978)
Legum C., Godel V., Nemet P.: Heterogeneity and pleiotropism in the Moebius syndrome. Clin. Genet. 20:254 (1981); thereto ibid 21:290 (1982)
Benney H., Kinzinger W.: Kinder mit Moebius-Syndrome... Pädiatr. Prax. 26:237 (1978)

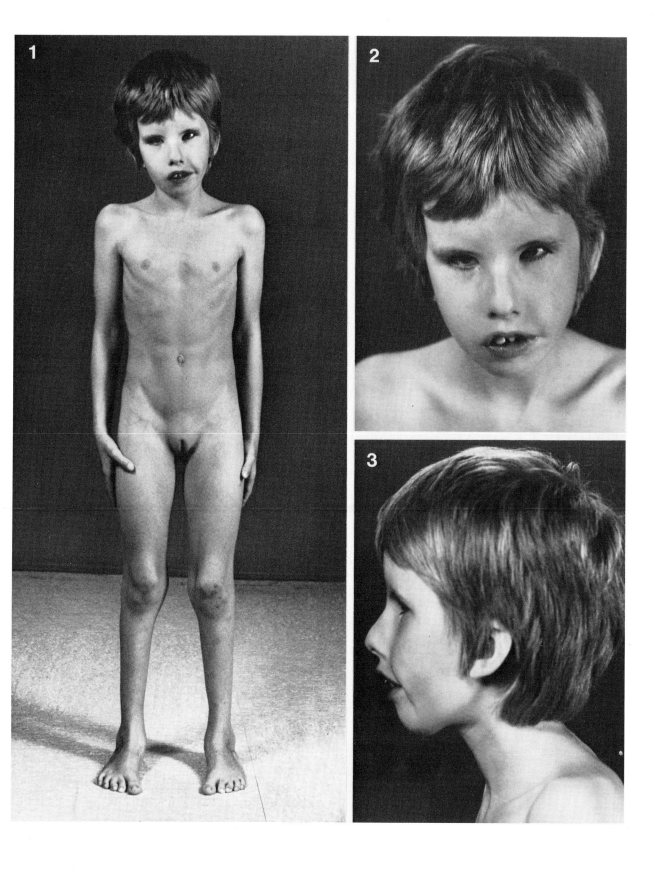

187. Smith–Lemli–Opitz Syndrome

A hereditary disorder comprising primordial growth deficiency, mental retardation with microcephaly, unusual facies, genital anomalies in males, and further abnormalities.

Main Signs:
1. Primordial growth deficiency (with failure to thrive and frequent emesis in infancy).
2. Microcephaly (possibly with a midfrontal ridge).
3. Facies: ptosis, epicanthi, possible strabismus; low-set or posteriorly rotated ears; anteverted nostrils with broad tip of the nose; micrognathia (3 and 4).
4. Hypospadias (9), small penis, possible cryptorchidism.
5. Syndactyly of the 2nd and 3rd toes (8); abnormal palmar creases (6), and dermatoglyphics.
6. Marked psychomotor retardation with anomalies of muscle tone (2).

Supplementary Findings: Possible prominent lateral palatine ridges (5) and cleft plate (5), abnormally positioned fingers (7), hip dysplasia, hernias, cardiac defect, and other anomalies.
Hyperexcitability. Low resistance to infections.

Manifestation: At birth (the majority from a breech presentation).

Aetiology: Hereditary defect, autosomal recessive.

Frequency: Low (about 65 cases have been reported in the literature).

Course, Prognosis: Unfavourable, especially considering the marked mental retardation. Frequently death in infancy as a result of pneumonia or other problems.

Treatment: Symptomatic. Genetic counselling of the parents.

Illustrations:
1–9 A 2-year-old child of young, healthy parents, born at term by breech delivery after an unremarkable pregnancy (birth measurements unknown). Present measurements: 76 cm; 6.4 kg; 43.5 cm head circumference; all well below the 2nd percentile. Typical facies. Median cleft palate. Asymmetry of the mamillae. Short metacarpal I; ulnar deviation of the 2nd and 3rd fingers; cutaneous syndactyly of the 2nd and 3rd toes to the middle phalanges bilaterally, dysplasia of the 3rd toes. Severe psychomotor retardation, marked muscular hypotonia with hyperirritability and attacks of dystonia (2). Severe failure to thrive; frequent vomiting. Abnormal EEG. Chromosome analysis (including banded preparations) negative.

References:
Garcia C. A., McGarry P. A., Voirol M., et al: Neurological involvement in the Smith-Lemli-Opitz syndrome…Develop. Med. Child Neurol. *15*:48 (1973)
Johnson V. P.: Smith-Lemli-Opitz syndrome: Review…Z. Kinderheilkd. *119*:221 (1975)
Fierro M., Martinez A. J., Harbison J. W., et al: Smith-Lemli-Opitz syndrome…Develop. Med. Child Neurol. *19*:57 (1977)
Kretzer F. L., Hittner H. M., Mehta R. S.; Ocular manifestations of the Smith-Lemli-Opitz syndrome. Arch. Ophthalmol. *99*:2000 (1981)

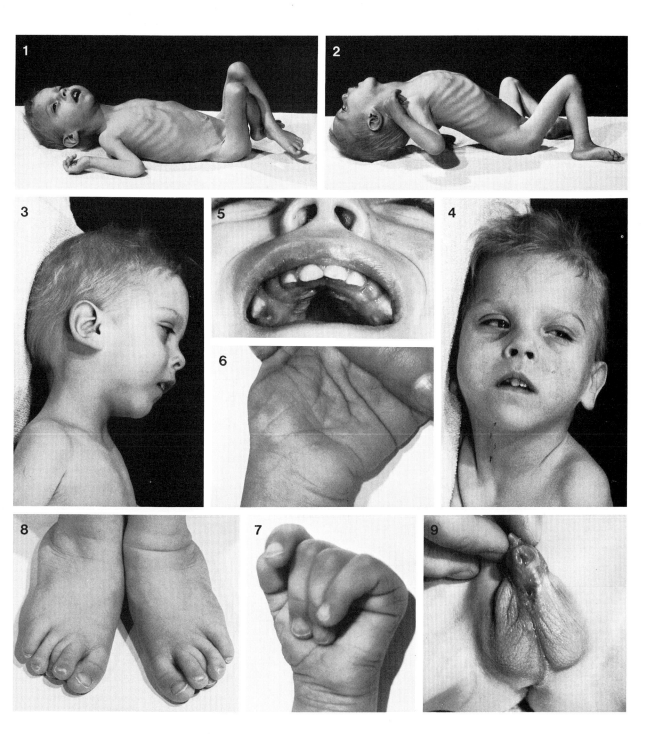

188. Congenital Form of Myotonic Dystrophy

(Dystrophia Myotonica Congenita)

A congenitally manifested form of myotonic dystrophy transmitted by an affected mother.

Main Signs:
1. Severe congenital generalised muscular hypotonia with symmetrical weakness of the facial musculature and ptosis (facial diplegia). Good tendon reflexes.
2. Frequent disorders of sucking, swallowing, and respiration, possibly of life-threatening severity, during the first days or weeks of life.
3. Delayed statomotor development and generally definite mental retardation.

Supplementary Findings: Mother affected by myotonic dystrophy (but possibly showing only very mild signs).
Very frequently pedes equinovari. Also high palate and other anomalies.

Manifestation: At birth – sometimes after a history of weak fetal movements during pregnancy and frequently with hydramnios.

Aetiology: Autosomal dominant hereditary disorder. For unexplained reasons, the congenital form is transmitted predominantly by the affected mother.

Frequency: Variable, depending on the gene frequency; not extremely rare in some areas.

Course, Prognosis: After survival of the early, possibly life-threatening phase, the muscle weakness is barely or not at all progressive and the myotonia scarcely or not at all noticeable. In subsequent years, muscle weakness and atrophy increase, especially in the face (languid, poorly expressive myotonic facies with triangular patulous mouth, **4**), at the neck anteriorly (sternocleidomastoids) and posteriorly, in the distal extremities (e.g., extensors of the hands and fingers, levators of the feet), and other areas. Generally impaired articulation. Tendon reflexes now usually decreased, myotonic signs now usually demonstrable to a moderate degree. The endocrine signs and cataracts of the adult form are not present in the first decade of life. Frequent mental retardation and increasing muscle atrophy cloud the prognosis.

Diagnosis, Differential Diagnosis: Motionless facies with mouth constantly open (**1–3**), general hypotonic asthenia, and hypokinesia yield an impressive picture that – together with signs of the disorder in the mother – make an early diagnosis possible. Otherwise, Möbius syndrome, Prader–Willi syndrome (pp.372 and 208 respectively), or others could initially be difficult to rule out.

Treatment: Symptomatic. Genetic counselling. Under certain – relatively infrequent – conditions, prenatal diagnosis can be carried out.

Illustrations: A girl with congenital myotonic dystrophy, the first-born child of her parents.
1   The patient as a newborn infant.
2 and 3   The patient at 4 weeks.
4   The patient at 16 months, together with her mother. The mother and one of her brothers and perhaps her father: myotonic dystrophy.
(By kind permission of Dr M. Bauer, Frau Dr A. Fuhrmann-Rieger, and Prof. Dr G. Neuhäuser, all of Gießen a. d. Lahn.)

References:
Any comprehensive paediatric or paediatric neurology textbook

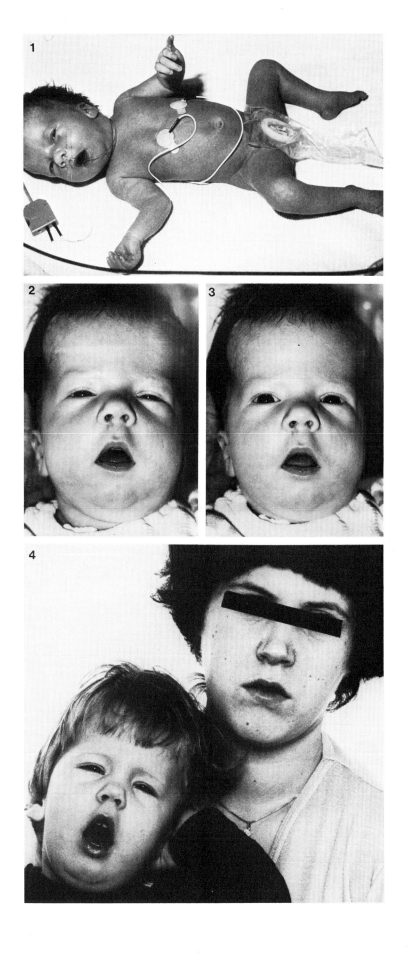

189. Myotonia Congenita, Type Becker

An autosomal recessive hereditary myotonia causing an increasing clinical handicap and associated with distinct hypertrophy of the musculature.

Main Signs:
1. Strong or sudden stimuli elicit a state of tonic contraction in the innervated striated muscles (especially in the extremities, but also the external eye muscles, etc.), the rigidity resolving only after a few seconds, becoming less, and finally no longer occurring when the same movement is carried out repeatedly. Onset of symptoms in the legs, then the hands and arms, later in the neck and the muscles of mastication, etc., becoming generalised by adulthood.
2. Distinct hypertrophy of the musculature (1–3), without increase in general strength.
3. Limitation of dorsiflexion of the hands and feet.

Supplementary Findings: Reflexes and sensation intact. Diagnostically, when the patient (by request) clenches his fist suddenly, he cannot release it immediately; tapping the thenar eminence, tongue, or biceps briefly with a reflex hammer elicits a persistent contraction depression as a myotonic reaction; characteristic myotonic pattern on EMG.

Manifestation: Generally in the course of the second half of the first decade of life (as described above).

Aetiology: Autosomal recessive hereditary disorder.

Frequency: About 1:50 000.

Course, Prognosis: A generalised, progressive disorder leading to increasing weakness and atrophy of the musculature.

Differential Diagnosis: In autosomal dominant myotonia congenita type Thomsen, pronounced muscle hypertrophy is an exception; the disorder runs a milder course and usually does not cause the patient to seek medical help.

Treatment: Protection from cold; avoidance of high calcium intake in the diet. In case of definite subjective complaints due to the myotonic reaction, treatment may be initiated with quinidine sulphate or procainamide, among other possibilities. Genetic counselling.

Illustrations:
1–3 A 12½-year-old boy, normally developed for his age and from a healthy family. Myotonia, manifest since age 7 years, was initially limited to his lower extremities (at first, disturbance of gait; difficulties with starts in sports) and is now generalised, including involvement of the m. levator palpebrae and orbicularis oculorum. Pronounced muscle hypertrophy and not quite adequate general strength. A myotonic reaction can be elicited mechanically on the tongue and thenar eminences; characteristic EMG findings.

References:
Zellweger H., Pavone L., Biondi A., et al: Autosomal recessive generalised myotonia. Muscle Nerv. *3*:176 (1980)
Any comprehensive paediatric, internal medicine, or neurology textbook

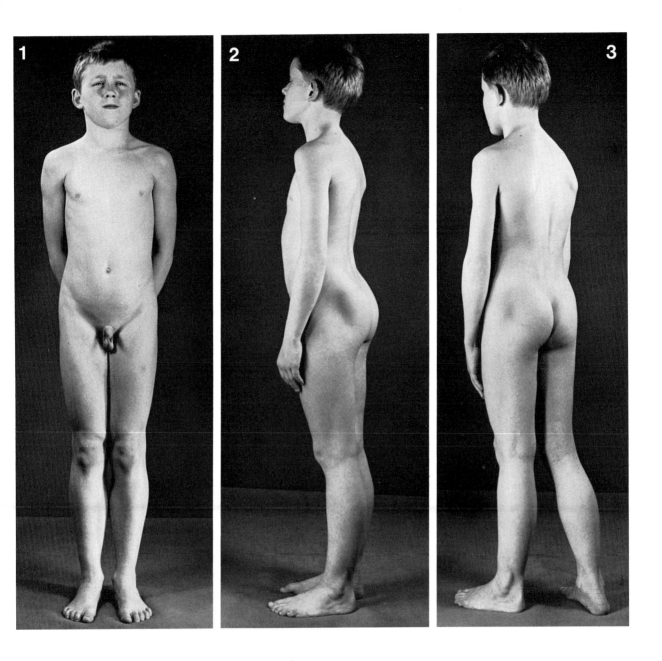

190. Catel–Schwartz–Jampel Syndrome

(Syndrome of Chondrodysplasia Myotonica)

A characteristic hereditary syndrome with postnatal development of signs of myotonia, typical facies, growth retardation, and osteoarticular disorders.

Main Signs:
1. Flat, full-cheeked face which appears small in relation to the normal-sized cranium, small-appearing mouth, small chin, and fixed expression. Eyes appear deep set; narrow palpebral fissures (possibly with slight antimongoloid slant) as a result of blepharospasm of variable severity. Tense to pinched, possibly snout-formed mouth which is difficult to open. The facial expression may be described as 'a frozen smile', but also 'sad' or 'like crying' and can hardly be relaxed (2 and 4).
2. Increasing growth deficiency; height often below the 3rd percentile, 'Trunk-dwarfism'; thus, the extremities appear too long relative to the short trunk (3 and 4).
3. Motor functions impeded, rapid fatigability due to 'stiffness' of the palpably firm, sometimes hypertrophied musculature of the trunk and extremities. (Myotonic reaction usually readily elicited on thenar eminences.) Early flexion contractures of more or less all large joints; corresponding changes of gait and posture.
4. Early complaints of pain, especially in the lower extremities. On X-ray especially, more or less marked dysplasia of the head of the femur (6); all in all, the picture of moderate spondyloepimetaphyseal dysplasia.

Supplementary Findings: Horizontal wrinkling of the brow and raised eyebrows brought about by the contracted facial musculature. Large, low-set ears (2). Sometimes multiple rows of eyelashes; ptosis in some patients; frequent myopia, which may be severe. Alae nasi sometimes hypoplastic; high palate; possible dimpled chin. High, nasal voice (occasionally stridor).

Short neck; elevated shoulders (3); pectus carinatum; increased dorsal kyphosis and lumbar lordosis; also scoliosis. Retarded bone age in some cases.

Electromyography shows: findings of myotonia. No characteristic abnormality of laboratory chemistries. Unaffected mental development.

Manifestation: As an exception, the growth retardation, pinched mouth, early blepharospasm, other 'muscle stiffness', and hip abnormalities may come to attention in infancy. But usually, slowing of motor development and growth, facial changes, and limited mobility of the extremities are not distinct until the 2nd year of life or later; pain and rapid fatigability appear more or less concomitantly with these.

Aetiology: Autosomal recessive hereditary disorder with variable expressivity. Basic defect unknown.

Frequency: Rare; about 40 cases were described by 1980.

Course, Prognosis: Life expectancy does not appear to be affected. The myotonic manifestations may remain stationary soon after appearing in early childhood; motor function may improve. However, further – as a rule slow – progression for years is just as likely.

Diagnosis, Differential Diagnosis: The signs of myotonia, and thus the diagnosis, may be easily overlooked in face of the growth deficiency, conspicuous osteoarticular signs, and 'peculiar' facies. Myotonia must be confirmed electromyographically. Signs of the Freeman–Sheldon syndrome (p.34) overlap considerably with those of the syndrome under discussion. However, the former is manifest at birth, does not show multiple bony dysplasias, does not have signs of myotonia on EMG, and as a rule shows an autosomal dominant mode of inheritance. Exclusion of myotonia congenita (p.378), paramyotonia, and myotonic dystrophy (p.376) should not be difficult.

Treatment: The known antimyotonic medications are apparently ineffective. All appropriate and adequate orthopaedic aids; ophthalmological care; psychological guidance. Increased precautions with regard to untoward anaesthetic incidents. Genetic counselling of the family.

Illustrations:
1 The patient as a young pre-school boy, before the characteristic facies were distinctly manifest;
2–5 The patient showing the full clinical picture at age 6½ years (a pigmented naevus is seen on his back).
6 Typical hip findings in the same child.

The first child of healthy parents. Manifestation of the disorder in the 2nd year of life (eyes closed slowly). Skin of the face smooth and shiny, with taut musculature. Blepharophimosis right > left; difficulty in opening his contracted, snout-formed mouth. High narrow palate. Stiffness, impaired mobility, and contractures; pain in his legs. Corresponding EMG findings. Small stature. Intellect normal. Eventual improvement of function.
(By kind permission of Prof. C.-G. Bennholdt-Thomsen, Prof. E. Gladtke, Prof. A. Rütt.)

References:
Rütt A.: Ein Beitrag zum Krankheitsbild der Chondrodystrophia tarda. Z. Orthop. 83:609 (1953)
Huffelen A.C., van, Gabreëls F.J.M., et al: Chondrodystrophic myotonia. Neuropädiatrie 5:71 (1974)
Pfeiffer R.A., Bauer H., et al: Das Syndrom von Schwartz-Jampel. Helv. Paediatr. Acta 32:251 (1977)

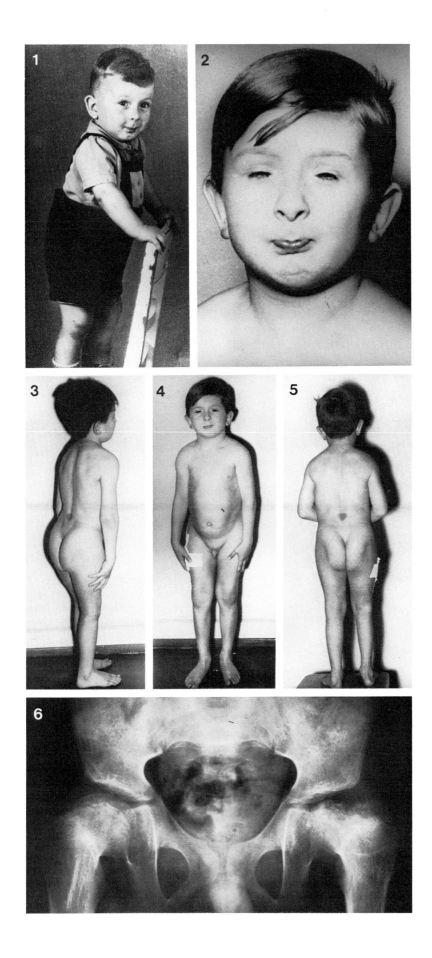

191. Syndrome of Blepharophimosis, Pterygium Colli, Flexion Contractures of the Fingers and Toes, and Osteodysplasia

A syndrome of distinctive facies, short neck with mild pterygium, and development of flexion contractures of the fingers and toes and of spondyloepiphyseal dysplasia.

Main Signs:
1. Facies: Round, with blepharophimosis, broad nasal root, epicanthus, and small mouth with very narrow prolabium (**1**). 'A congenital strabismus syndrome of microstrabismus convergens with bilateral dissociated vertical squint and rotary nystagmus.' Left-sided amblyopia.
2. Short neck; somewhat low posterior hairline; slight pterygium colli (**1** and **2**).
3. Flexion contractures of – the very long – fingers II–V bilaterally, especially of the proximal interphalangeal joints, and of all toes (**3** and **4**) with subluxation of the terminal joints of II–V bilaterally.
4. Somewhat small stature (around the 10th percentile) with the extremities being relatively too long. Dysgenesis of vertebral bodies and epiphyses (see below).

Supplementary Findings: Free mobility of the large joints Scapulae alatae. Slight pectus carinatum; S-formed scoliosis. Crura valga. Flat feet.

On X-ray, slight flattening of the vertebral bodies dorsally, yielding a slightly ovoid configuration. Flattening of both femoral heads with in part irregularly honeycombed, in part markedly sclerotic changes, left > right (**5**), at times resembling the picture in Perthes disease. Coxae varae. Slight flattening of the epiphyses of the knee joints; somewhat lumpy-appearing structure of the patella. Varus deformity of the toes bilaterally (**6**).

Normal intellectual development. No evidence of a neurological or muscular disorder. Laboratory chemistries unremarkable. Normal female karyotype.

Manifestation: Partly at birth (facies); partly, later in infancy and early childhood (flexion contractures of the fingers and toes; osteodysplasia).

Aetiology: Uncertain. Genetic basis may be assumed (the unusual appearance, with narrow palpebral fissures and narrow lips is also present in the child's mother and maternal grandfather; on the other hand, the – deceased – paternal grandmother and her mother are said to have suffered from severely twisted toes. The appearance of the proband's father is quite unremarkable.

Comment: The proband's clinical picture shows certain superficial similarities to diverse disorders such as arthro-ophthalmopathy (Stickler syndrome, p.404), myotonic chondrodysplasia (Cartel–Schwartz–Jampel syndrome, p.380), and the Ullrich–Turner syndrome (p.128), none of which is present here.

Illustrations:
1–6 The proband at barely 9 years of age. The 2nd child of young, healthy, nonconsanguineous parents; older brother unremarkable. Normal birth and early development. Later in early childhood, contractures of the fingers and toes became manifest; these have remained stationary since and do not handicap the patient. At about the same time, hip dysplasia – especially on the left – became apparent, associated with pain in the left leg, which tired easily and which she favoured. Subsequent relief of the hip joints by bilateral intertrochanteric osteotomy with realignment. Patient now free of pain.
(In part, by kind permission of Prof. J. Shaub, Kiel.)

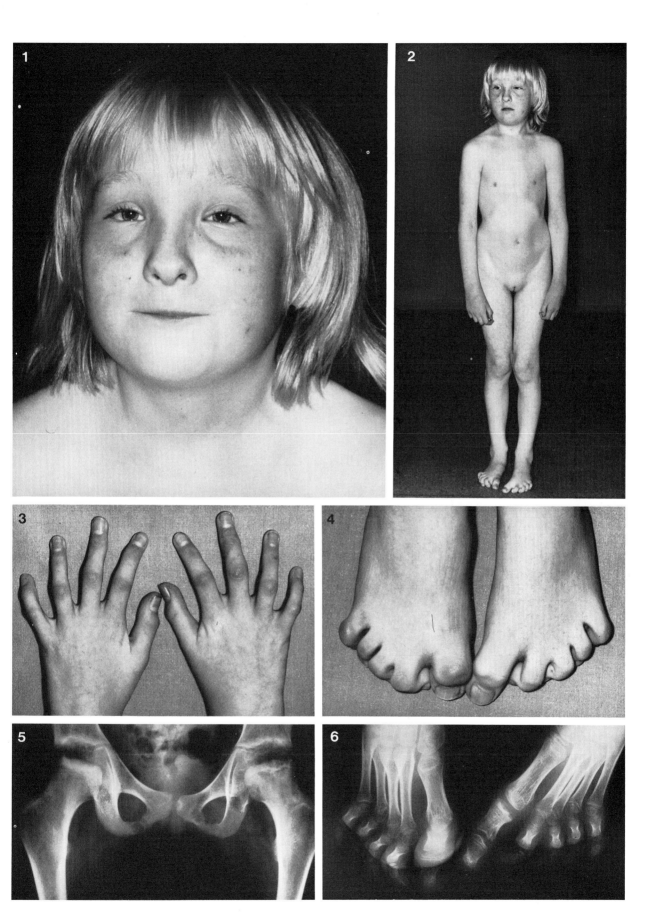

192. Zellweger Syndrome

(Cerebro-hepato-renal Syndrome)

A recessively inherited lethal malformation–retardation syndrome (with evidence of a metabolic disorder), consisting of characteristic facies, extreme muscular hypotonia, hepatomegaly, and practically no psychomotor development.

Main Signs:
1. Characteristic facies with high forehead, hypertelorism, flat root of the nose, possible slight mongoloid slant of the palpebral fissures and epicanthi, 'full' cheeks, and micrognathia. Wide open fontanelles and cranial sutures, persisting frontal stuture; high palate (1 and 3).
2. Extreme muscular hypotonia (4) with absent tendon reflexes and weak sucking and swallowing reflexes. Cerebral seizures.
3. Extremely little psychomotor development.
4. Hepatomegaly (fibrosis, cirrhosis), occasionally also splenomegaly, abnormal liver functions.
5. Retarded growth.

Supplementary Findings: Corneal clouding, glaucoma, cataract, nystagmus, pallor of the optic discs.

Cubitus valgus, contractures of the finger joints, simian crease; club feet. Clitoral hypertrophy or cryptorchidism, hypospadias.

Renal cortical cysts, albuminuria.

Cardiovascular anomalies.

Spotty calcifications of the skeleton on X-ray (2), similar to those in chondrodysplasia punctata (p.154).

Anomalies of the central nervous system.

Frequent elevation of serum iron and copper levels, siderosis of the reticuloendothelial system. Elevated pipecolic acid levels in the serum and cerebrospinal fluid, as well as further abnormal biochemical findings.

Manifestation: At birth (hepatomegaly usually later).

Aetiology: Autosomal recessive hereditary disease (with the significant preponderance of females still unexplained).

Frequency: Rare; since the first description in 1964, about 75 cases have become known.

Course, Prognosis: Death usually within the first half-year of life. (Elevated serum iron levels and the siderosis of the reticuloendothelium system are usually demonstrable in younger patients, whereas liver fibrosis and cirrhosis are found primarily in the somewhat older patients.)

Treatment: Unknown. Genetic counselling.

Illustrations:
1–4 An affected female infant who died at age 6 months. Serum iron in the first months of life markedly elevated on several occasions; follow-up determination in the 6th month of life normal. The transaminase level, at first markedly elevated, also showed a tendency to fall with increasing age. Hypoprothrombinaemia, no icterus. Cerebral seizures. No psychomotor development. Autopsy: arhinencephaly, moderate hydrocephaly; fibrosis of the liver; renal cortical cysts.

References:
Danks D.M., Tipett P., Adams C., et al: Cerebro-hepato-renal syndrome of Zellweger; a report of 8 cases with comments on the incidence, the liver lesion and a fault in pipecolic acid metabolism. J.Pediatr. 86:382 (1975)
Gilchrist K.W., Gilbert E.F., Goldfarb St., et al: Studies of the malformation syndromes of man XI B: The cerebro-hepato-renal syndrome of Zellweger: Comparative pathology. Z.Kinderheilkd. 121:99 (1976)
Hittner H.M., Kretzer F.L.: Zellweger syndrome. Lenticular opacities indicating carrier status...Arch.Ophthalmol. 99:1977 (1981)
Govaerts L., Monnens L., Tegelaers W., et al: Cerebro-hepato-renal syndrome of Zellweger: Clinical symptoms and relevant laboratory findings in 16 patients. Eur.J.Pediatr. 139:125 (1982)

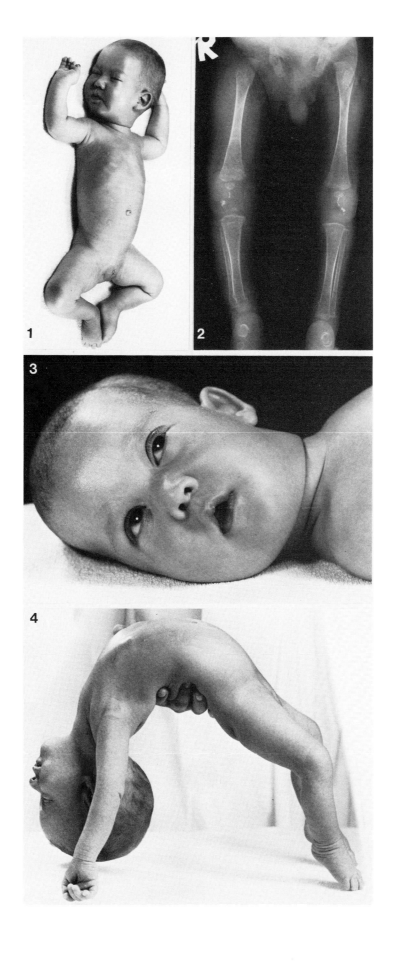

385

193. Werdnig–Hoffmann Syndrome

(Progressive Spinal Muscular Atrophy of Infants)

A characteristic picture with onset of progressive muscular hypotonia and atrophy in infancy, disappearance of tendon reflexes, and appearance of further signs of denervation, with intelligence, clear sensorium, sensation, and sphincter function being preserved.

Main Signs:
1. Symmetrical hypotonia, weakness and decreased motion at first of the pelvic girdle and leg muscles, then of all remaining large muscle regions. Lower extremities flaccid, externally rotated; upper extremities 'handle-like', flaccid, abducted. Almost exclusively diaphragmatic breathing; long, narrow, bell-shaped thorax. Little facial expression (1–3).
2. Disappearance of the tendon reflexes. Sensorium intact; absence of pain. Sensation, sphincter function, and intelligence unaffected.
3. Fascicular twitching (most readily recognised on the tongue; 5).

Supplementary Findings: Abundant fatty infiltration.
Development of contractures of the large joints, kyphoscoliosis, deformity of the thorax (4).
Pattern of neurogenic atrophy on EMG.

Manifestation: During infancy. In some cases the mother may note weak movements or a gradual decrease in movements of her unborn child, and the diagnosis can be established shortly after birth.

Aetiology: Autosomal recessive inherited disease.

Frequency: Not rare.

Course, Prognosis: Unfavourable. Not infrequently, death occurs in infancy, otherwise usually within the first years of life, often after the onset of signs of bulbar paralysis, frequently of hypostatic or aspiration pneumonia. Occasional patients survive longer, eventually becoming completely paralysed (4).

Differential Diagnosis: Congenital early form of myotonic dystrophy (p.376), Prader–Willi syndrome (p.208), Zellweger syndrome (p.384).

Treatment: Symptomatic: Physical therapy; prevention of contractures. High protein diet; prevention of obesity. Protection against infections. Intellectual furtherance. Psychological guidance. Genetic counselling.

Illustrations:
1–3   Patient 1 at barely 4 months: At 4 weeks of age noted to have rapidly progressive muscle weakness and paralysis. Exclusively diaphragmatic respiration; deformity of the thorax. Contractions of the knee and hip joints. Generalised areflexia. Complete reaction of degeneration. Little facial expression. Mental development normal for her age. Soon thereafter death from respiratory paralysis. Diagnosis confirmed histopathologically. A similarly affected sibling died at age 2 months.
4 and 5   Patient 2 at 8 and barely 11 years: Diagnosed clinically and by muscle biopsy in infancy. With optimal care, survival of multiple episodes of pneumonia. Extreme muscle atrophy. Funnel breast, kyphoscoliosis, joint contractures; absolutely no head control; little facial expression; intellectual responses normal for age. Signs of denervation. Puffy deformity of the tongue with marked fasciculations.

References:
Any paediatric textbook

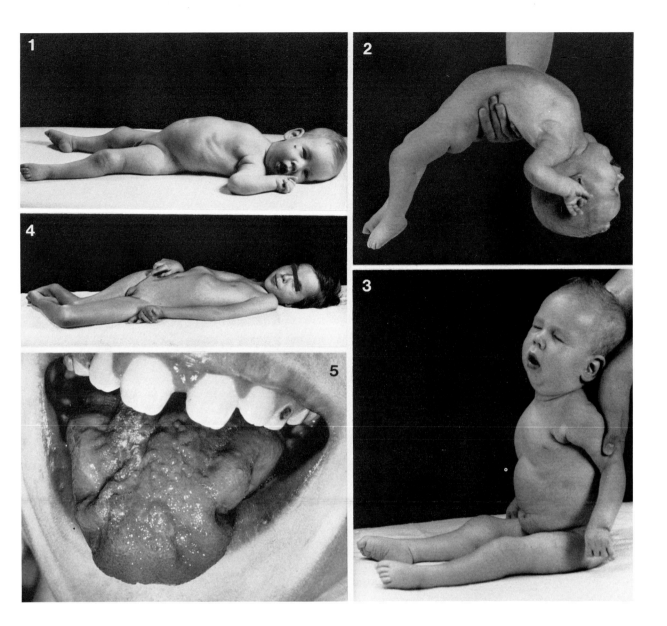

194. Syndrome of Duchenne Muscular Dystrophy

(Infantile Progressive Muscular Dystrophy of the Duchenne Pseudohypertrophic Type)

A quite characteristic hereditary syndrome in males, with onset in early childhood of 'ascending' muscle atrophy, beginning at the pelvic basin and thigh region, at first masked by fatty infiltration, and associated with progressive decrease of performance (with simultaneous slowing of mental development in about one-third of cases).

Main Signs:
1. After learning to walk, with delay and difficulty and frequent falls, the child develops a rocking, weaving, or waddling gait; difficulty getting up from a horizontal position, in the final process 'climbing up on himself' (Gowers' sign; 1).
2. Hyperlordosis with protruding abdomen (1c, 3). Wide-based stance (1–3). Protruding, 'loose' shoulders (2 and 3a).
3. Pseudohypertrophy (fatty infiltration) especially of the calves, also of the thigh and buttock musculature (1–3), less frequently of other muscle regions.
4. Starting with the musculature of the pelvic girdle and thigh, ascending degeneration of the musculature, clinically involving that of the remaining trunk, then that of the shoulder girdle, upper arm, and other regions. Tendency for contractures to develop, especially in the lower extremities: relatively early tendency to develop talipes equinus and toe-walking.
5. Mental retardation in about 30% of cases.

Supplementary Findings:
Absence of unusual pain, disorder of sensation, or denervation phenomena. Gradual weakening and eventual loss of tendon reflexes. Myocardial involvement frequently demonstrable on ECG.

Frequent development of scoliosis; coxa valga. Secondary obesity not unusual.

Very marked increase of serum creatine phosphokinase activity (also of some other enzyme activities to a lesser degree), especially in the initial stages of the process.

Manifestation: First few years of life.

Aetiology: Sex-linked recessive hereditary disorder; thus practically exclusively males affected. Frequently new mutations.

Frequency: With at least 1 in 4000 male newborns, not extremely rare.

Course, Prognosis: Unrelenting progression. Invalidism (wheelchair) usually about the end of the first decade of life, and death in the course of the second.

Differential Diagnosis: Other forms in the large group of muscular dystrophies as well as other types of diseases ('pseudomyopathic') are usually not difficult to exclude by careful observation of the onset, the clinical picture, and the course; in all cases of doubt, EMG, enzyme, and in some cases muscle biopsy findings should make differentiation possible.

Treatment: Furtherance and conservation of physical mobility as far as possible. Physical therapy measures, swimming, prophylaxis of contractures, avoidance of any unnecessary bed confinement or inactivity. Promotion of intellectual and social contacts. Psychological guidance. Recognition of female heterozygotes can be achieved by the combined use of enzyme determinations, EMG, and muscle biopsy. Prenatal diagnosis in case of pregnancy in such a 'carrier'.

Illustrations:
1–3 Three typically affected patients aged, 6, 7½, and 8 years, showing pseudohypertrophy, Gowers' sign (1), hyperlordosis, scapulae alatae, waddling gait, inability to climb stairs. Mental retardation in two of the boys.

References:
Any comprehensive paediatrics or neurology textbook

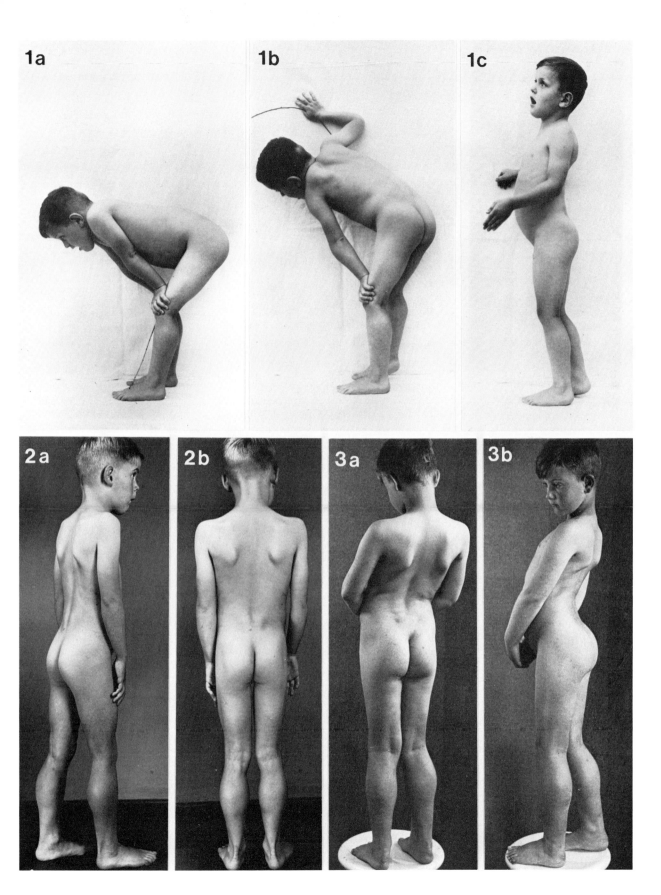

195. Syndrome of Progressive Diaphyseal Dysplasia

(Camurati–Engelmann Syndrome)

Hereditary systemic hyperostosis and sclerosis of the diaphyses of the long bones and the cranium with hypoplasia of the skeletal musculature.

Main Signs:
1. Waddling or dragging gait and rapid fatigability especially of the lower extremities; also complaints of pain in the limbs after exertion.
2. Unusual proportions, with relatively short trunk and exceptionally long, very slender (thin muscles, little subcutaneous fat) extremities (**1**).
3. Radiologically, widening and thickening of the diaphyses of the long bones (**4–8**) due to endosteal and periosteal proliferation; also sclerosis of the skull (**2** and **3**), basis > calotte.

Supplementary Findings: Neurologically unremarkable as a rule.

Possible slight – usually transitory – short stature in early childhood.

The cranium may protrude in the occipito-frontal areas (**1**); possible slight exophthalmos.

Delayed sexual maturity not unusual.

Manifestation: Variable, often in early childhood. Not infrequently delay in learning to walk; then abnormal gait (see above), and general failure to thrive. Later, various degrees of decrease in general vitality; in this respect, possible spontaneous remission during or after adolescence. Mild cases of the syndrome may be recognised only as an incidental finding on X-ray.

Aetiology: Hereditary disorder, autosomal dominant; frequently distinct intrafamilial differences of expression.

Frequency: Rare; somewhat more than 120 cases described in the literature.

Prognosis: Life expectancy not affected. Late complications due to cranial nerve compression – impaired sight or hearing, facial paralysis – are infrequent.

Treatment: Definite improvement with long-term corticosteroid treatment has been observed repeatedly. Genetic counselling.

Illustrations:
1 An 11-year-old boy.
2 and 4–7 His X-rays.
3 Skull X-ray of the same patient at age 32 years; later, optic nerve damage in the optic canal.
8 and 9 Progression of the changes after 15 and after 21 years, respectively.

References:
Wiedemann H.-R.: Systematisierte sklerotische Hyperostose des Kindesalters mit Myopathie. Z. Kinderheilkd. *65*:346 (1948)
Hansen H. G.: Progressive diaphysäre Dysplasie. Handbuch der Kinderheilkunde, Band 6, p.356 ff, Heidelberg, Springer 1967
Spranger J. W., Langer L. O. jr, Wiedemann H.-R.: Bone Dysplasias. An Atlas of Constitutional Disorders of Skeletal Development, Stuttgart and Philadelphia, G. Fischer and W.B. Saunders 1974
Kuhlencordt F., Kruse H.-P., Hellner K.-A., et al: Diaphysäre Dysplasie (Camurati-Engelmann-Syndrom) mit fortschreitendem Visusverlust. Dtsch. Med. Wochenschr. *106*:617 (1981)
Sheldon J., Reeve J., Clayton B.: Engelmann's disease (progressive diaphyseal dysplasia). A review and presentation of two cases with abnormal phosphate retention. Metab. Bone Dis. Rel. Res. 2:307 (1981)

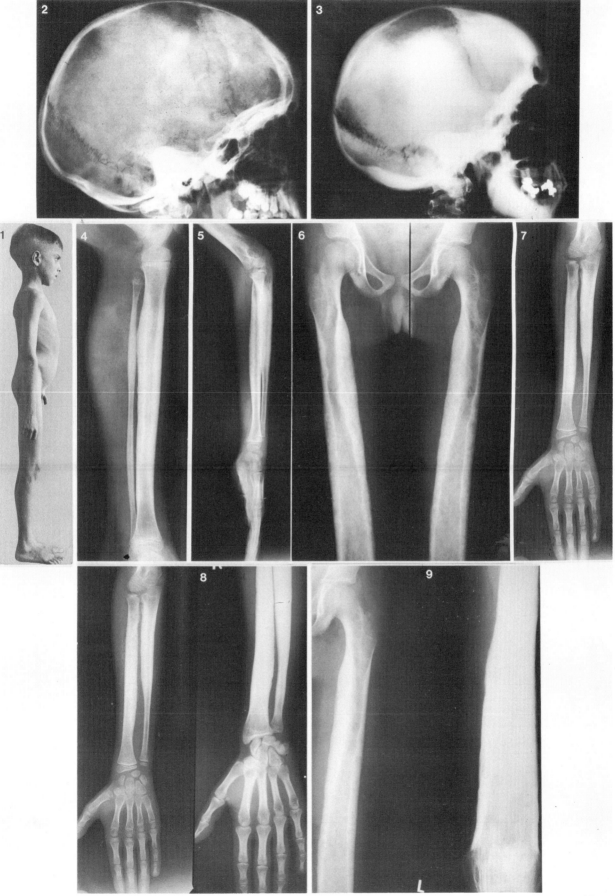

196. Lesch–Nyhan Syndrome

A hereditary syndrome in males who show a cerebral disorder with dystonia, choreoathetosis, mental retardation, and marked tendency to self mutilation, associated with hyperuricaemia (and its eventual typical sequelae) due to an X-chromosomal recessive enzyme defect.

Main Signs:
1. Cerebral disorder manifest as spastic paralysis, choreoathetotic hyperkinesia with severe dysarthria (if not anarthria), and concomitant severe mental defect (1).
2. Pathognomonic bizarre, aggressive behaviour with fits of biting and scratching especially in the form of self mutilation [biting through or picking apart the lips (2 and 3), fingers, and toes; scratching the eyelids, etc., until severely damaged].
3. Development of all the signs of gout (with hyperuricaemia, haematuria, crystaluria, kidney stones, progressive nephropathy, and – usually much later – tophi and recurrent attacks of acute arthritis).

Supplementary Findings: Growth retardation.
Regularly macrocytic anaemia, usually of moderate severity.

Manifestation: First year of life and thereafter. (Initial generalised hypotonia gradually develops into generalised spasticity. Mental retardation. Failure to thrive. Choreoathetosis from the second year of life; then, from about the third year of life, aggressive tendencies with fits of biting and scratching, principally as self mutilation.)

Aetiology: X-chromosomal recessive hereditary disease with variable expressivity. Thus, exclusively males are affected. (Absence of the enzyme hypoxanthine-guanine phosphoribosyl transferase = HGPRT, with consequent disorders of purine synthesis and purine body catabolism.)

Frequency: Rare.

Course, Prognosis: Patients may be severely compromised by nutritional problems, resulting from choreoathetotic dysphagia and frequent vomiting, and by the renal involvement. Before the introduction of allopurinol treatment, patients rarely survived the 5th year of life.

Diagnosis: In rare, exceptional cases, mental deficiency and (auto-) aggressive tendencies may be absent.

Treatment: Allopurinol, on a long-term basis, is very effective in the treatment of hyperuricaemia and all of its direct (=gouty) sequelae. However, it can neither prevent nor mitigate the cerebral disorder. Best possible protection from automutilation. Genetic counselling. Recognition of heterozygotes possible. Prenatal diagnosis.

Illustrations:
1–3 A 2¼-year-old boy, his parents' 1st child, with the typical clinical picture. Diagnosis, and the heterozygotic status of the mother, established by determining the rate of incorporation of ^{14}C-hypoxanthine. In the second pregnancy, prenatal recognition of an affected male fetus; confirmation of the diagnosis after interruption of the pregnancy. The 3rd pregnancy, again with a male fetus, resulted in the birth of a healthy child after prenatal exclusion of the disorder. (By kind permission of Prof. W. Fuhrmann. Gießen a. d. Lahn.)

References:
Leiber B., Olbrich G.: Lesch-Nyhan-Syndrom. Monatschr. Kinderheilkd. *121*:42 (1973)
Letts R. M., Hobson D. A.: Special devices as aids in the management of child selfmutilation in the Lesch-Nyhan syndrome. Pediatrics *55*:852 (1975)
Francke U., Felsenstein J., Gartler S. M., et al: The occurrence of new mutants in the…Lesch-Nyhan disease. Am. J. Hum. Genet. *28*:123 (1976)
Schneider W., Morgenstern E., Schindera I.: Lesch-Nyhan-Syndrom ohne Selbstverstümmelungstendenz. Dtsch. Med. Wochenschr. *101*:167 (1976)
Manzke H.: Variable Expressivität der Genwirkung beim Lesch-Nyhan-Syndrom. Dtsch. Med. Wochenschr. *101*:428 (1976)
Christie R., Bay C., Kaufman I. A., et al: Lesch-Nyhan disease: Clinical experience with nineteen patients. Develop. Med. Child Neurol. *24*:293 (1982)

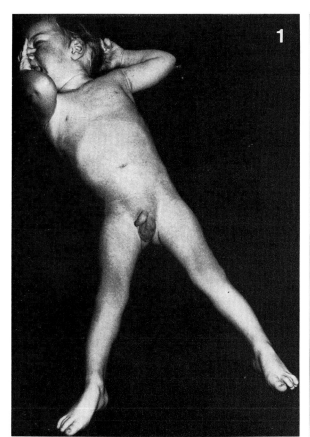

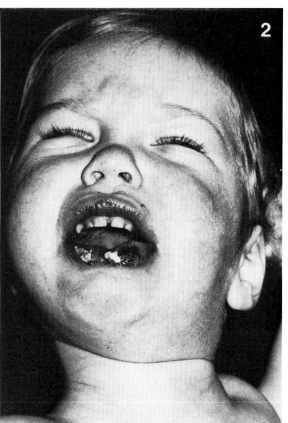

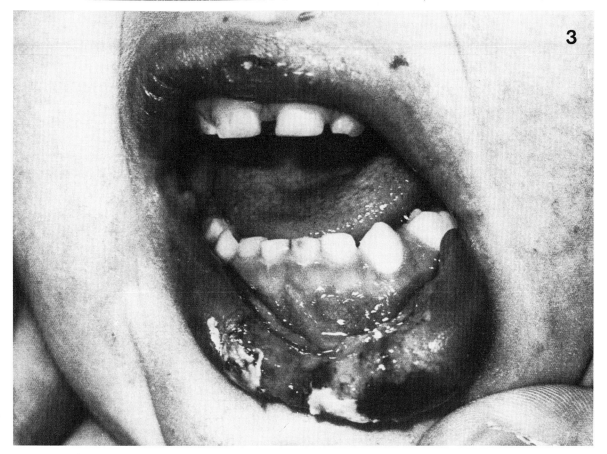

197. Syndrome of Ataxia Telangiectasia

(Louis–Bar Syndrome)

A characteristic hereditary syndrome with neurological, cutaneous, and immunopathological manifestations.

Main Signs:
1. Progressive static and locomotor cerebellar *ataxia* (beginning in infancy) (**1**). Subsequent choreoathetosis, later dyssynergia and intention tremor. Deterioration of speech, disturbance of eye movements; lax, apathetic to masklike facial expression (**2**), with slow development of a smile. Salivation. Stooped posture. Occasionally myoclonus. Mental involvement beginning about the end of the first decade of life and increasing with age.
2. *Telangiectasia* (usually appearing in the preschool child), at first mainly in the light-exposed parts of the bulbar conjunctiva (**3**), later possibly also on the lids, in a butterfly-like distribution on and alongside the nose, on the ears (**4 and 5**), palate, neck and chest, elbows and knees, back of the hands and feet. The vessels, which are initially delicate and attenuated, giving the impression of mere conjunctival hyperaemia in the eye, become increasingly dilated and tortuous. Areas most exposed to sunlight are generally affected. Within a few years, the ears become inelastic, the skin of the face becomes stretched and taut with loss of adipose tissue. Affected areas of skin develop pigmentation disorders (areas of hyper- and depigmentation side by side) and become atrophic; the patients show signs of seborrhoeic dermatitis. Also, frequently café-au-lait spots.
3. *Immune deficiency* (dysplasia of the thymolymphatic system) determines frequent or 'constant' signs of respiratory tract infection (sinobronchitis, frequent progressive bronchiectasis, pneumonias).

Supplementary Findings: Growth deficiency regularly present (although usually first noticeable in the toddler or pre-school child).

Dystrophy. Later, disorders of sexual maturation and other endocrinological anomalies.

Possible lymphocytopenia. Serologically, deficiency of mainly IgA and IgE, as also particularly IgG_2 and IgG_4.

Increased levels of α-fetoprotein.

Chromosome analysis shows a pathological frequency of chromosome breakage. The syndrome carriers show an increased disposition to develop lymphoreticular malignancies.

Manifestation: Onset of ataxia at about the beginning of the 2nd year of life or later, appearance of telangiectases usually between the 3rd and 5th years; mental deterioration, when occurring, often not apparent until the disease is in an advanced stage.

Aetiology: Autosomal recessive hereditary disease.

Frequency: Relatively rare (somewhat over 100 cases in the literature in 1963; a decade later, over 150 cases reported).

Course, Prognosis: Progressive. Patients usually confined to a wheelchair by about the middle of the second decade of life. Most do not complete their 3rd decade; the patients succumb to the sequelae of chronic pulmonary infection, to the neurological affliction itself, or to a malignancy.

Diagnosis: Unmistakable when telangiectases are present.

Treatment: Symptomatic. Qualified health care (including careful physiotherapy); timely antibiotic therapy for acute bacterial infections. Genetic counselling. Recently, prenatal diagnosis possible.

Illustrations:
1–5 A 10-year-old girl, no longer able to stand unsupported. Completely unremarkable development until the age of 1½ years; since then, manifestation and progression of ataxia. Telangiectases on the conjunctiva, eyelids, ears, and arms. Mask-like fixed facial expression; frequent episodes of extrapyramidal dyskinesia, usually with torsion of the head to the right. Short stature, dystrophy, lymphocytopenia.

References:
Hereitani D. M.: Das Louis-Bar-Syndrom. Pädiatr. Prax. *14*:327 (1974)
Bar R. S., Levis W. R., Rechler M. M., et al: Extreme insulin resistance in ataxia telangiectasia. Defect in affinity of insulin receptors. N. Engl. J. Med. 1164 (1978)
Oxelius V.-A., Berkel A. I., Hanson L. A.: IgG_2 deficiency in ataxia telangiectasia. N. Engl. J. Med. *306*:515 (1982)
Shaham M., Voss R., Becker Y., et al: Prenatal diagnosis of ataxia telangiectasia. J. Pediatr. *100*:135 (1982)

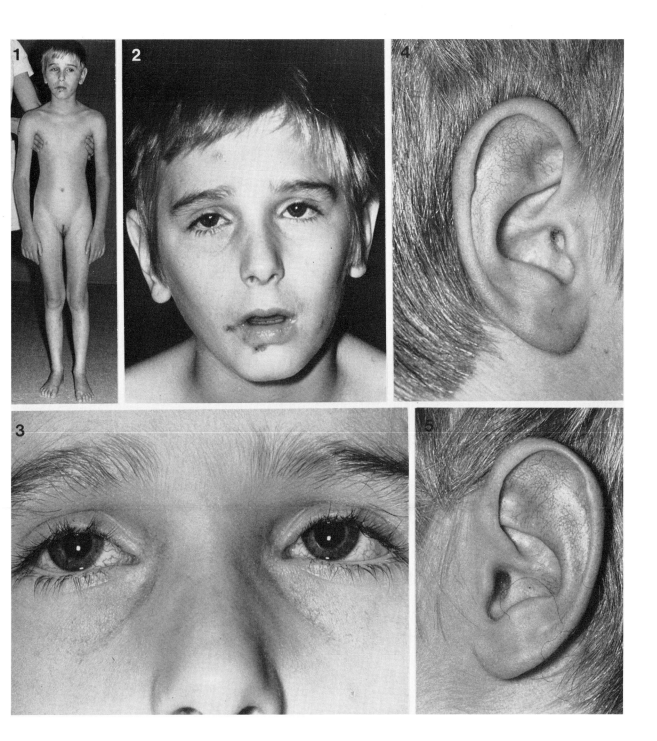

198. Marinesco–Sjögren Syndrome

(Hereditary Cerebellolenticular Degeneration with Mental Retardation)

A syndrome of early manifested cataract, mental retardation, ataxia, and small stature.

Main Signs:
1. Cerebellar ataxia with more or less marked motor impairment such as, e.g., severe delay in and difficulty with walking.
2. Primary mental retardation of various grades of severity.
3. 'Congenital' cataract.
4. Moderate growth deficiency.

Supplementary Findings: Dysarthria, strabismus, nystagmus.
Possible development of scoliosis:

Manifestation: First years of life.

Aetiology: Autosomal recessive hereditary disease.

Frequency: Rare; up to 1975, only about 50 cases had been described.

Course, Prognosis: Very dependent on the severity and possible progression of the ataxia and on the degree of mental retardation.

Differential Diagnosis: Other ataxia syndromes should not be difficult to rule out, especially in view of the cataracts.

Treatment: Symptomatic. Ophthalmological care is especially important. Genetic counselling.

Illustrations:
1–3 A 15-year-old girl, the 2nd child of healthy parents with no evidence of consanguinity. Cataracts operated on in the 1st year of life. Primary mental retardation. Early manifestation of ataxia. Height 1.56 m. Strabismus, little change of facial expression. Micrognathia of the lower jaw; crura valga.
4–6 The 21-year-old sister of the proband, height 1.60 m, with quite similar development; however, this patient is not yet dependent on crutches. Both girls have a basically whiny disposition.

References:
Andersen B.: Marinesco-Sjögren syndrome: Spinocerebellar ataxia congenital cataract, somatic and mental retardation. Dev. Med. Child Neurol. 7:249 (1965)
Alter M., Kennedy W.: The Marinesco-Sjögren syndrome. Minn. Med. 51:901 (1968)

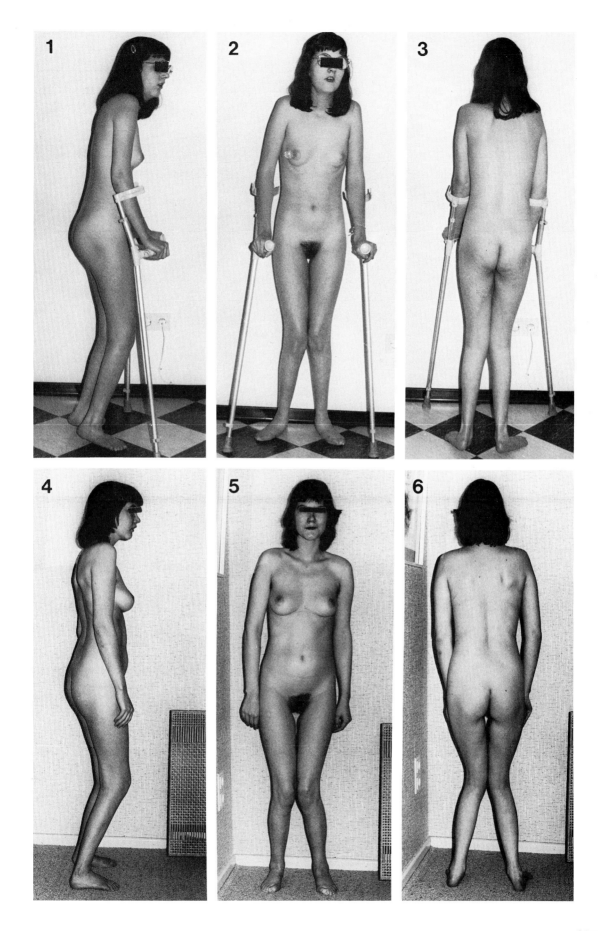

397

199. Mitochondrial Cytopathy

(Kearns-Sayre Syndrome)

A syndrome of chronic, progressive external ophthalmoplegia and further neuromuscular signs, intracardial conduction defect, tapetoretinal degeneration, and characteristic general appearance.

Main Signs:
1. Chronic and progressive external ophthalmoplegia (**1** and **2**).
2. Defect of intracardial conduction or complete heart block.
3. Retinitis pigmentosa.
4. Characteristic appearance, in particular, typical facies (**1** and **2**).

Supplementary Findings: Possibly, multiple defects of the central or peripheral nervous system: optic atrophy, hearing impairment and vestibular defects, cerebellar ataxia, pareses, and pyramidal tract signs, myopathy of the proximal skeletal muscles; increase of protein and sometimes of cell count in the CSF, and EEG changes. In some cases signs of spongy degeneration of the brain on CCT.

Mental retardation or deterioration not infrequent.

Possible signs of hypogonadism and/or hypoparathyroidism and diabetes mellitus.

Electromyographic evidence of a generalised myopathy; characteristic (but nonspecific) muscle biopsy findings of 'ragged-red fibres' (= special mitochondrial changes with paracristalline inclusions, which can be demonstrated in other organs).

Often considerable growth deficiency. This and the drooped posture, meagre musculature, frequent secondary kyphoscoliosis and/or hyperlordosis, frequent wasting, and typical facies all contribute to the characteristic general appearance (**1** and **2**).

Manifestation: Possibly in the 1st year of life (ptosis). More likely, onset toward the end of the first decade of life or later. Progressive paralysis of the external eye muscles; in some cases progressive facial paresis, decreased hearing for high tones, dysphonia, dysphagia, ataxia, spasticity, mental decline, signs of congestive cardiomyopathy, and other signs.

Aetiology: Not completely clear. The majority of cases described have been sporadic. However, familial occurrence has been demonstrated and autosomal dominant inheritance with variable expressivity is probable. But other modes of inheritance have also been considered.

Frequency: Not extremely rare; from the time of the first description until 1981, about 70 'complete' (and probably about the same number of 'incomplete') cases had been described.

Course, Prognosis: Apparently, the earlier the disease is manifest, the less favourable the prognosis. Even with the very best cardiac care, more or less sudden deterioration and (cardiac or brain stem) death must be expected.

Treatment: Symptomatic. Careful cardiac follow-up with early or even preventative implantation of a pacemaker. Possible surgery for severe ptosis. Follow-up of hearing. Physical therapy and orthopaedic measures. In some cases hormone substitution. Genetic counselling.

Illustrations:
1 and **2** A 15¾-year-old girl, the 4th child of healthy parents after 3 healthy siblings. Primary delay of statomotor development; bilateral ptosis at 4 years (multiple operations). Total ophthalmoplegia, retinitis pigmentosa, hypoacusis, dysphagia, complete left bundle branch block (preventative implantation of a pacemaker), myopathy especially of the musculature of the proximal extremities, ataxia, short stature below the 3rd percentile, mental retardation, wasting.
(In part, by kind permission of Prof. H.-G. Hansen, Lübeck and Prof. P. Heintzen and Frau D. E. Stephan, Kiel.)

References:
Kearns T. R., Sayre G. P.: Retinitis pigmentosa, external ophthalmoplegia and complete heart block. Arch. Ophthalmol. *60*:280 (1958)
Schnitzler E. R., Robertson W. C., jr: Familial Kearns-Sayre syndrome. Neurology *29*:1172 (1979)
Dobiasch H., Krause K.-H.: Das Kearns-Sayres-Syndrom. Nervenarzt. *51*:55 (1980)
Voisin M., Marty-Double C., Grolleau R., et al: Syndrome de Kearns. Arch. Fr., Pédiatr. *37*:119 (1980)
Coulter D. L., Allen R. J.: Abrupt neurological deterioration in children with Kearns-Sayre syndrome. Arch. Neurol. *38*:247 (1981)
Egger J., Lake B. D., Wilson J.: Mitochondrial cytopathy... Arch. Dis. Childh. *56*:741 (1981)

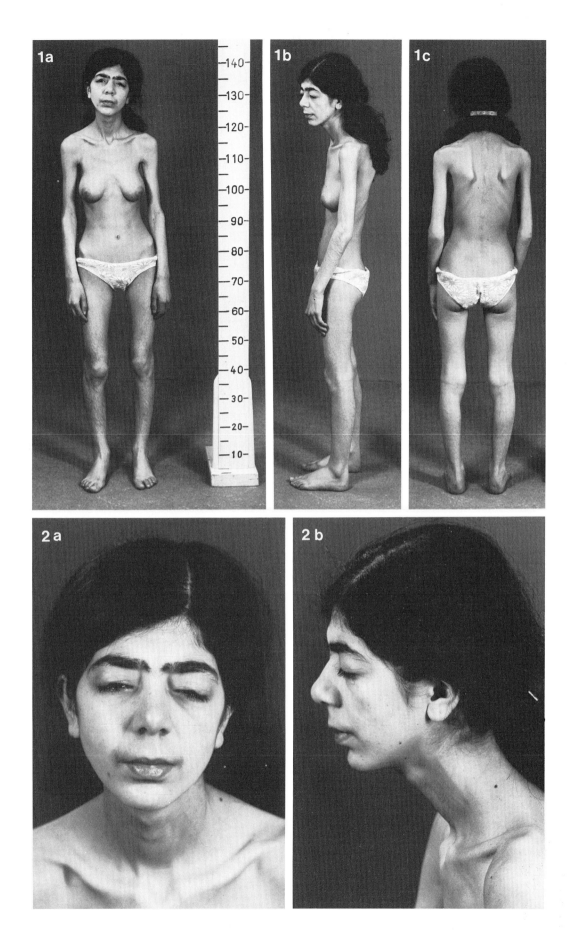

200. Syndrome of Rubella Embryofetopathy

(Extended Gregg Syndrome)

A more or less extensive and characteristic syndrome of embryo and/or fetal damage due to the rubella virus.

Main Signs:

1. *Syndrome of defects in older children* (Gregg syndrome [previous early designation]) (**1–3, 5–7,** and **9**): Cararact, uni- or bilaterally, frequently with microphthalmos (and retinitis pigmentosa). Inner ear hearing impairment or deafness, uni- or bilaterally, frequently with signs of defective vestibular function. Small size, microcephaly in relation to height (usually mild), and psychomotor retardation (mild to severe, with or without neurological signs). Cardiovascular anomalies: most frequently persistent ductus arteriosis or pulmonary stenosis.

2. *Spectrum of disease and damage in newborns and infants* (**4** and **8**): Usually congenital small size, failure to thrive, and problems with rearing. Cataract at birth or possible manifestation in the first weeks of life. Secondary glaucoma with corneal clouding may be present at birth or develop in the following weeks. Additionally, the optional signs noted in **8**: thrombocytopenic purpura, hepatosplenomegaly, hepatitis, myocarditis, meningoencephaloretinitis, etc.

Supplementary Findings: Possible hypoplastic anaemia. X-ray evidence of metaphyseal lesions of the long bones during the first months of life.

Demonstration of rubella-specific IgM in the child's serum.

Possibility of demonstration of rubella virus in tissues, body fluids (CSF!), and excretions of the child for months post partum!

Manifestation: Birth and early infancy.

Aetiology: Embryofetal infection with rubella virus.

Frequency: Variable – depending on 'genius epidemicus' or the extent to which young women have been immunised.

Course, Prognosis: Dependent on the type and extent of damage as well as on the intensity and quality of rehabilitating measures. Fatal outcome in the first months not rare.

Differential Diagnosis: Microphthalmos, microcephaly, central nervous system signs, and deafness may also occur with embryofetal cytomegalic virus infection or fetal toxoplasmosis – the broad spectrum of congenital signs of fetal rubella may resemble those of fetal sepsis from other pathogens.

Treatment: Urgent treatment of glaucoma. Removal of cataracts generally after the 6th month of life. Operative correction of a cardiac defect at the appropriate time. Early hearing aids in case of hearing impairment. All other appropriate aids for the handicapped. Prednisone recommended for thrombocytopenic purpura and hypoplastic anaemia.

Illustrations:

1, 7, and **9** A 4-year-old patient; maternal rubella in months I/II. Low birth weight, rearing problems; congenital cataracts and microphthalmos bilaterally; deafness; slight microcephaly, mental retardation, amblyopic motoricity and athetosis; small stature.

2 A 9-year-old patient; cataract, microphthalmos, debility, PDA, club foot, dysodontiasis.

3 and **6** A 4-year-old patient; microphthalmos and cataract on the right, retinopathy on the left; inner ear hearing defect left > right; slight microcephaly, debility; PDA.

4 A 6-week-old patient; cataract, microphthalmos and corneal clouding bilaterally; PDA and ASD; hepatosplenomegaly, icterus, anaemia, thrombocytopenia; muscular hypotonia; prenatal dystrophy. Maternal rubella months III/IV.

5 A 9-month-old patient; microcephaly, cataract, microphthalmos, amblyopia, cardiac defect, growth deficiency.

8 Possible signs of rubella embryopathy in newborns and infants.

References:
Cooper L. Z., Ziring P. R., Ockerse A. B., et al: Rubella: clinical manifestations and management. Am. J. Dis. Child. *118*:18 (1969)
Macfarlane D. W., Boyd R. D., Dodrill C. B., et al: Intrauterine rubella, head size, and intellect. Pediatrics *55*:797 (1975)

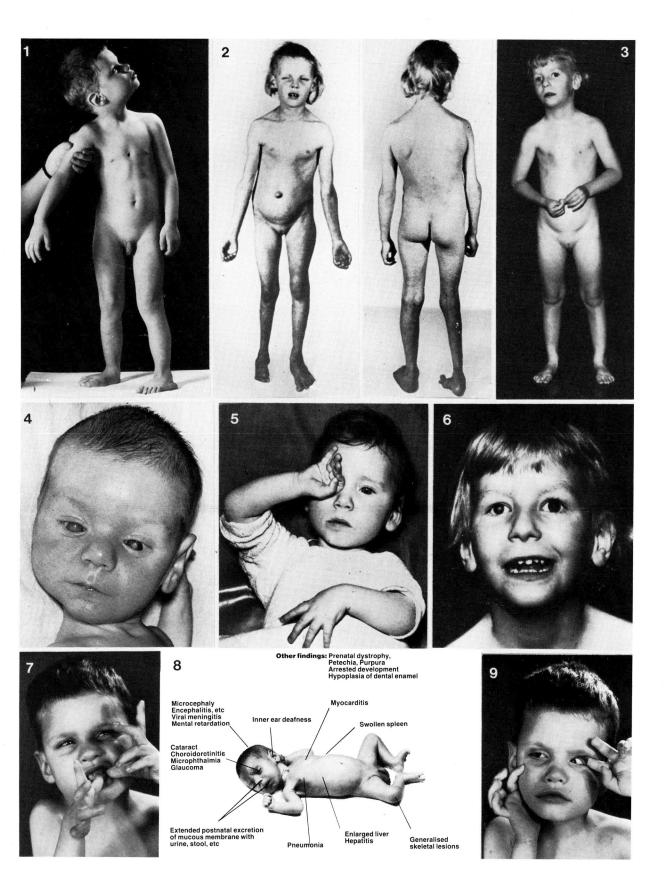

Other findings: Prenatal dystrophy,
Petechia, Purpura
Arrested development
Hypoplasia of dental enamel

Microcephaly
Encephalitis, etc
Viral meningitis
Mental retardation

Inner ear deafness

Myocarditis

Swollen spleen

Cataract
Choroidorotinitis
Microphthalmia
Glaucoma

Extended postnatal excretion
of mucous membrane with
urine, stool, etc

Pneumonia

Enlarged liver
Hepatitis

Generalised
skeletal lesions

201. Hallermann–Streiff–François Syndrome

(Oculo-mandibulo Dyscrania with Hypotrichosis)

A highly characteristic syndrome of dyscrania with hypotrichosis, facial and, especially, eye anomalies, and growth deficiency.

Main Signs:
1. Dyscrania (frontal and/or occipitoparietal bossing, delayed closure of the sutures and fontanelles; relatively small face with flat orbits, hypoplasia of the jaws, and micrognathia) (1–5).
2. Microphthalmos, congenital (or becoming manifest in the early postnatal period) cataracts.
3. Small, narrow nose, which becomes increasingly beaklike.
4. Congenital teeth and other dental anomalies; high narrow palate.
5. Atrophy of the skin, especially over the nose and along the cranial sutures; hypotrichosis, especially of the cranium, eyebrows, and eyelashes (3–5).
6. Proportional growth deficiency.

Supplementary Findings: Mental development normal as a rule, but exceptions not rare. In many cases (amblyopia-) nystagmus, strabismus, occurrence of blue sclerae.

On X-ray, hypoplasia of the ascending ramus of the mandible and anterior displacement of the temporomandibular joint.

Occurrence of funnel breast, winged scapulae, and other skeletal anomalies. Possible right heart anomalies and hypogenitalism.

Manifestation: At birth.

Aetiology: Genetic basis beyond a doubt, but more details are needed to clarify the situation. Almost all cases occur sporadically (perhaps as a new mutation of an autosomal dominant gene; however, evidence also for possible autosomal recessive transmission. Heterogeneity?).

Frequency: Rare; about 100 cases described in the literature up to 1980.

Course, Prognosis: In early infancy, glossoptosis or related anomalies may cause feeding and respiratory problems. Later, eye defects present the greatest problem (apropos: spontaneous resorption of the cataracts not rare!); vision often very markedly decreased. Adult height in females somewhat over 150 cm, in males somewhat over 155.

Differential Diagnosis: Progeria (p.194) and progeroid syndromes (p.196, 200) are not difficult to rule out; even less difficult: mandibulofacial dysostosis (p.36), cleidocranial dysostosis (p.22), and pyknodysostosis (p.136).

Treatment: Ophthalmological and dental care very important. Growth hormone not indicated. Genetic counselling.

Illustrations:
1–5 A 1½-year-old boy with the fully expressed syndrome. Congenital cataracts, congenital teeth. Mental development normal for age. Height below the 3rd percentile. Cataract operation at age 5 months; vision well corrected with contact lenses.

References:
Steele R. W., Bass J. W.: Hallermann-Streiff syndrome. Am. J. Dis. Child. 20:462 (1970)
Suzuki Y., Fujii T., Fukuyama Y.: Hallermann–Streiff syndrome, Develop. Med. Child Neurol. 12:496 (1970)
Dinwiddie R., Gewitz M., Taylor J. F. N.: Cardiac defects in the Hallermann–Streiff syndrome. J. Pediatr. 92:77 (1978)
Ronen S., Rozenmann Y., Isaacson M., et al: The early management of a baby with Hallermann Streiff François syndrome. J. Pediatr. Ophthalmol. Strab. 16/2: 119 (1979)

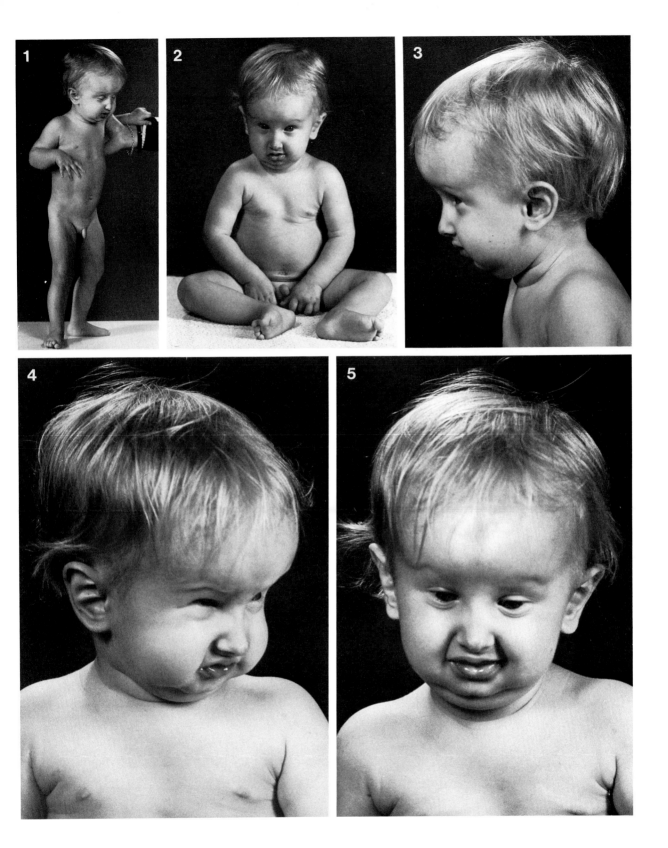

202. Arthro-ophthalmopathy

(Stickler Syndrome)

A relatively frequent, important, autosomal dominant hereditary disorder of orofacial signs and changes of the eyes, skeleton, and joints.

Main Signs:
1. Flat face with more or less low nasal root and nose (**1, 4**), epicanthal folds, midface or mandibular hypoplasia (**1 and 4; 3**), cleft palate (hard and/or soft palate; possibly with bifid uvula), often with fully expressed Robin anomaly (see p.52).
2. Early myopia of marked to extreme severity with changes of the eyegrounds, possibly with glaucoma, cataract, retinal detachment, and retinoschisis on to blindness.
3. Possible marfanoid characteristics (**1, 2, and 4**). Hypotonic, moderately developed musculature, hyperextensibility of the large prominent (possibly also the smaller) joints; in some cases mild, rheumatoid, but also severe arthropathies in childhood. Hip and knee joints then the most severely affected. These arthropathies are inconstant and the least important sign.

Supplementary Findings: Hearing impairment not infrequent (conductive or inner ear defect). Dental anomalies.

Possible development of kyphosis or scoliosis; deformities of the thorax; genua valga (**1**), etc.

On X-ray, the picture of mild spondyloepiphyseal dysplasia with flattening of the vertebral bodies reminiscent of the picture in Scheuermann disease, narrow diaphyses and broad-appearing metaphyses of the long bones and changes of the knee and other joints (e.g., subluxation of the hips).

Manifestation: Birth (orofacial signs as well as possible conspicuous bony prominence of the large joints, especially the ankle, knee, and wrist joints) and later. Myopia usually manifest in early childhood; retinal detachment usually not until the 2nd decade or later.

Aetiology: Autosomal dominant hereditary disorder (in the form of a generalised disorder of supporting tissues) with very variable expressivity of individual signs, even within a family. Polyallelism possible.

Frequency: Not rare. Stickler syndrome should be considered and myopia sought in every case of isolated cleft palate and in every case of Robin anomaly.

Course, Prognosis: Normal life expectancy. As a rule normal intelligence and height. Handicap due to impaired vision or possible joint disorders may be expected, usually starting in the second decade (or even earlier).

Differential Diagnosis: Marfan's syndrome and homocystinuria (pp.88, 92), spondyloepiphyseal dysplasia (e.g., p.174), and osteodysplasia type Kniest (p.176) or perhaps the Ehlers–Danlos syndrome (p.272) are more or less easy to rule out.

Treatment: Paediatric care for Robin anomaly. From infancy, regular check-ups by a qualified ophthalmologist; treatment of glaucoma in some cases; operation for cataracts or specific treatment for retinal detachment. Closure of cleft palate and speech therapy as required. Audiometric check-ups. Avoidance of physical strain. Genetic counselling.

Illustrations:
1–4 A child and adolescents from a large sibship with Stickler syndrome. In **1** and **4**, midface hypoplasia is prominent; in **3**, micrognathia.
(By kind permission of Prof. G. B. Stickler, Rochester.)

References:
Herrmann J., France Th. D., Spranger J. W., et al: The Stickler syndrome (hereditary arthroophthalmopathy). Birth Defects XI/2:76 (1975)
Hanson J. W., Graham C. B., Smith D. W.: Early diagnosis of the Stickler syndrome presenting as Robin anomalad. Birth Defects 13/3C: 235 (1977)
Blair N. P., Albert D. M., Liberfarb R. M., et al: Hereditary progressive arthroophthalmopathy of Stickler. Am. J. Ophthalmol. 88:876 (1979)
Liberfarb R. M., Hirose T., Holmes L. B.: The Wagner-Stickler syndrome…22 families. J. Pediatr. 99:394 (1981)
Meinecke P.: Das Stickler Syndrom. Pädiatr. Prax. 24:705 (1980/81)

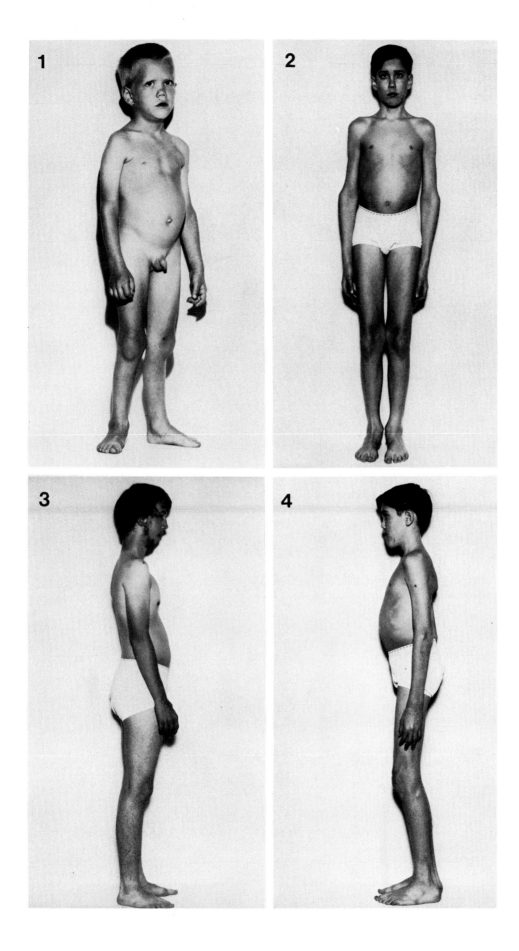

203. An Unfamiliar Malformation–Retardation Syndrome with Haemorrhagic Diathesis

A syndrome of eye and skeletal anomalies, haemorrhagic diathesis, and mental retardation.

Main Signs:
1. Ptosis, more severe on the right than the left (1), with deep-set eyes and myopia on the right. Loss of roundness of the iris on the right, typical coloboma of the iris on the left. Large coloboma of the choroid beneath the optic disc bilaterally. Large ears with simple configuration (1 and 2).
2. Scoliosis, lumbar hyperlordosis (2); clinodactyly of the index and fifth fingers bilaterally (3); bilateral pes cavus.
3. Haemorrhagic diathesis since age 6 years with palm-size haematomas.
4. Psychomotor retardation (IQ 66 at age 11 years) – uncertain whether primary or as a result of unilateral akinetic cerebral focal seizures which occurred from early infancy until about the end of nursery school age.

Supplementary Findings: On X-ray, somewhat large, coarse 1st rays of the hands and feet (4 and 5). Very coarse epiphyses of the terminal phalanges of the big toes as well as malformation of the proc. unguiculares; atypia of the middle and end phalanges of the other toes also (5). Slight clinodactyly of the 5th fingers; very pronounced pseudoepiphyses in the metacarpals II (4).

Haematologically, occasional borderline thrombocyte counts; prolonged periods of leucopenia; normoerythraemia. Somewhat cell-poor bone marrow without definite pathological findings. Good global thrombocyte function. No evidence of defective plasmic clotting. (Haemoglobin analysis negative. No erythrocyte enzyme defects demonstrable.)

Manifestation: Birth and later.

Aetiology: Unknown.

Course, Prognosis: Apart from the mental deficiency, apparently favourable. At 14½ years, no further bleedings, thrombocyte count normal; still slight ('constitutional') leucopenia.

Comment: The patient had no cardiac defect (cf. Reference), no basis for Fanconi anaemia syndrome (p.338), nor for a cat-eye syndrome (p.56), etc.

Treatment: Symptomatic.

Illustrations:
1–5 The same boy (4 at 7 years, 1–3 and 5 at 9 years), the 3rd child of young, healthy, nonconsanguineous parents after 2 healthy brothers. Pregnancy and delivery normal (3600 g, 51 cm). No hyperpigmentation. Very good continuous growth (at age 14½ years 11 cm above average height). Normal head circumference. Normal genitalia and normal sexual maturation for age. Heart negative; renal pyelogram negative. Normal male karyotype and no increased chromosome breakage.

Reference:
Ho C.K., Kaufman R.L., Podos S.M.: Ocular colobomata, cardiac defect, and other anomalies. A study of seven cases including two sibs. J.Med.Genet. *12*:289 (1975)

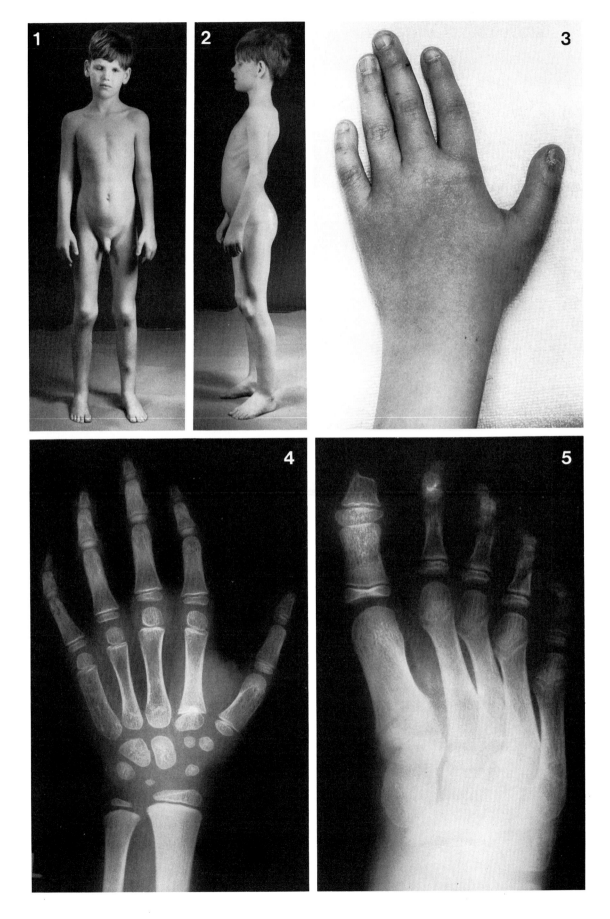

204. Klinefelter Syndrome

(XXY Syndrome)

A hypogonadism syndrome in males with an additional X chromosome.

Main Signs:
(A) *In childhood:*
1. Frequently very tall with slightly eunuchoid body proportions (exceptionally long lower extremities).
2. Below average intelligence or slight retardation (optional), sometimes with behavioural disorders.
3. Possible delay of onset of puberty; gynaecomastia.
(B) *In adolescence and adulthood:*
1. Eunuchoid proportions with (moderately) tall stature. Possibly more or less pronounced gynaecomastia. Frequent development of obesity.
2. Below average intelligence with immature personality or slight to moderate mental retardation (see above); possibly impulsive behaviour or other psychological aberrations.
3. Normally developed penis with small, firm testes and possibly weakly developed secondary male characteristics.

Supplementary Findings: Increased disposition to varicosities of the lower legs and leg ulcers.
(Azoospermia; infertility.)
Demonstration of 'X chromatin-positivity' in a simple screening test; confirmation of the anomalous sex chromosome constitution by chromosome analysis.

Manifestation: Clinically in early childhood by tall stature due to unusually long legs (possibly combined with below average intelligence or slight retardation).

Aetiology: The syndrome expresses a chromosomal aberration in the form of an extra X, resulting from abnormal chromosome separation during oogenesis or spermatogenesis.

Frequency: About 1:500 newborn males.

Course, Prognosis: Normal life expectancy. Not infrequently poor social adjustment. Infertility.

Differential Diagnosis: Other forms of male hypogonadism.

Treatment: Androgen substitution if endocrinological testicular insufficiency is demonstrated. In some cases surgical treatment of marked gynaecomastia. Psychological guidance. Prevention of obesity.

Illustrations:
1 A boy with Klinefelter syndrome at 8½ years. Height 18.5 cm above average; mental retardation, severe behavioural problems; anomalous EEG.
4, 5 and 8 Same case as in **1** at 26 years.
2, 3, 6 and 7 Another boy at 14¼ years: 176.5 cm (above the 97th percentile); left testis 2 ml, right 3 ml, firm; moderate mental retardation. Both cases confirmed by chromosome analysis.
(Case 2 by kind permission of Prof P. Heintzen, Kiel.)

References:
Any comprehensive paediatrics or internal medicine textbook

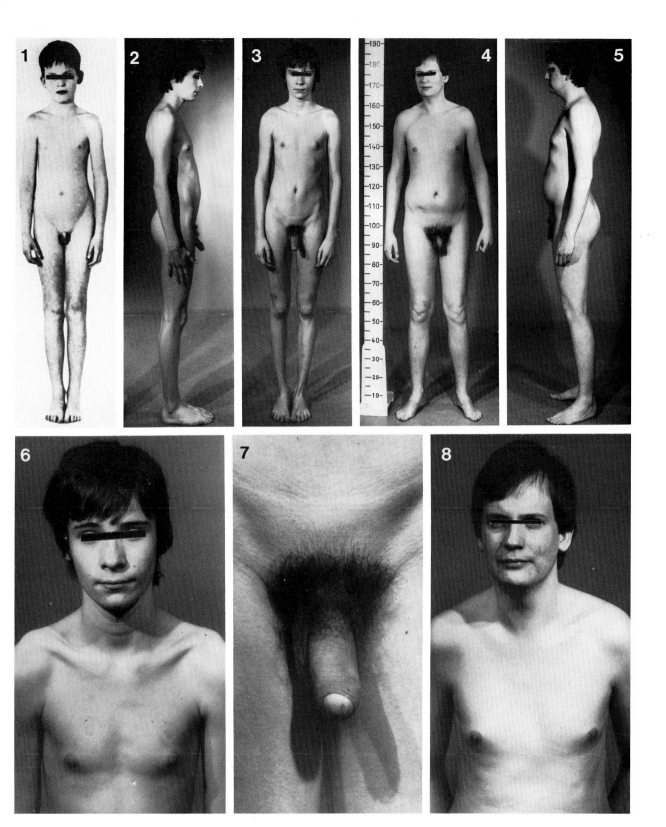

Index